The FOOD and DRUG INTERACTION GUIDE

Brian L. G. Morgan, Ph.D.

A Fireside Book
Published by Simon and Schuster, Inc.
New York

First Fireside Edition, 1986
Published by Simon & Schuster, Inc.
Simon & Schuster Building
Rockefeller Center
1230 Avenue of the Americas
New York, New York 10020

FIRESIDE and colophon are registered trademarks of Simon & Schuster, Inc.
Manufactured in the United States of America
10 9 8 7 6 5 4 3 2

Library of Congress Cataloging in Publication Data

ISBN: 0-671-61776-1 (Pbk.)
ISBN: 0-671-52430-5

*To the readers of this book, that they may all be
healed and enjoy the best of health,*

*and to my parents, for everything they have done to
bring light and love into my life.*

Acknowledgments

In a book of this nature and size, very little can be accomplished without a lot of help. Therefore I would like to thank warmly the following people, who gave either their time, their effort, or their expertise to help make this book a reality:

John Gallagher, for his invaluable help in the conception and planning of this volume.

Hugh Howard, for his organizational and editing work, and his advice.

My editor, Fred Hills, for his tremendous support and for having the vision to see the need for such a book.

My wife, Roberta, for her patience and many helpful suggestions.

Dr. Myron Winick, director of the Institute of Human Nutrition, College of Physicians and Surgeons, Columbia University, for his never-failing support and friendship, and for his professional guidance throughout my career.

My agent, friend, and trusted adviser, Glen Cowley, for his support and help.

And to the experts in this field, including those listed in the bibliography, without whom it would have been impossible to compile this book.

Contents

Containing alphabetically arranged entries
describing over 300 generic drugs, these pages
identify the brand names, the action of the drug,
and the family to which each drug belongs; the
possible adverse side effects, and the groups of
people at highest risk of experiencing these
effects; foods to avoid while taking the drug; and
instructions on how to take it. In addition,
possible nutritional interactions—and methods of
prevention and treatment for them—are
enumerated at length in the body of the entry.

Preface

The purpose of this book is to explain the effects of prescription and nonprescription medications on your body's nutritional status. Conversely, this book will also explain how the nutrients themselves can change the effectiveness of certain drugs.

Before using this book, however, there are a few important points you should understand. First of all, though this book is a valuable, in fact necessary, tool for anyone taking any of the drugs cited in its pages, it is not meant to be a substitute for your physician and his advice. If a specific medication has been prescribed for you by your doctor, you should always ask him if there are any special precautions you should take regarding its use. His special knowledge of your condition and medical history gives him a great advantage in advising you.

Second, you will notice that in certain entries supplementation with specific nutrients has been advised. The amounts indicated are totally adequate, and you should not take more than the stated amount (that is, once again, unless you are otherwise directed by your doctor). Too much of some supplements can decrease the effectiveness of certain drugs.

Third, you will find that the drug-specific entries that constitute the bulk of this book will be most helpful to you if you are familiar with the basics of food and drug interactions. To that end, it is advised that you read the introduction that follows this preface.

Fourth, you should be aware as you read about the drugs you are taking that the text of each description addresses not only the potential problems but also the likelihood that they will occur. Terms like "conceivable" and "likely" and "highly unlikely" are used. When the interaction has been termed "likely," the drug is usually nutrient-antagonistic, either because of its direct effect on the nutrient or because of a physical effect that disturbs the body's supply of that nutrient, even when the drug is taken over a short period of time. The term "conceivable" indicates essentially the same thing, save that in these cases, either the drug-nutrient interaction requires a more lengthy use of the drug to cause the same effect, or the effect is found only in users of the drug who start out with a poor nutritional status. Interactions that are termed "unlikely" occur only if the patient is either severely deficient in the particular nutrient involved or is taking another drug that compounds the effect. These complications are indicated where applicable in each of the entries.

There are, of course, no absolutes in life. It is conceivable that an interaction that is listed as being likely may not affect certain people. However, to be on the safe side— and since the dietary adjustments indicated cannot harm you and can only promote better health—you should follow the recommendations indicated in each drug entry.

Fifth, and perhaps most important of all, regardless of the drug you are taking or the potential interactions indicated, you should be sure your nutrient intake is adequate. A simple outline to follow is that you should consume, on a daily basis, the following:

2 servings of protein; 4 to 6 servings of fruit and vegetables (one of which should be a green, leafy vegetable, one a citrus fruit); 4 to 6 servings of breads and cereals; 2 servings of milk and dairy products; 6 to 8 glasses of fluid.

It is my hope that this book will help you maintain the best physical health possible, along with a good nutritional status, no matter what type of drug or drugs you are taking.

B.L.G.M.
New York

Introduction

In this age of increasing awareness of the importance of nutrition, we have come to believe more than ever the old maxim, "You are what you eat."

By the same token, for the 75 million Americans who regularly take prescription or over-the-counter medications, there is a crucially important corollary: "How your body handles what you eat is what you are."

There is a dynamic relationship between the food we consume and the drugs we take. Only in recent years have we come to recognize that most of the drugs we consume alter the way in which our bodies handle essential nutrients. If the drugs we take can relieve our pains, calm us down or perk us up, dry our sinuses, induce sleep, and generally promote better health, they can also create unintended consequences, ranging from mild discomfort to serious, even life-threatening, problems.

From common aspirin to rarely used prescription medications, every drug on the market interacts in our bodies in one way or another with the food we eat. In the following pages, we will look at the ways in which this occurs. We will see how a food can interact with a drug to enhance its effect or to reduce it, to speed up its action or prolong it. We will see how, in some cases, the drug can be rendered entirely useless by what we eat with it.

We will also look at other interactions that are extremely important: drug-induced nutrient deficiencies, cases in which medication reduces the value of the food we eat.

The interactions are numerous and complex. But the message is simple: How our bodies handle what we put into them has a great deal to do with how healthy we are.

FOOD ABSORPTION

Drug-induced nutrient deficiencies are the principal concern of this book. The drugs we take often rob our food of a significant portion of its nutritive value, usually by interfering with our body's absorption processes.

Different drugs create different malabsorption problems. Primary malabsorption occurs when the drug itself has a direct effect on absorption; secondary malabsorption, a more frequent problem, occurs when a drug interferes with the absorption or metabolism of certain nutrients and so causes a deficiency.

A good example of a drug that creates a primary absorption problem is mineral oil. A familiar laxative, mineral oil causes the malabsorption of the fat-soluble vitamins— A, D, E, and K—by imposing a physical barrier between the vitamins and the wall of the intestine where the nutrients are ordinarily absorbed. Denied absorption through the intestine, the vitamins simply dissolve in the nonabsorbable mineral oil and, as captured nutrients, are passed through the intestines and out in the stool.

Most drug-nutrient interactions are somewhat more complex. An example is the antibiotic neomycin, which creates a primary absorption problem by damaging the wall of the intestine and, as a result, prevents the absorption of fat, protein, milk sugar, sodium, potassium, calcium, iron, and vitamin B_{12}. If this drug is taken for two weeks or longer, deficiencies can result in any or even all of these nutrients.

An example of a drug that creates a secondary absorption problem is phenytoin, most commonly known by its brand name, Dilantin. It accelerates the rate at which the liver breaks down vitamin D, a vitamin upon which calcium depends for its absorption. If you are taking Dilantin, much of the vitamin D in your body will be used inefficiently. This can lead to two separate deficiencies—one of vitamin D, the other of calcium. In the absence of the efficient absorption of vitamin D, the body will liberate whatever calcium it needs from the bones, leading to a condition known as osteomalacia. A demineralization of the bones will occur, in some cases weakening them

to such a degree that they will become brittle and may even fracture.

All of these examples point to the crucial issue here: that your body is an operating system that will malfunction if it suffers the loss of an important nutrient.

There are other examples, as well. Some drugs cause the excretion of abnormally large amounts of minerals. A good example is the family of drugs known as diuretics, which are mainly prescribed for the treatment of hypertension. Diuretics will reduce the body's water retention, as well as its salt content. However, this can also reduce the amount of the mineral potassium, which is essential for the proper functioning of the kidneys, heart, and muscles, and the secretion of the stomach juices. Consequently, on depletion of the potassium stores in the body, the potential problems the chronic user of diuretics faces are irregular heartbeat, heart attack, and kidney failure. Potassium depletion can also sensitize a patient to a drug such as digitalis (prescribed for heart disease) and create the possibility of digitalis intoxication, leading to heart failure.

Other problems occur with the chronic use of antacids. Phosphate, which helps form teeth and bones, and is needed in the functioning of several B vitamins, is depleted in people who chronically use the antacids aluminum hydroxide and magnesium hydroxide. The dietary phosphate combines with these antacids to form aluminum and magnesium phosphate, compounds which are not absorbable and are passed out in the stool. In the event of a reduced supply of dietary phosphate, the body will, once again, turn to the bones to fulfill its mineral needs, and osteomalacia (weak bones) can result.

The effectiveness of the vitamins and minerals we take in through our foods can be threatened by a wide variety of drugs that either increase their excretion or interfere with their metabolism. The following are a few examples: Anti-coagulants make vitamin K less effective; oral contraceptives increase the need for vitamin B_6; nitrous oxide, an anesthetic, destroys vitamin B_{12}.

DRUG ABSORPTION

More of a drug is likely to be absorbed the longer it remains in your system. Since digesting a meal takes time, a drug taken with, say, a five-course dinner has more time to be dissolved by the gastric acid. The result is that when the drug is presented to the intestine, where most of the absorption takes place, it is in a form that can be readily absorbed.

While more of whatever drug we are taking is likely to be used by our bodies when we take it on a full stomach, there is a price to be paid: Certain foods taken with particular drugs will cause a slowed or, in some cases, impaired absorption of the drug from the intestine. For example, tetracycline, an antibiotic, binds to the calcium in milk and forms an insoluble substance that is not absorbed by the body. Further, since foods high in fat and protein are digested more slowly than others, there can be a delay in the emptying of the stomach, so that drugs consumed with a meal high in fat or protein are slower to arrive in the small intestine for absorption.

OTHER DRUG INTERACTION PROBLEMS

The opposite problem can also occur: Instead of being unable to metabolize a drug, your body can succeed in metabolizing it, but may have difficulty in getting rid of it. For example, if the often used anti-anxiety drug Valium is taken with alcohol, the alcohol will not inhibit the body's ability to use the drug, for it will still sedate you. But the body will not be able to rid itself of the drug as it normally does, and a toxic buildup of Valium can result.

A similar situation occurs with such drugs as the antibiotic quinine or the anti-protozoal agent quinacrine. Dosages of quinacrine are calculated with the expectation that the drug will be used by the body and then excreted. However, this drug and a number of others will not be passed out with the urine as expected if the urine is alkaline. So, people who eat a diet high in alkaline foods—milk, buttermilk, cream, and most fruits and vegetables—risk a considerable increase in the potency of the drug, and exaggerated side effects.

Nonnutrient food substances also play a role in drug breakdown. Substances called indoles (present in brussels sprouts and cabbage) and a substance called flavonoid (found in citrus fruits) will increase the breakdown of some drugs, as will the charcoal broiling of beef. Another factor in metabolism is intestinal bacteria, since they aid in the degradation or breakdown of drugs. Changes in the composition of the diet can alter the intestinal bacteria and therefore the effectiveness of the drug.

This is by no means a comprehensive list of the ways in which the drugs we take are able or unable to accomplish their desired result because of dietary factors. In the individual drug entries that follow, you will discover many more.

WHEN FOODS AND DRUGS ARE INCOMPATIBLE

Severe adverse reactions to drugs can be caused by specific foods or alcoholic beverages. Some reactions, if left unchecked, can be life-threatening.

In 1961, a variety of side effects were noted in patients receiving drugs from the MAO-inhibitor drug family (monoamine-oxidase inhibitors). While the drugs effectively relieved severe depression, they also seemed to cause high blood pressure, headaches, palpitations, nausea, and vomiting. When the circumstances were studied more closely, it was determined that many of the patients ate a diet rich in foods containing a substance called tyramine.

Tyramine is found in many foods, but in especially high quantities in pickled herring, chicken livers, certain cheeses, and Chianti wine. Tyramine is now known to cause an alarming increase in blood pressure, but its effects are usually counteracted by the MAO enzymes in the body. However, in patients taking MAO-inhibitor drugs, these enzymes are inactivated.

Alcohol is also frequently a problem for proper drug utilization. For example, it is always rapidly absorbed and causes a decreased production of glucose by the liver, tending to lower blood glucose (sugar) levels. A diabetic who takes a drug intended to encourage insulin production should not drink alcohol, because the pancreas will overproduce insulin and bring the blood glucose level down dramatically. Alcohol in combination with many other drugs has a great variety of different—and all too often dangerous—interactions.

Clearly, there are many interactions between foods and drugs—some to be avoided at all costs. It is the purpose of this book to help you become aware of the problems you may face when taking a given drug and to help you deal with those problems.

WHO IS AT RISK?

Not everyone is subject to the same risk for a drug-induced nutrient deficiency. We all handle drugs and nutrients differently. However, the special nutritional requirements of the following groups make them particularly vulnerable to side effects: the elderly; women in general, but especially those who are pregnant, lactating, or have reached menopause; vegetarians; heavy drinkers; the 30 million undiagnosed hypertensives; those on a severe weight loss, low-protein diet; and the countless number of people on a low sodium (salt-free) diet. Heavy smokers also tend to have special nutritional requirements. They usually have lower levels of vitamins B_6 and B_{12}, which may indicate an increased need for these nutrients. It has been estimated that they also need up to one-and-a-half times the vitamin C required by nonsmokers, meaning that their daily requirements are 90 to 100 mg daily. Smoking also tends to deplete the body's calcium.

In other words, everyone—but particularly members of these special groups—should be aware of all the nutritional consequences involved with the drugs they are taking.

HOW TO USE THIS BOOK

This book describes more than 300 generic drugs and their nutritional interactions. Organized alphabetically, the drugs (prescription and over-the-counter) are those most commonly used. The entry for each drug opens with general information—the drug family, the common brand names by which the drug is known, how to take the drug, foods to avoid, possible adverse side effects, the action of the drug, and the groups to whom the drug represents the greatest risk.

The major portion of each entry describes the likely interactions between each drug and the foods we eat. The symptoms of each interaction are described, as well as the long- and short-term effects. Most important, the methods of prevention or treatment are detailed.

It is recommended that you first read the entry for the drug you are taking and then follow the cross-references to the tables at the back of the book for further information on the best food sources of certain nutrients, and on supplements.

The Food and Drug Interaction Guide is a unique nutritional and pharmaceutical reference volume. It is designed to help you understand not only the way your body uses the drugs you take and how they are affected by what you eat, but also how the nutrients in the food you consume can help you live a healthier life.

Food and Drug Interactions

ACETAMINOPHEN

DRUG FAMILY: Analgesic

BRAND NAMES: Apap with Codeine; Acetaco; Acetaminophen Elixir; Acetaminophen with Codeine Phosphate; Algisin; Amacodone; Amaphen; Amaphen with Codeine; Anacin-3; Anatuss with Codeine; Anoquan; Apap 300 mg with Codeine; Apap with Codeine Elixir; Aspirin-Free Arthritis Pain Formula; Bancap; Bancap c̄ Codeine; Bancap HC; Capital with Codeine; Children's Panadol; Chlorzone Forte; Chlorzoxazone with APAP; Codalan; Co-Gesic, Colrex; Compal; Comtrex; Congespirin; CoTylenol; Darvocet-N, Di-Gesic; Dristan Ultra Colds Formula; Dristan, Advanced Formula; Duradyne DHC; Empracet with Codeine Phosphate; Esgic; Espasmotex; Excedrin; Excedrin P.M.; Extra-Strength Datril; G-1; G-2; G-3; Gemnisyn; Hycodaphen; Hycomine; Hyco-Pap; Korigesic; Maximum Strength Panadol; Midrin; Migralam; Oxycodone Hydrochloride and Acetaminophen; Pacaps; Parafon Forte; Percocet; Percogesic; Phenaphen w/Codeine; Phenaphen; Phenate; Phrenilin; Propoxyphene and Apap; Protid; Repan; SK-APAP with Codeine; SK-Oxycodone with Acetaminophen; SK-65 APAP; Sedapap-10; Sine-Aid; Singlet; Sinubid; Sinulin; Stopayne; Supac; T-Gesic; Talacen; Two-Dyne; Tylenol acetaminophen; Tylenol, Extra-Strength; Tylenol, Maximum-Strength; Tylenol, Regular Strength; Tylenol w/Codeine; Tylox Capsules; Vanquish; Vicodin; Wygesic

HOW TO TAKE ACETAMINOPHEN: At mealtimes or with milk

FOODS TO AVOID: Vitamin C supplements greater than 500 mg; alcoholic beverages

POSSIBLE ADVERSE SIDE EFFECTS: Diarrhea; sodium depletion; kidney damage

ACTION OF ACETAMINOPHEN: This analgesic is prescribed for the relief of mild to moderate pain, with or without fever. However, it does not have significant anti-inflammatory effects and is not effective for the treatment of rheumatic pain.

HIGH-RISK GROUPS: The elderly

NUTRITIONAL INTERACTIONS

GASTROINTESTINAL DISTURBANCES: In rare instances, long-term abuse of acetaminophen can lead to kidney damage, which results in the inability of the body to conserve sodium. Further salt loss, through episodes of diarrhea, can bring on a condition called hyponatremia (abnormally low blood sodium levels). It leads to anorexia, nausea, vomiting, and muscle weakness. If the blood sodium levels drop extremely low, your senses may be impaired, and seizures may occur.

Very high doses of vitamin C (several grams per day) can prevent the body from excreting acetaminophen. In the habitual user, this can lead to a toxic buildup, and damage the kidneys and liver.

Prevention and Treatment: People taking this drug, especially older people whose kidney function may be declining, should be careful to follow the dosage instructions.

Chronic users of acetaminophen should not take more than 500 mg of vitamin C per day.

If the drug has a tendency to cause an upset stomach, it should be taken with milk or at mealtimes.

ACETOHEXAMIDE

DRUG FAMILY: Anti-diabetic

BRAND NAME: Dymelor

HOW TO TAKE ACETOHEXAMIDE: Just before meals with a glass of water

FOODS TO AVOID: All foods or beverages containing alcohol

POSSIBLE ADVERSE SIDE EFFECTS: Hypoglycemia, hyperglycemia, flatulence, loose stools, diarrhea

ACTION OF ACETOHEXAMIDE: This drug is a member of the sulfonylurea family and is prescribed to reduce blood glucose levels by stimulating the pancreas to produce insulin.

HIGH-RISK GROUPS: The elderly, heavy drinkers

NUTRITIONAL INTERACTION

HYPOGLYCEMIA AND HYPERGLYCEMIA: Too much or too little acetohexamide can lead to hyperglycemia or hypoglycemia. Hypoglycemia is conceivable in those who do not eat regularly or who exercise without consuming extra calories to account for the extra energy expenditure. Hypoglycemia is a condition in which there is too little sugar (glucose) in the blood. If your blood sugar levels drop to below 30 mg/100 ml of blood (a normal level is 100 mg/100ml), you may become mentally confused due to a lack of glucose reaching the brain. Other early symptoms are headaches, hunger, and a general sensation resembling mild drunkenness. Below 10 mg/100 ml, you could go into a diabetic coma. If the situation is not corrected within a few minutes, permanent brain damage may occur.

If too little acetohexamide is taken, you will experience the opposite condition, hyperglycemia, from too much sugar in the blood, though this is unlikely. This condition results because insufficient amounts of the drug cause the pancreas to release amounts of insulin insufficient to allow the cells in the body to absorb glucose, which starves the cells of the energy they need. In this instance, as well, coma can eventually result.

Alcohol and aspirin enhance the blood-glucose-lowering activity. They can cause the glucose levels to drop so low that the brain is starved of glucose and energy, and you can go into a coma.

Prevention and Treatment: If you are diabetic, you should carefully monitor your food intake to avoid an excess of carbohydrates in the form of simple sugars, such as cookies, candies, sodas, honey, and table sugar. These foods are absorbed very rapidly and will increase your blood sugar to very high levels. If you are diabetic, such high blood sugar levels are dangerous because the limited amount of insulin produced by the pancreas may not be sufficient to bring the levels back into the normal range. A preferred diet is low in fats, but with plenty of complex carbohydrates, such as starches, cereals, and vegetables. (See table of Simple and Complex Carbohydrate Foods, page 305.) It is important that the diabetic eat regularly and match his food intake to his caloric output. Thus, when he increases his energy output, as when he takes part in some sporting activity, he must also increase his caloric intake, and when he reduces one, he must reduce the other.

Recent studies have demonstrated that a high-fiber diet may cause a slower and more sustained release of glucose from the gastrointestinal tract into the bloodstream, preventing the wide swings in blood sugar levels. High-fiber diets also increase the efficiency with which glucose is absorbed. For the diabetic, it is recommended that you remain physically active and exercise daily, because by doing so the cells are made more susceptible to the insulin available. Finally, a change in eating schedule from the standard three meals per day to five or six smaller meals will also help keep blood sugar levels within normal range.

HYPOGLYCEMIA: Acetohexamide is sometimes prescribed for nondiabetics suffering from Parkinson's disease, a nervous disorder involving a rhythmic tremor, rigidity of muscle action, and slowing of body motion. The elderly seem to be sensitive to this drug, and it is conceivable, particularly in elderly patients taking this or other sulfonylurea drugs, that hypoglycemia will occur. In extreme cases, patients have succumbed to coma.

Prevention and Treatment: If you are an elderly patient, you should carry sugar cubes or candy in the event you experience hypoglycemia.

OTHER ADVICE: Acetohexamide could conceivably irritate your gastrointestinal tract and cause flatulence, loose stools, or diarrhea. It is recommended that it be taken just before meals, to minimize gastric irritation.

Acetohexamide inhibits the breakdown of acetaldehyde, which is produced when alcohol is broken down in the body. This causes a number of unpleasant symptoms. If alcohol is consumed after this drug is taken, severe headaches, flushing, nausea, vomiting, hypertension, weakness, vertigo, blurred vision, and convulsions may occur. The reaction begins within 5 to 10 minutes of one's drinking the alcohol and in sensitive people may be caused by only a few sips. As a result, even wine vinegar, sauces containing wine, or desserts containing liquor may cause such a reaction.

ALLOPURINOL

DRUG FAMILY: Anti-gout

BRAND NAMES: Lopurin; Zyloprim

HOW TO TAKE ALLOPURINOL: Directly after meals, with a glass of water

FOODS TO AVOID: The following should not be eaten in large quantities: meat, fish, poultry, eggs, cheese, peanut butter, bacon, nuts, bread, candies, crackers, macaroni, spaghetti, noodles, cakes, cookies, Brazil nuts, filberts, walnuts, tea (including herbal types); also coffee, cola beverages, and alcoholic beverages, especially beer.

POSSIBLE ADVERSE SIDE EFFECTS: Iron deficiency; kidney stones, gastrointestinal disturbances

ACTION OF ALLOPURINOL: This drug is prescribed for patients with gout and, in some instances, as a chemical agent in cancer therapy. Gout is an arthritis-type disease caused by deposits of uric acid crystals in the joints. It usually occurs in single joints, most often the big toe, in painful episodes that last only a few days but are likely to recur. Gout most often afflicts middle-aged men. Allopurinol helps the body excrete the uric acid in the normal manner.

Your doctor is likely to recommend a special diet low in purine-rich foods in addition to prescribing this or another of the anti-gout medications. That diet is a crucial part of the treatment, since the purines in foods are broken down by your body to produce uric acid. (See table of Purine-Rich Foods, page 303.)

HIGH-RISK GROUPS: Anyone who takes this drug

NUTRIONAL INTERACTIONS

IRON DEFICIENCY: Since allopurinol impairs iron absorption, it is conceivable that, while taking allopurinol, you will develop an iron deficiency. Iron is especially important to the oxygen-carrying cells of the blood and muscles, which consume two thirds of the iron your body requires. Thus, an iron shortage reduces the blood's oxygen-carrying capacity, and the result is an anemia signaled by such symptoms as tiredness, general feelings of malaise, irritability, decreased attention span, pale complexion, rapid heart rhythm, headaches, the loss of concentration, and breathlessness on exertion. A mild iron deficiency will also impair the functioning of your immune system.

For iron to be absorbed from any vegetable source, it must first be converted to another form by the action of the hydrochloric acid produced in the stomach. Many elderly people secrete less hydrochloric acid than normal, so they absorb iron poorly even under normal circumstances. The diets of many Americans lack adequate quantities of this mineral for their normal needs. For example, 10 percent of American women suffer from an iron deficiency, and up to 30 percent have inadequate iron stores, giving them less to draw upon in times of shortage. Other people who are at significant risk for an iron deficiency are women who have had several pregnancies and those whose menstrual periods are heavy.

The shortage of iron in many diets is due not only to the selection of foods that are poor sources of iron, but also to the switch from cast-iron cookware to aluminum, stainless steel, and nonstick surfaces. Iron used to be leached from iron pots and pans by the acids in foods, and became available as dietary iron.

Prevention and Treatment: To counteract an iron deficiency, iron-rich foods should be included in your diet: liver, whole grain products, oysters, dried apricots, prunes, peaches, leafy green vegetables, and, occasionally, lean red meat. (See table of Iron-Rich Foods, page 299.)

Other foods and drugs have a considerable impact on the way your body absorbs (or does not absorb) iron. There are two kinds of iron in food sources: heme iron in meat and ionic iron in vegetables. Up to 30 percent of the iron from meat, fish, and poultry is absorbed, but less than 10 percent is absorbed from eggs, whole grains, nuts, and dried beans. Only 10 percent of iron is absorbed from vegetable sources, with as little as 2 percent being absorbed from spinach. Antacids will interfere with iron absorption in vegetables, as will commercial black and pekoe tea, taken in substantial quantities, because of its tannin content. Coffee also seems to decrease iron absorption, but not to the same degree as tea. Vitamin C supplements or citrus fruit juices increase the absorption of iron from vegetable sources by two to three times if taken simultaneously.

If your diet is rich in high-fiber foods, you will have impaired iron absorption, because the fiber will bind with the iron and pass it out in the stool. This same action contributes to the poor absorption of iron from vegetable sources. Foods high in phosphorus (e.g. meat) interfere with iron absorption, which explains why only 30 percent of the iron in meat is captured. (However, meat and fish facilitate iron absorption from vegetables.) For that matter, any use of large quantities of mineral supplements, such as zinc, will impair iron absorption. Because iron can be leached from vegetables if they are cooked in large amounts of water, it is preferable to steam them.

Iron supplements should not be taken without a physician's recommendation, because an accumulation of too much iron can lead in extreme cases to such serious problems as anemia, malfunctioning of the pancreas and the heart, cirrhosis of the liver, a brown cast to the skin, and depression.

KIDNEY STONES AND OTHER COMPLICATIONS: Allopurinol could conceivably lead to the production of kidney stones. The chances of this are increased by foods that cause acidic urine. When purine-rich foods are a part of the diet, they are normally excreted as uric acid, but this drug may cause an unusual buildup of uric acid in the kidneys, leading to the formation of uric acid crystals, a form of kidney stones. A difficulty in urinating and blood in the urine may signal the development of kidney stones.

Prevention and Treatment: To prevent the formation of kidney stones, it is advised you drink no fewer than 8 glasses or 5 to 6 pints of liquid every 24 hours, particularly at night when the urine becomes concentrated. To keep your urine alkaline or nonacidic, consume a diet rich in alkaline foods such as milk, cream, buttermilk, almonds, chestnuts, coconut, all vegetables except corn and lentils, and all fruits except cranberries, prunes, and plums. You should also cut down on foods that make the urine acidic, including meat, fish, poultry, eggs, cheese, peanut butter, bacon, Brazil nuts, filberts, peanuts, walnuts, bread, crackers, macaroni, spaghetti, noodles, cakes, and cookies.

OTHER ADVICE: Avoid tea, coffee, or cola beverages in large quantities because they are likely to reduce the effectiveness of allopurinol. Also avoid alcohol, especially beer, and simple sugars (see table of Simple and Complex Carbohydrates, page 305) because they can raise the blood uric-acid level and impair the drug's ability to manage chronic gout. Avoid herbal teas, since they contain phenylbutazone, which raises blood uric-acid levels.

This drug causes gastrointestinal disturbances in many patients and is better tolerated if taken after meals.

If obese, the gout sufferer should also achieve ideal body weight by gradual weight reduction (1 to 2 pounds per week). All sufferers should decrease their animal fat intake and increase their complex carbohydrate intake.

ALUMINUM ANTACIDS

DRUG FAMILY: Antacids

BRAND NAMES: [GENERIC/Brand] ALUMINUM HYDROXIDE/Camalox; Delcid; Di-Gel; Gaviscon; Gelusil-M; Gelusil-II; Maalox; Maalox Plus; Maalox TC; Nephrox; Tempo; WinGel; ALUMINUM HYDROXIDE GEL/ALternaGEL; Aludrox; Amphojel; Di-Gel; Gelusil; Mylanta; Mylanta-II; Simeco; ALUMINUM HYDROXIDE GEL, DRIED/Aludrox; Amphojel; Ascriptin; Ascriptin A/D; Gaviscon; Gaviscon-2; Mylanta, Mylanta-II, ALUMINUM HYDROXIDE PREPARATIONS/Kolantyl; Magnatril

HOW TO TAKE ALUMINUM ANTACIDS: On an empty stomach between meals and at bedtime, with a glass of water

FOODS TO AVOID: Large amounts of acidic foods such as fruit juice, coffee, tea, chocolate, and cola

POSSIBLE ADVERSE SIDE EFFECTS: Phosphate and calcium deficiencies, kidney stones, constipation and, rarely, deficiencies of vitamins A, C, D, B_1, and folacin, magnesium, and iron

ACTION OF ALUMINUM ANTACIDS: These drugs are commonly prescribed to reduce stomach acid levels and to reduce blood phosphate levels for patients with kidney disease

HIGH-RISK GROUPS: The elderly, heavy drinkers, young women, smokers, teenagers, pregnant women, lactating women, vegetarians

NUTRITIONAL INTERACTIONS

PHOSPHATE AND CALCIUM DEFICIENCIES: Prolonged use of antacids containing aluminum hydroxide is likely to cause phosphate and, to a lesser degree, calcium depletion from the body. The aluminum hydroxide in these drugs reacts with phosphate in your diet to form aluminum phosphate, which is passed out in the stool. On rare occasions, hypophosphatemia, or dangerously low blood phosphate levels, can also develop. It is difficult to diagnose, because it is indicated by confusion and a slow development of weakness, common symptoms of many metabolic disorders in the elderly.

To replace the lost phosphate, your body withdraws the mineral from the bones to maintain optimal blood phosphate levels. As phosphate cannot be withdrawn from the bones without removing calcium, there is also a loss of calcium, and the attendant risk, over a protracted period of time, of osteomalacia or osteoporosis.

Osteomalacia is a weakening of the bones that results from a uniform and steady calcium loss. Prominent symptoms are bone pain in the back, thighs, shoulder region, or ribs; difficulty in walking; and weakness in the muscles of the legs. The condition is reversible once calcium blood levels are raised.

Long-term calcium deficiencies can also lead to osteoporosis, an unexplained and rapid loss of calcium from the bones. Backache, loss of height, and periodontal disease are often the first signs of the disease. Fractures of the vertebrae, hip, and wrist are also common.

If aluminum antacids are given to children, a condition known as rickets can result. Rickets causes the bones to become bent or malformed. Children under four years of age may also develop pigeon breast, bowlegs, a protruding abdomen (due to a weakness of stomach muscles), and poorly formed teeth that tend to decay.

Antacids may also lead to kidney stones. Therefore, people known to suffer from osteomalacia or osteoporosis, or who have a history of kidney stones, should not take these medications on a regular basis.

Prevention and Treatment: In order to guard against hypophosphatemia, plenty of phosphate-rich foods should be eaten, such as liver, nuts, beans, peas, whole grains, and refined cereals. (See table of Phosphorus-Rich Foods, page 302.)

The phosphate-rich foods in your diet should include foods containing magnesium, such as leafy green vegetables. No vitamin supplements are needed, provided a well-balanced diet based on the four food groups is followed. People with a poor diet will need a one-a-day vitamin supplement containing the Recommended Dietary Allowance.

OTHER ADVICE: Though much less likely, there can be other side effects of using these antacids. They can reduce the absorption of vitamins A, C, and D; magnesium; iron; thiamine; and folacin. They may also cause constipation, but an increased consumption of the bulk in leafy green vegetables can help relieve that problem.

If taken in excess, aluminum antacids may also lead to dementia. This is especially a factor in kidney patients, who have difficulty in excreting the aluminum, which then builds up in the body, including the brain.

Malnutrition can result from excessive self-medication with antacids, as a result of malabsorption of nutrients. It should be emphasized that nutrient depletion from antacid use is gradual, and evidence of malnutrition does not make its appearance until nutrient stores are exhausted.

People taking antacids therapeutically should avoid large amounts of acid-containing foods, such as fruit juices and foods containing caffeine, which irritate the stomach wall.

AMINOPHYLLINE

DRUG FAMILY: Anti-asthmatic

BRAND NAMES: Aminophyllin; Mudrane; Somophyllin

HOW TO TAKE AMINOPHYLLINE: Immediately after meals with a strong-tasting beverage such as fruit juice

FOODS TO AVOID: None

POSSIBLE ADVERSE SIDE EFFECTS: Gastrointestinal distress

ACTION OF AMINOPHYLLINE: This drug relaxes the muscle in the airways in the lungs, enabling asthmatics to breathe more easily. The drug is also used in treating bronchitis and emphysema.

HIGH-RISK GROUPS: Anyone who takes this drug

NUTRITIONAL INTERACTIONS

GASTROINTESTINAL DISTRESS: This drug can cause gastrointestinal discomfort. It also has a bitter aftertaste.

Prevention and Treatment: Aminophylline should be taken after meals, with fruit juice or some other strong-tasting fluid.

AMOXICILLIN

DRUG FAMILY: Antibiotic

BRAND NAMES: Amoxicillin Trihydrate; Amoxil; Polymox; Trimox; Wymox

HOW TO TAKE AMOXICILLIN: Between meals, with a large glass of water

FOODS TO AVOID: None

POSSIBLE ADVERSE SIDE EFFECTS: Nausea, vomiting, and diarrhea

ACTION OF AMOXICILLIN: This broad-based antibiotic is often prescribed for infections of the skin and of other soft tissues, and of the respiratory and urinary tracts.

HIGH-RISK GROUPS: People with a history of abdominal distress

NUTRITIONAL INTERACTIONS

GASTROINTESTINAL DISTRESS: For maximum effectiveness, amoxicillin should be taken on an empty stomach, with a large volume of water. However, it is likely that this drug will cause nausea, vomiting, and diarrhea.

Prevention and Treatment: If you experience stomach upset after taking amoxicillin, take it with a glass of milk or a meal. However, food slightly reduces the rate of absorption, so its effects will be slowed.

AMPHETAMINES

DRUG FAMILY: Appetite suppressant

BRAND NAMES: [GENERIC/Brand] AMPHETAMINE SULFATE/Obetrol-10; Obetrol-20; DEXTROAMPHETAMINE SULPHATE/Dexedrine; Obetrol-10; Obetrol-20

HOW TO TAKE AMPHETAMINES: With meals or milk

FOODS TO AVOID: Tyramine- and dopamine-rich foods such as aged cheeses, raisins, avocados, liver, bananas, eggplant, sour cream, alcoholic beverages, salami, meat tenderizers, chocolate, yeast, and soy sauce

POSSIBLE ADVERSE SIDE EFFECTS: Addiction; high blood pressure; nausea; diarrhea; vomiting, and stomachache

ACTION OF AMPHETAMINES: Amphetamines are prescribed as appetite suppressants for use in the treatment of obesity.

HIGH-RISK GROUPS: Hypertensives, heart patients

NUTRITIONAL INTERACTIONS

AMPHETAMINE ADDICTION: Like many antidepressant drugs, amphetamines inhibit the action of monoamine oxidase (MAO) in the brain, which breaks down the chemical messengers (neurotransmitters) responsible for making one feel uplifted. If you are already being treated with an anti-depressant, the use of this drug is likely to result in serious side effects due to an excess of the uplifting chemical messengers. The flooding of the brain in this way with chemical messengers can permanently alter the brain's chemistry and lead to a long-term need for an excess of these substances to maintain a normal state of mind. In short, these drugs are addictive.

Prevention and Treatment: Amphetamines should not be taken habitually, because they are addicting; they should be used with caution, especially by patients taking other anti-depressants.

TYRAMINE-RICH FOODS: Tyramine, a food substance, is likely to cause an alarming increase in blood pressure when taken in significant quantities at the same time as amphetamines. The ingested tyramine is usually converted in the liver to an inactive form through the action of monoamine oxidase (MAO). However, drugs in the MAO-inhibitor class leave tyramine in its active form. As a result, the tyramine remains in the blood and can increase blood pressure to dangerous levels. In some people, migraine headaches also result.

Prevention and Treatment: Tyramine-containing foods must be restricted while you are being treated with amphetamines. Tyramine is common in many foods, but it is found in the greatest amounts in high-protein foods that have undergone some decomposition, such as aged cheese. Tyramine is also found in chicken and beef livers, bananas, eggplant, sour cream, alcoholic beverages, salami, meat tenderizers, chocolate, yeast, and soy sauce. (See table of Tyramine-Rich Foods, page 307.) Raisins and avocados should also be avoided, because they contain dopamine, which has the same effect as tyramine.

WEIGHT-REDUCTION PROGRAMS: Amphetamines are addictive and should be used only as a short-term aid to weight loss. A reasonable and moderate weight-reduction program should aim at a manageable 1 or 2 pound loss per week. An intake reduction of 500 calories per day, for a weekly total of 3,500 calories, will result in the loss of 1 pound per week regardless of your present weight. Two eggs and a milk shake, 1½ cups of tuna salad, 4 ounces of a roast, 3 frankfurters, 2 cups of ice cream, or 2 pieces of cheesecake all represent approximately 500 calories.

The Weight Watchers exercise and behavior modification program is among those that offer a sensible balance of proper nutrition, exercise, and support in making a dietary change.

OTHER ADVICE: The chronic and extensive use of amphetamines could conceivably result in the development of unwanted side effects, including such gastrointestinal disorders as nausea, diarrhea, vomiting, and stomachache, more good reasons not to use amphetamines. These effects can be limited by taking the drugs with meals or milk.

AMPICILLIN

DRUG FAMILY: Antibiotic

BRAND NAMES: Amcill; Ampicillin Trihydrate; Ampicillin-Probenecid; Omnipen; Omnipen-N; Principen; Principen with Probenecid; SK-Ampicillin; SK-Ampicillin-N; Polycillin; Polycillin-N; Polycillin-PRB

HOW TO TAKE AMPICILLIN: With water, on an empty stomach 1 hour before or 2 to 3 hours after eating

FOODS TO AVOID: Fruit juices and other acid-containing foods such as soda and wine

POSSIBLE SIDE EFFECTS; Diarrhea

ACTION OF AMPICILLIN: This broad-based antibiotic is prescribed primarily for urinary, respiratory, and gastrointestinal-tract infections. In children, it is also used to treat ear infections and meningitis.

HIGH RISK GROUPS: People with a history of abdominal distress

NUTRITIONAL INTERACTIONS

GASTROINTESTINAL DISTRESS: Ampicillin frequently causes diarrhea. If you experience this reaction, you should inform your doctor, and he will switch you to an alternative antibiotic such as amoxicillin.

Prevention and Treatment: This drug should be taken on an empty stomach 1 hour before or 2 to 3 hours after eating. In addition to reducing the likelihood of diarrhea, this will maximize the effectiveness of the drug, since its potency may be reduced by as much as 50 percent if it is taken with meals. Fruit juices inactivate the drug and should not be taken with it.

ANABOLIC STEROIDS

DRUG FAMILY: Sex hormones

BRAND NAMES: [GENERIC/Brand] ETHYLESTRENOL/Maxibolin; NANDROLONE DECANOATE/Deca-Durabolin; Kabolin; NANDRO-LONE PHENPROPIONATE/Durabolin; OXANDROLONE/Anavar; OXYMETHOLONE/Anadrol-50; STANOZOLOL/Winstrol; TESTOLACTONE/Teslac

HOW TO TAKE ANABOLIC STEROIDS: In tablet form, just before or with meals

FOODS TO AVOID: Salty foods such as anchovies, dill pickles, sardines, green olives, canned soups and vegetables, TV dinners, soy sauce, processed cheeses, and salty snack foods such as potato chips and cold cuts

POSSIBLE SIDE EFFECTS: Edema and irregular heartbeat

ACTION OF ANABOLIC STEROIDS: These drugs are used mainly to stimulate muscle growth in a wide assortment of conditions, from recovery after an operation to recuperation from a long-term debilitating disease. They are also used to suppress lactation and to treat breast cancer.

HIGH-RISK GROUPS: Heart patients, kidney patients

NUTRITIONAL INTERACTIONS

EDEMA: These drugs can lead to water and salt retention, which will tend to cause swelling (called edema) in your legs, ankles, feet, and breasts, and around your eyes. An increase in sodium and water retention will also increase the volume of blood in the body, which places an added strain on the heart and tends to elevate blood pressure.

Prevention and Treatment: While taking these drugs, you should restrict your consumption of sodium to 2 grams, or 1 teaspoon, of salt per day. In particular, those foods listed in the table of Sodium-Rich

Foods (see page 306) should be avoided, or consumed in small quantities. You should add no salt at the table and no more than ½ teaspoon in cooking.

Many people are unaware of how much salt their diet contains. The average American, in fact, consumes some 15 pounds of salt a year. This amounts to 3 to 4 teaspoons per day. Even if you do not salt your food while preparing or eating it, you consume quantities of salt in such foods as anchovies, dill pickles, sardines, green olives, canned soups and vegetables, so-called TV dinners, soy sauce, processed cheeses, many snack foods, cold cuts, and catsup. Other sources of sodium such as monosodium glutamate should be avoided.

To sharpen your awareness of the sodium content of food products, read the list of ingredients that appears on the labels of all packaged foods. If sodium is one of the first ingredients on the label, it is present in significant quantities. If sodium is at the lower end of the list, then the food contains very little sodium.

OTHER ADVICE: Some 10 percent of patients taking anabolic steroids develop very high blood calcium levels, which can cause heart arrhythmias. To avoid the problem, drink at least 6 to 8 glasses of liquid every day while taking this drug.

ANDROGENS

DRUG FAMILY: Hormone

BRAND NAMES: [GENERIC/Brand] TESTOSTERONE/BayTestone-50; BayTestone-100; TESTOSTERONE ANANTHATE/Ditate-DS; Tes-taval 90/4; TESTOSTERONE CYPIONATE/Depo-Testosterone: T-Cypionate 200; METHYLTESTOSTERONE/Android-5 Buccal; Android-10; Android-25; Estratest H.S.; Estratest; Metandren; Oreton Methyl; Premarin w/Methyltestosterone; Primotest Forte; Primotest; Testred; Virilon; FLUOXYMESTERONE/Android-F; Fluoxymesterone; Halotestin; DANAZOL/Danocrine

HOW TO TAKE ANDROGENS: Between meals

FOODS TO AVOID: Salty foods such as anchovies, dill pickles, sardines, green olives, canned soups and vegetables, TV dinners, soy sauce, processed cheeses, salty snack foods like potato chips and cold cuts

POSSIBLE SIDE EFFECTS: Edema

ACTION OF ANDROGENS: Androgen therapy is used primarily in androgen-deficient males for the development or maintenance of secondary sexual characteristics such as well-developed muscles and a full beard. Androgens are also used to accelerate growth in children, and to treat endometriosis and certain types of anemia.

HIGH-RISK GROUPS: Heart patients, kidney patients

NUTRITIONAL INTERACTIONS

EDEMA: These drugs can lead to water and salt retention, which will tend to cause swelling (called edema) in your legs, ankles, feet, and breasts, and around your eyes. An increase in sodium and water retention will also increase the volume of blood in the body, which places an added strain on the heart and tends to elevate blood pressure.

Prevention and Treatment While taking these drugs, you should restrict your consumption of sodium. In particular, those foods listed in the table of Sodium-Rich Foods (see page 306) should be avoided, or consumed in small quantities. You should add no salt at the table and use no more than a ½ teaspoon per day in cooking.

Many people are unaware of how much salt their diet contains. The average American, in fact, consumes some 15 pounds of salt a year. This amounts to 3 to 4 teaspoons a day. Even if you do not salt your food while preparing or eating it, you consume quantities of salt in such foods as anchovies, dill pickles, sardines, green olives, canned soups and vegetables, so-called TV dinners, soy sauce, processed cheeses, many snack foods, cold cuts, and catsup. Other sources such as monosodium glutamate should be avoided.

To sharpen your awareness of the sodium content of food products, read the list of ingredients that appears on the labels of all packaged foods. If sodium is one of the first ingredients on the label, it is present in significant quantities. If sodium is at the lower end of the list, then the food contains very little sodium.

ANTHRAQUINONE CATHARTICS

DRUG FAMILY: Laxative

BRAND NAMES: [GENERIC/Brand] CASCARA SAGRADA/Aromatic Cascara Fluidextract; Milk of Magnesia–Cascara; Peri-Colace; DANTHRON/Doxidan; Modane Plus; Modane; SENNA/Perdiem; Senokot; Senokot-S; X-Prep; Herbal Laxative; HerbLax Laxative; Swiss Kriss Herbal Laxative

HOW TO TAKE ANTHRAQUINONE CATHARTICS: Before bedtime

FOODS TO AVOID: None

POSSIBLE SIDE EFFECTS: Potassium deficiency

ACTION OF ANTHRAQUINONE CATHARTICS: These drugs give a laxative effect in 6 to 8 hours. They act by increasing the action of the muscles lining the large intestine and so reduce the time required for food to pass through the intestinal tract. They also act partly by causing secretion of water into the large intestine, which increases the bulk of the stools.

HIGH-RISK GROUPS: Heart patients, the elderly

NUTRITIONAL INTERACTIONS

POTASSIUM DEFICIENCY: It is conceivable that frequent use of one of these drugs will lead to a potassium deficiency. These laxatives cause the excretion of body potassium into the digestive tract, from where it is excreted in the stool. Potassium regulates the amount of water in the cells of the body and is essential for the proper functioning of the kidneys and the heart muscle, and the secretion of stomach juices. The most alarming symptom of a potassium deficiency is an irregular heartbeat, which can lead to heart failure.

Low blood levels of potassium, called hypokalemia, are especially prevalent among elderly people, who often consume diets low in potassium and take laxatives daily. Common symptoms of potassium deficiency are weakness, loss of appetite, nausea, vomiting, dryness of the mouth, increased thirst, listlessness, apprehension, and diffuse pain that comes and goes.

Diuretics, commonly prescribed for people with heart disease, decrease the level of body potassium, as do cortisone-containing drugs. Therefore, the risk of a deficiency is significantly increased if they are taken concurrently with this drug.

Prevention and Treatment: Potassium depletion can be avoided by including potassium-rich foods in your diet, such as tomato juice, lentils, dried apricots, asparagus, bananas, peanut butter, chicken, almonds, and milk. (See table of Potassium-Rich Foods, page 302.)

Potassium supplements should never be taken unless prescribed by a physician. They can cause anemia by interfering with the absorption of vitamin B_{12}. Just a few grams can also drastically increase the risk of heart failure. If you experience difficulty in swallowing while taking potassium supplements, consult your physician immediately. If supplements are prescribed, be aware that the absorption of the supplements potassium iodide and potassium chloride is decreased by dairy products, and that both are gastric irritants and should be taken with meals.

Too much salt in your diet can also compromise your body's supply of potassium.

ANTIHISTAMINES

DRUG FAMILY: Antihistamines

BRAND NAMES: [GENERIC/Brand] CARBINOXAMINE/Clistin; Brexin; Cardec DM; Rondec; Rondec-DM; Rondec-TR; CHLORCYCLIZINE HYDROCHLORIDE/Perazil; CYCLIZINE/Marezine; DEXCHLORPHENIRAMINE/Polaramine Repetabs; DIPHENHYDRAMINE HYDROCHLORIDE/Allerdryl 50; Ambenyl; Benadryl; Benylin; Bromanyl; Compoz Nighttime Sleep-Aid; Dytuss; Miles Nervine Nighttime Sleep Aid; Nytol; Sleep-eze 3; Sleepinal; Sominex 2; DIPHENYLPYRALINE HYDROCHLORIDE/Hispril; HYDROXYZINE HYDROCHLORIDE/Atarax; Durrax; Marax; Neucalm 50; T.E.H.; T.E.P.; Theozine; Vistaril; METHDILAZINE/Tacaryl; PHENIRAMINE MALEATE/Citra Forte; Fiogesic; Poly-Histine-D; Ru-Tuss; S-T Forte; Triaminic; Tussagesic; Triaminicol; Ursinus Inlay-Tabs; PROMETHAZINE HYDROCHLORIDE/Compal; Dihydrocodeine Compound; Mepergan; Phenergan; Phenergan VC; Remsed; Stopayne; PROMETHAZINE/Dihydrocodeine; Promethazine DM; Promethazine w/Codeine; Promethazine VC; Promethazine VC w/Codeine; TRIMEPRAZINE TARTRATE/Temaril; TRIPELENNAMINE HYDROCHLORIDE/PBZ HYDROCHLORIDE; PBZ-SR; TRIPELENNAMINE/PBZ; TRIPROLIDINE/Triafed; TRIPROLIDINE HYDROCHLORIDE/Actidil; Actifed; Actifed-C; Triafed-C; Trifed; Tripodrine

HOW TO TAKE ANTIHISTAMINES: These drugs can be taken at any time with a nonalcoholic beverage, except for tripelennamine antihistamines, which should be taken with meals.

FOODS TO AVOID: Large quantities of alkaline foods such as milk, buttermilk, cream, almonds, chestnuts, coconuts, all vegetables except corn and lentils, all fruits except cranberries, prunes, and plums; alcoholic beverages

POSSIBLE SIDE EFFECTS: Inability to concentrate; dizziness; drowsiness; and impaired coordination. In the case of tripelennamine-containing drugs, an upset stomach can also occur.

ACTION OF ANTIHISTAMINES: These drugs prevent the secretion of histamine and are used in the treatment of allergies, nausea, and motion sickness, to relieve congestion, cough, and itching, and as a tranquilizer and local anesthetic. The drug is also the preferred treatment in seasonal allergies and is sometimes used in the treatment of asthma.

HIGH-RISK GROUPS: People with a history of abdominal distress

NUTRITIONAL INTERACTIONS

ALKALINE URINE: The action of this drug can be prolonged if your urine is alkaline, as the residue of the drug is excreted at a normal rate only if your urine is acidic. If the quantity of alkaline foods in your diet is high, your urine will lose its acidity, and the excretion of this drug will be slowed. A hazardous buildup could conceivably result. The symptoms of such a buildup or overdose are an inability to concentrate, dizziness, poor coordination, drowsiness, and a dry mouth. Fruits, vegetables, and dairy products tend to be alkaline, and high-protein foods tend to be acidic.

Prevention and Treatment: Foods causing the production of alkaline urine, such as milk, buttermilk, cream, almonds, chestnuts, coconuts, all vegetables except corn and lentils, and all fruits except cranberries, prunes, and plums, can increase the potency of this drug by as much as two times,

further increasing the risk of adverse side effects.

Anatacids that neutralize the acid in the stomach will also neutralize the acid in the urine, making it alkaline. Therefore, avoid antacids when taking this drug.

GASTROINTESTINAL DISTRESS: In the case of tripelennamine, gastric irritation may result from its use.

Prevention and Treatment: To minimize the gastric discomfort, these varieties should be taken with meals.

OTHER ADVICE: These drugs speed up the degradation of digitoxin, rendering it less effective if the two are taken together.

Antihistamines may bring about dizziness, an inability to concentrate, and reduced coordination, making it unwise to drive while using them. Alcohol exacerbates these effects and should never be combined with these drugs.

ASPARAGINASE

DRUG FAMILY: Anti-cancer

BRAND NAMES: Elspar

HOW TO TAKE ASPARAGINASE: Injection

FOODS TO AVOID: None

POSSIBLE SIDE EFFECTS: Loss of appetite

ACTION OF ASPARAGINASE: This drug is used in combination with other drugs to induce remission in children with Hodgkin's disease.

HIGH-RISK GROUPS: Children

NUTRITIONAL INTERACTIONS

WEIGHT LOSS: This drug is likely to cause anorexia (loss of appetite) and weight loss.

Prevention and Treatment: As this drug is usually used for periods of up to one month, special precautions are not usually taken. However, if weight loss is a problem, your doctor may decide intravenous feeding is necessary.

ASPIRIN

DRUG FAMILY: Anti-inflammatory

BRAND NAMES: A.P.C. with Codeine; Anacin Analgesic; Anacin; Arthritis Bayer; Arthritis Pain Formula; Arthritis Strength Bufferin; Ascriptin; Ascriptin with Codeine; Axotal; Bayer Aspirin; Buff-A Comp; Bufferin; Bufferin with Codeine; Cama Arthritis; Congespirin; Cosprin; Cosprin 650; Darvon with A.S.A.; Darvon-N with A.S.A.; Di-Gesic; Dihydrocodeine Compound; Easprin; Ecotrin; Empirin with Codeine; Equagesic; Excedrin; 4-Way Cold; Fiorinal; Gemnisyn; Hyco-Pap; Mepro Compound; Methocarbamol with Aspirin; Midol; Norgesic and Norgesic Forte; Oxycodone Hydrochloride, Oxycodone Terephthalate & Aspirin; Percodan; Percodan-Demi; Propoxyphene Compound 65; Robaxisal; SK-Oxycodone with Aspirin; SK-65 Compound; Supac; Synalgos-DC; Talwin Compound; Vanquish; Verin; Zorprin

HOW TO TAKE ASPIRIN: Regular aspirin should be taken with milk or meals. Buffered aspirin may be taken at any time with any nonalcoholic beverage.

FOODS TO AVOID: Alcoholic beverages

POSSIBLE SIDE EFFECTS: Gastric bleeding. In frequent users, deficiencies of the following may occur: iron, folacin, and vitamins A and B_1. On rare occasions, vitamin K deficiencies may also occur.

ACTION OF ASPIRIN: A widely used and effective analgesic and anti-inflammatory agent, aspirin is commonly used for the relief of headache, insomnia, nervousness, hangover, cold, cough, sore throat, and pain or discomfort. The elderly most often use aspirin to relieve pain associated with arthritic and other musculoskeletal disorders.

The elderly also take aspirin on medical advice to prevent heart attacks and strokes. Just as aspirin prevents platelets (small blood cells) from sticking together to form a clot when you cut yourself, so it prevents the clotting in the body that can lead to the blocking of blood vessels. It also tends to reduce the production of prothrombin, another blood-clotting factor.

HIGH-RISK GROUPS: The elderly, users of oral contraceptives, heavy drinkers, menstruating women, children, pregnant women, smokers, lactating women, teenagers, vegetarians

NUTRITIONAL INTERACTIONS

IRON DEFICIENCY: Of those people who take 1 to 3 grams of unbuffered aspirin daily, some 70 percent experience gastrointestinal bleeding. One characteristic sign is black stools. This loss of blood is likely to lead to an iron deficiency.

Iron is particularly important to the oxygen-carrying cells of the blood and muscles, which consume two thirds of the iron your body requires. An iron shortage reduces the blood's oxygen-carrying capacity, and the result is anemia, signaled by such symptoms as tiredness, general feelings of malaise, irritability, decreased attention span, pale complexion, rapid heart rhythm, headaches, loss of concentration, and breathlessness on exertion. A mild iron deficiency will also impair the functioning of your immune system.

For iron to be absorbed from any vegetable source, the mineral must be converted to another form by the action of the hydrochloric acid produced in the stomach. Many of the elderly secrete less hydrochloric acid than normal, so they absorb iron poorly even under normal circumstances. The diets of many Americans lack adequate quantities of this mineral for their average needs. For example, 10 percent of American women suffer from an iron deficiency, and up to 30 percent have inadequate iron stores. Other people who are at significant risk of an iron deficiency are women who have had several pregnancies and those whose menstrual periods are heavy.

Many diets are short on iron not only because of the selection of foods that are poor sources of the nutrient, but also because of the switch from cast-iron cookware to aluminum, stainless steel, and nonstick surfaces. The acids in the foods being prepared used to leach the mineral from the iron pots and pans, which then became available as dietary iron.

Prevention and Treatment: To counteract an iron deficiency, iron-rich foods should be included in your diet: liver, whole grain products, oysters, dried apricots, prunes, peaches, leafy green vegetables, and occasionally, lean red meat. (See table of Iron-Rich Foods, page 299.)

Other foods and drugs have a considerable impact on the way your body absorbs (or does not absorb) iron. There are two kinds of iron in food sources: heme iron in meat and ionic iron in vegetables. Up to 40 percent of the iron from meat, fish, and poultry is absorbed, but less than 10 percent is absorbed from eggs, whole grains, nuts, and dried beans. Only 10 percent of ionic iron is absorbed from vegetable sources, with as little as 2 percent being absorbed from spinach.

Antacids will interfere with iron absorption from vegetables, as will commercial black and pekoe tea, taken in substantial quantities, because of its tannin content. Coffee also seems to decrease iron absorption, but not to the same degree as tea. Vitamin C supplements or citrus fruit juices increase the absorption of iron from vegetable sources by two to three times if taken simultaneously. If your diet is high in fiber-containing foods, you will have impaired iron absorption because the indigestible fiber will bind to the iron and pass it out in the stool. This same action contributes to the poor absorption of iron from vegetable sources. Foods high in phosphorus (e.g., meat) interfere with iron absorption, which explains why only 30 percent of the iron in meat is captured. (However, meat and fish facilitate iron absorption from vegetables.) For that matter, any use of large quantities of mineral supplements, such as zinc, will impair iron absorption. Because iron can be leached from vegetables if they are cooked in large amounts of water, it is preferable to steam them.

You should not take iron supplements without your physician's recommendation because an accumulation of too much iron can lead in extreme cases to such serious problems as anemia, malfunctioning of the pancreas and the heart, cirrhosis of the liver, a brown cast to the skin, and depression.

FOLIC ACID DEFICIENCY: Chronic use of aspirin is likely to increase the rate of loss of folacin in the urine, leading to a deficiency. Often the first sign of a folic acid or folacin deficiency is inflamed or bleeding gums. The symptoms that follow are a sore, smooth tongue; diarrhea; forgetfulness; apathy; irritability; anemia; and a reduced resistance to infection. Despite the fact that folacin is found in a variety of foods, folacin deficiency is still the most common vitamin deficiency in the United States.

In adults, deficiencies are limited almost exclusively to the elderly and women, almost a third of whom have intakes below the Recommended Dietary Allowance, while at least one out of twenty also has severe anemia. There are several factors that account for this, but one of the most obvious reasons is that oral contraceptive use decreases the absorption of folic acid. Constant dieting also limits folacin intake, while alcohol interferes both with the body's use of folic acid and its absorption. Folacin is not stored by the body in any appreciable amounts, so an adequate supply must be consumed on a daily basis.

Pregnant women should be especially careful, since folate deficiencies cause fetal abnormalities. Folic acid is also crucial to the normal metabolism of proteins.

Prevention and Treatment: To counteract a deficiency in folic acid, your diet should contain liver, yeast, and leafy vegetables such as spinach, kale, parsley, cauliflower, brussels sprouts, and broccoli. The fruits that are highest in folic acid are oranges and cantaloupes. To a lesser degree, folacin is found in almonds and lima beans, corn, parsnips, green peas, pumpkins, sweet potatoes, bran, peanuts, rye, and whole grain wheat. (See table of Folacin-Rich Foods, page 297.) Approximately one half of the folic acid you consume is absorbed by your body.

Since normal cooking temperatures (110 to 120 degrees for 10 minutes) destroy up to 65 percent of the folacin in your food, your daily diet should include some raw vegetables and fruits. Cooking utensils made out of copper speed up folacin's destruction.

The recommended daily consumption of folacin is 400 mcg, but since screening for folacin blood levels is difficult and few laboratories conduct such tests, lactating women should assume a daily need of 1,200 mcg. Pregnant women and oral contraceptive users should consume 800 mcg daily.

VITAMIN C DEFICIENCY: Aspirin causes the body to retain less of the dietary vitamin C. If you take twelve or more aspirins a day, as may well be the case if you suffer from arthritis, this dosage is likely to lead to a vitamin C deficiency, which is usually indicated by bleeding gums and bruising.

With an adequate vitamin C intake, the body normally maintains a fixed pool of the vitamin and rapidly excretes any excess in the urine. Ordinarily, 60 to 100 mg of vitamin C per day will fulfill the body's needs.

However, with an inadequate intake, the reservoir becomes depleted at the rate of up to 3 percent per day, and even more quickly in users of this drug. Obvious symptoms of a vitamin C deficiency do not appear until the available vitamin C has been reduced to about one fifth of its optimal level, and this may take two months to occur.

Other signs of a deficiency are slightly swollen wrists and ankles, and capillaries that break under the skin, producing pinpoint hemorrhages around the hair follicles on the arms and legs.

Vitamin C is important to the functioning of your bodily systems in a number of ways. When your body is deficient in Vitamin C, your white blood cells are less able to detect and destroy invading bacteria. On the other hand, megadoses of the vitamin (over 2 grams daily) can also impair this ability. Vitamin C also helps your body guard itself against such pollutants as known cancer-causing agents nitrites and nitrosamines, and protects vitamins A and E from degradation. It also aids in iron absorption, speeds up wound healing, and strengthens blood vessels. Other well-known effects are that, in some people, vitamin C reduces the symptoms of a cold by one third, and is important in preventing plaque formation on the teeth, which reduces the likelihood of gum disease and tooth decay.

Prevention and Treatment: Patients taking aspirin should be sure to get 100 mg per day of vitamin C. Vitamin C-rich foods include citrus fruits, broccoli, spinach, cabbage, and bananas. (See table of Vitamin-C Rich Foods, page 313.) In preparing foods rich in vitamin C, you should keep in mind that it is readily oxidized (when exposed to the air during both food processing and storage). Copper and iron cooking utensils will speed up the oxidation; also, the longer the food is cooked and the higher the temperature, the greater the vitamin loss. Large amounts of water used in cooking will wash out the vitamin. Vitamin C is also destroyed when fruit or vegetables are cut or bruised.

Supplements can be taken, although, once again, the body tends to eliminate any surplus of the vitamin, so supplements of more than 100 mg a day are unnecessary. In fact, megadoses can cause nausea, abdominal cramps, and diarrhea, among other undesirable side effects. Supplements are especially important for oral contraceptive users and for smokers, who need one and a half times the Recommended Dietary Allowance.

VITAMIN B₁ DEFICIENCY: While taking aspirin regularly, it is conceivable that you will develop a deficiency of thiamin, as aspirin increases its excretion.

Vitamin B_1, or thiamin as it is also known, can be destroyed by antacids consumed at mealtimes. Heart palpitations may result, along with mental confusion, moodiness, and tiredness. Other symptoms of a B_1 deficiency are difficulty in walking, weight loss, and water retention, especially at the ankles. Heavy consumers of alcohol tend to be deficient in this vitamin and therefore are at higher risk.

Older Americans are also frequently found to be marginally deficient in this vitamin. A severe deficiency in this age group can be the cause of symptoms resembling senility, which are reversible when the supply of B_1

is replenished. This vitamin is also said to stimulate appetite.

Prevention and Treatment: To avoid a thiamin deficiency, significant food sources of the vitamin should be included in your diet, such as whole grain cereals, oatmeal, nuts, peas, lima beans, oysters, liver, pork (especially ham), beef, lamb, poultry, and eggs. (See table of Vitamin B₁(Thiamin)-Rich Foods, page 309.)

The presence of baking soda in cooking will destroy both vitamins B_1 and B_{12}, so it should be avoided when possible. High temperatures too are very destructive to B_1. Blackberries, brussels sprouts, beets, red cabbage, and spinach contain the enzyme thiaminase, which inactivates the vitamin. Large quantities of these foods should not be consumed raw.

VITAMIN K DEFICIENCY: Although highly unlikely, a vitamin K deficiency may also develop. Since vitamin K helps the liver produce blood-clotting substances, a deficiency could result in hemorrhaging in the body.

Prevention and Treatment: To safeguard against such a deficiency, include some good sources of the vitamin in the diet, such as kale, spinach, cabbage, cauliflower, leafy green vegetables, liver (especially pork liver), and fish. (See table of Vitamin K-Rich Foods, page 315.)

OTHER ADVICE: People using aspirin on a regular basis should always prefer buffered aspirin. Regular aspirin should be taken with meals or milk to prevent gastric irritation bleeding.

ATENOLOL

DRUG FAMILY: Anti-hypertensive

BRAND NAME: Tenormin

HOW TO TAKE ATENOLOL: One hour before or 2 to 3 after meals, on an empty stomach with a nonalcoholic beverage

FOODS TO AVOID: Large amounts of tyramine- and dopamine-containing foods: aged cheeses, raisins, avocados, liver, bananas, eggplant, sour cream, alcoholic beverages, salami, meat tenderizers, chocolate, yeast, soy sauce, and others; licorice candy

POSSIBLE SIDE EFFECTS: On rare occasions: dizziness; fatigue; diarrhea and nausea

ACTION OF ATENOLOL: This drug is prescribed for the management of high blood pressure.

HIGH-RISK GROUPS: Anyone who takes this drug

NUTRITIONAL INTERACTIONS

TYRAMINE-RICH FOODS: Foods that are high in tyramines, a food substance, elevate blood pressure when consumed in quantity. Consequently they are likely to make this drug less effective.

Prevention and Treatment: Tyramine-containing foods should be restricted while you are being treated with this drug. Tyramine is common in many foods, but it is found in the greatest amounts in high-protein foods that have undergone some decomposition, like aged cheese. Tyramine is also found in chicken and beef livers, bananas, eggplant, sour cream, alcoholic beverages, salami, meat tenderizers, chocolate, yeast, and soy sauce. (See table of Tyramine-Rich Foods, page 307.) Raisins and avocados should also be avoided, because they contain dopamine, which has the same effect as tyramine.

Licorice candy that is made with natural extract contains glycyrrhizic acid, which also can elevate blood pressure by causing sodium and water retention. As little as 3 ounces is enough to induce such a reaction, so it is best to avoid eating it when taking atenolol.

POTENCY: This drug has been shown to be less effective when consumed with food.

Prevention and Treatment: Atenolol should be taken on an empty stomach, 1 hour before or 2 to 3 after meals.

ATROPINE

DRUG FAMILY: Anti-muscarinic

BRAND NAMES: Diphenoxylate & Atropine; Espasmotex; Trac Tabs; Trac Tabs 2X; Festalan; Antrocol; Arco-Lase Plus; Atropine Sulfate; Comhist; Diphenoxylate Hydrochloride & Atropine Sulfate; Probocon; Ru-Tuss; SK-Diphenoxylate; Urised

HOW TO TAKE ATROPINE: One-half hour before meals, with some nonalcoholic beverage

FOODS TO AVOID: Large amounts of alkaline foods such as milk, buttermilk, cream, almonds, chestnuts, coconuts, all vegetables except corn and lentils, and all fruits except cranberries, prunes, and plums

POSSIBLE SIDE EFFECTS: Dry mouth

ACTION OF ATROPINE: This drug interferes with the transmission of nerve impulses to smooth muscles, causing them to relax and also causing various glands to reduce their rate of secretion.

Among its numerous applications, atropine is used in the following ways: to treat diarrhea associated with diverticulosis and dysenteries; to control extensive salivation associated with Parkinson's disease and heavy metal poisoning; to reduce secretion in the nasal passages and lungs due to hay fever and colds; to regulate heart rate; to treat motion sickness; to relax the bladder; locally to dilate the pupil of the eye and put the eye muscle at rest prior to an eye examination or eye surgery; and to inhibit gastrointestinal motility and reduce gastric acid secretion, as an adjunct to therapy for peptic ulcer patients. It is also used in aerosol form by asthma patients to dilate the air passages in their lungs.

HIGH-RISK GROUPS: Anyone who takes this drug

NUTRITIONAL INTERACTIONS

ALKALINE URINE: The action of atropine is prolonged by alkaline urine. If the quantity of alkaline foods in your diet is high, your urine will lose its acidity, and the excretion of this drug will be slowed. A hazardous buildup could conceivably result. The symptoms of such a buildup or overdose are blurred vision, dry mouth, difficult urination, and a flushing or dryness of the skin.

Prevention and Treatment: Fruits, vegetables, and dairy products tend to be alkaline, and high-protein foods tend to be acidic. Foods causing the production of alkaline urine include milk, buttermilk, cream, almonds, chestnuts, coconuts, all vegetables except corn and lentils, and all fruits except cranberries, prunes, and plums.

Antacids that neutralize the acid in the stomach will also neutralize the acid in the urine, causing it to turn alkaline. Therefore, you should avoid antacids when taking this drug.

OTHER ADVICE: Significant doses of atropine increase the absorption of digoxin, so be sure your doctor is aware that you are taking both drugs.

This drug can also cause a dry mouth sensation, so be sure you drink plenty of fluids, which means at least 6 to 8 glasses per day.

Atropine should be taken one-half hour before meals, since it is best absorbed and therefore most effective on an empty stomach.

AZATHIOPRINE

DRUG FAMILY: Immune system suppressing agent

BRAND NAME: Imuran

HOW TO TAKE AZATHIOPRINE: At the end of meals, with a beverage

FOODS TO AVOID: None

POSSIBLE SIDE EFFECTS: Nausea, vomiting, and other gastrointestinal distress

ACTION OF AZATHIOPRINE: This drug is used for the prevention of rejection in renal transplantation. It is also used in treating severe rheumatoid arthritis that does not respond to rest or to steroidal anti-inflammatory drugs.

HIGH-RISK GROUPS: Anyone who takes this drug

NUTRITIONAL INTERACTIONS

GASTROINTESTINAL DISTURBANCES: Slightly more than 1 in 10 patients taking this drug report nausea and vomiting or other gastrointestinal distress.

Prevention and Treatment: In order to reduce the chances of such discomfort, the drug should be taken at the end of meals.

BARBITURATES

DRUG FAMILY: Anti-anxiety

BRAND NAMES: [GENERIC/Brand] AMOBARBITAL/Amytal; AMOBARBITAL SODIUM/Amytal Sodium; Tuinal; APROBARBITAL/Alurate; BARBITURATE PREPARATIONS/Alurate; Buff-A Comp; Buff-A Comp No. 3; Donnatal; G-1; G-2; G-3; Kinesed; Levsin/Phenobarbital; Levsinex/Phenobarbital; Lotusate; Mebaral; Nembutal Sodium; Repan; BUTABARBITAL/Pyridium Plus; Quibron Plus; Tedral-25; BUTALBITAL/Amaphen; Amaphen with Codeine No. 3; Anoquan; Axotal; Bancap; Bancap c̄ Codeine; Buff-A Comp; Buff-A Comp No. 3; Butalbital Compound; Esgic; Fiorinal; Fiorinal w/Codeine; G-1; G-2; G-3; Pacaps; Phrenilin; Phrenilin Forte; Repan; Sedapap-10; Two-Dyne; MEPHOBARBITAL/Mebaral; METHARBITAL/Gemonil; METHOHEXITAL SODIUM/Brevital Sodium; SECOBARBITAL SODIUM/Seconal Sodium; Tuinal;

TALBUTAL/Lotusate; THIAMYLAL SODIUM/ Surital

HOW TO TAKE BARBITURATES: With a non-alcoholic beverage at any time

FOODS TO AVOID: All alcoholic beverages. Very sweet foods rich in simple sugars, such as cookies, candies, cake, and soft drinks containing sugar, should not be consumed in large quantities.

POSSIBLE SIDE EFFECTS: Vitamin C deficiency

ACTION OF BARBITURATES: These drugs decrease anxiety and tension, and can also be used in the treatment of insomnia. However, barbiturates have been largely replaced by the safer benzodiazepines, since barbiturates both depress the brain to a greater degree than the benzodiazepines, and involve a higher risk of overdosage and toxicity.

HIGH-RISK GROUPS: Smokers, users of oral contraceptives, heavy drinkers, the elderly (especially those taking diuretics), vegetarians

NUTRITIONAL INTERACTIONS

VITAMIN C AND MINERAL DEFICIENCIES: Barbiturates increase vitamin C requirements and could conceivably lead to a deficiency. With an adequate vitamin C intake, the body normally maintains a fixed pool of the vitamin and rapidly excretes any excess in the urine. Ordinarily, 100 mg of vitamin C per day is sufficient to provide for the body's needs, except perhaps in the case of smokers, who may need a little more.

However, with an inadequate intake, the reservoir becomes depleted at the rate of up to 3 percent per day, and even more quickly in barbiturate users. Obvious symptoms of a vitamin C deficiency do not appear until the available vitamin C has been reduced to about one fifth of its optimal level, and this may very well take two months to occur.

The earliest signs of deficiency are spongy or bleeding gums, slightly swollen wrists and ankles, capillaries that break under the skin, producing pinpoint hemorrhages around the hair follicles on the arms and legs, and a decreased resistance to infection. Inadequate dietary levels of vitamin C, potassium, magnesium, and zinc all lead to an increased potency of the drug, due to a slower rate of drug degradation. Hence, to avoid drug toxicity, adequate amounts of vitamin C, zinc, magnesium, and potassium should be included in the diet. This is especially important in patients concurrently taking diuretics that tend to deplete the body's supply of these minerals.

Antacids should never be taken with barbiturates, because they delay the absorption of barbiturates and nullify their affect. Vegetarians may need to take higher doses of barbiturates for them to be effective, since dairy products, vegetables, and fruit, which cause the urine to be alkaline, help excrete the drug more rapidly than normal. Alcohol alarmingly enhances the effects of barbiturates.

Prevention and Treatment: Patients using barbiturates should be sure to get the Recommended Dietary Allowance of zinc, potassium, and magnesium in their diet, along with 100 mg per day of vitamin C. Rich sources of vitamin C include citrus fruits, tomatoes, cantaloupe, strawberries, broccoli, cabbage, peppers, and potatoes.

Animal foods are good sources of zinc, with the richest being oysters, herring, milk, and egg yolks. Among plant foods, whole grains are richest in zinc, but it is not as well absorbed from them as from meat. In cereal grains too the absorption of zinc is reduced, since the fiber and phytic acid (a substance found in vegetable fiber) in the cereal grains hinders the absorption of zinc. The recommended intake of 15 mg a day for adults is probably easily met by the diet of the average middle-class person, but a deficiency is likely if animal protein is underemphasized. As a rule of thumb, two small servings of animal protein a day will provide sufficient zinc.

Potassium-rich foods include bananas, orange and many other fruit juices, potatoes, tomatoes, and many other vegetables. Recommended intakes of magnesium are 300 to 350 mg a day for adult males and 250 to 300 mg for females. Good food sources include nuts, legumes, cereal grains, dark green vegetables, seafoods, chocolate, and cocoa.

Alcohol should not be taken concurrently with barbiturates since it increases the depressant effect of the drug on the brain. Very sweet foods should be limited because they speed up the rate of degradation of the drug, making it less effective.

BELLADONNA

DRUG FAMILY: Anti-muscarinic

BRAND NAMES: Bellergal; Bellergal-S; Chardonna-2; Belladenal; Belladenal-S; Comhist LA; Donnagel; Donnagel PG; Donnatal; Donnazyme; Kaolin, Pectin, Belladonna Mixture; Kinesed; Trac Tabs; Wyanoids HC

HOW TO TAKE BELLADONNA: With a nonalcoholic beverage one-half hour before meals

FOODS TO AVOID: Large amounts of alkaline foods such as milk, buttermilk, cream, almonds, chestnuts, coconuts, all vegetables except corn and lentils, and all fruits except cranberries, prunes, and plums

POSSIBLE SIDE EFFECTS: Dry mouth

ACTION OF BELLADONNA: Belladonna is an anti-muscarinic drug that relaxes smooth muscles and reduces glandular secretion. Belladonna acts by interfering with the transmission of nerve impulses to the muscles in the walls of the intestines and is used in treating patients with ulcerative colitis, to reduce gastrointestinal motility as a means of controlling diarrhea. It is also used in the treatment of motion sickness.

HIGH-RISK GROUPS: Anyone who takes this drug

NUTRITIONAL INTERACTIONS

ALKALINE URINE: The action of belladonna is prolonged by alkaline urine. If the quantity of alkaline foods in your diet is high, your urine will lose its acidity, and the excretion of this drug will be slowed. A hazardous buildup could conceivably result. The symptoms of such a buildup or overdose are a tingling and numbness of the feet and hands, blurred vision, palpitations, dry mouth, decreased sweating, urinary retention, rapid heart rate, flushing, and drowsiness.

Prevention and Treatment: Fruits, vegetables, and dairy products tend to be alkaline, and high-protein foods tend to be acidic. Foods causing the production of alkaline urine include milk, buttermilk, cream, almonds, chestnuts, coconuts, all vegetables except corn and lentils, and all fruits except cranberries, prunes, and plums.

Antacids that neutralize the acid in the stomach will also neutralize the acid in the urine, causing it to turn alkaline. Therefore, you should avoid antacids when taking this drug.

OTHER ADVICE: Significant doses of belladonna increase the absorption of digoxin, so be sure your doctor is aware you are taking both drugs.

This drug can also cause a dry mouth sensation, so be sure you drink plenty of fluids. This means at least 6 to 8 glasses a day.

Belladonna should be taken one-half hour before meals for maximum absorption and effectiveness.

BENZODIAZEPINES

DRUG FAMILY: Anti-anxiety

BRAND NAMES: [GENERIC/Brand] ALPRAZOLAM/Xanax; CHLORDIAZEPOXIDE/Libritabs; Limbitrol; Menrium; CLORAZEPATE DIPOTASSIUM/Tranxene; Tranxene-SD; DIAZEPAM/Valium; Valrelease; LORAZEPAM/Ativan; OXAZEPAM/Serax; PRAZEPAM/Centrax

HOW TO TAKE BENZODIAZEPINES: With meals

FOODS TO AVOID: All alcoholic beverages

POSSIBLE SIDE EFFECTS: Weight gain, diarrhea, nausea, vomiting, and stomach cramps

ACTION OF BENZODIAZEPINES: These drugs are sedatives and are used as anti-anxiety agents, anti-convulsants, muscle relaxants, and anesthetics, and in the treatment of insomnia.

HIGH-RISK GROUPS: Heavy drinkers, the elderly

NUTRITIONAL INTERACTIONS

WEIGHT GAIN: It is conceivable that you will find the use of one of the benzodiazepines will cause a significant increase in your appetite, which can lead to weight gain.

Prevention and Treatment: You must carefully watch your weight while taking these drugs. If you seem to be gaining weight, you should make a special effort to prevent yourself from eating more than usual.

If you have already gained weight, you should cut back on the carbohydrate component of your diet, remembering that a reasonable and moderate weight-reduction program should aim at a manageable loss of 1 to 2 pounds per week. An intake reduction of 500 calories per day, for a weekly total of 3,500 calories, will result in the loss of 1 pound per week regardless of your present weight. Two eggs and a milk shake, 1½ cups of tuna salad, 4 ounces of a roast, 3 frankfurters, 2 cups of ice cream, or 2 pieces of cheesecake all represent approximately 500 calories.

The Weight Watchers exercise and behavior modification program is among those that offer a sensible balance of proper nutrition, exercise, and support in making a dietary change. Remember that you need to cut down by 500 calories a day (or 3,500 calories a week) to lose 1 pound. You must never attempt to lose more than 2 pounds a week, however.

OTHER ADVICE: Alcohol intensifies the effects of these drugs and increases the length of time during which they are effective, especially in the elderly. This can lead to varying degrees of light-headedness, lassitude, increased reaction time, poor coordination, poor mental functions, confusion, loss of memory, slurred speech, dry mouth, and a bitter taste. (The same symptoms are experienced if one takes one of these drugs to combat insomnia.) In short, while you are taking any of the benzodiazepines, you should not consume alcohol.

Diarrhea, nausea, vomiting, and stomach cramps are relatively common side effects. In order to prevent stomach cramps and allied gastrointestinal complaints, you should take these drugs with meals.

BENZTROPINE MESYLATE

DRUG FAMILY: Anti-Parkinsonism

BRAND NAME: Cogentin

HOW TO TAKE BENZTROPINE MESYLATE: Best taken after meals

FOODS TO AVOID: None

POSSIBLE SIDE EFFECTS: Constipation

ACTION OF BENZTROPINE MESYLATE: This anti-Parkinsonism drug helps to control tremor.

HIGH-RISK GROUPS: The elderly

NUTRITIONAL INTERACTIONS

CONSTIPATION: The use of benztropine mesylate could conceivably cause constipation.

Prevention and Treatment: An increase in the bulk in the diet is usually the safest remedy to constipation. This means consuming larger servings of any of the following: dried or fresh fruits (especially unpeeled apples or pears), salad vegetables, radishes, oatmeal, and whole grain foods (brown rice, whole wheat breads, and cereals). It is not necessary to purchase products that claim "extra fiber" has been added to them.

Persistent constipation may also be relieved by doubling the amount of fluid consumed each day. Bran, if used, should be added to the diet gradually, and fluid should be increased by at least ¾ cup per teaspoon of bran. (See table of Dietary Fiber-Rich Foods, page 293.)

BORIC ACID

DRUG FAMILY: Local antiseptic

BRAND NAMES: Clear Eyes; Collyrium; Collyrium with Ephedrine; Murine Plus; Wyanoids HC

HOW TO TAKE BORIC ACID: Applied externally

FOODS TO AVOID: None

POSSIBLE SIDE EFFECTS: Riboflavin (vitamin B_2) deficiency

ACTION OF BORIC ACID: Boric acid inhibits bacterial growth and is used in rectal suppositories for hemorrhoids, in ophthalmic ointments, in vaginal deodorants, and in talcum powder.

HIGH-RISK GROUPS: Users of oral contraceptives

NUTRITIONAL INTERACTIONS

RIBOFLAVIN DEFICIENCY: Boric acid increases the rate at which riboflavin is excreted from the body, and a deficiency state could conceivably occur.

The symptoms most likely to appear will be dry skin around the nose and lips, cracks in the corners of the mouth, and sore lips and tongue. Discomfort in eating and swallowing may result. The eyes may burn, itch, be more sensitive than usual to light, and tend to be bloodshot. However, be aware that any B vitamin deficiency can cause similar symptoms.

Riboflavin helps the body transform protein, fats, and carbohydrates into the energy needed to maintain body tissues and to protect the body against common skin and eye disorders. Oral contraceptive users have an increased requirement for riboflavin and so are more likely than normal to develop a deficiency of this vitamin.

Prevention and Treatment: Good sources of riboflavin should be included in the diet. Milk usually contributes about 50 percent of our riboflavin intake, meat about 25 percent, and dark green leafy vegetables and enriched cereals and breads the rest. The need for riboflavin provides a major reason for including milk in some form in every day's meals; no other food that is commonly eaten can make such a substantial contribution to meeting our daily riboflavin needs. People who don't use milk products can substitute a generous serving of dark green leafy vegetables, because a cup of greens such as collards provides about the same amount of riboflavin as a cup of milk. (See table of vitamin B$_2$(Riboflavin)-Rich Foods, page 310.)

Among the meats, liver is the richest source, but all lean meats, as well as eggs, can provide some riboflavin. Riboflavin is light-sensitive; it can be destroyed by the ultraviolet rays of the sun or fluorescent lamps. For this reason, milk is seldom sold, and should not be stored, in transparent glass containers. Cardboard or plastic containers protect the riboflavin in the milk from ultraviolet rays.

BROMPHENIRAMINE MALEATE

DRUG FAMILY: Antihistamine

BRAND NAMES: Bromfed-PD; Bromfed; Bromphen Compound; Bromphen DC; Dimetapp; Dura Tap-PD; E.N.T.; Poly-Histine-DX; Tamine S.R.

HOW TO TAKE BROMPHENIRAMINE MALEATE: With meals

FOODS TO AVOID: All alcoholic beverages; large amounts of alkaline foods such as milk, buttermilk, cream, almonds, chestnuts, coconuts, all vegetables except corn and lentils, and all fruits except cranberries, prunes, and plums

POSSIBLE SIDE EFFECTS: Loss of appetite, nausea, vomiting, stomach cramps, constipation, diarrhea, increased urination, dry mouth

ACTION OF BROMPHENIRAMINE MALEATE: This drug is used in the treatment of seasonal allergies and motion sickness.

HIGH-RISK GROUPS: Heavy drinkers

NUTRITIONAL INTERACTIONS

GASTROINTESTINAL DISTRESS: One side effect of brompheniramine maleate that you might conceivably experience is gastrointestinal distress, which may include a loss of appetite, nausea, vomiting, stomach cramps, constipation, diarrhea, increased urination, and dryness of the mouth.

Prevention and Treatment: These drugs should be taken with meals to avoid the gastric symptoms. To prevent dehydration due to excess urination, at least 6 to 8 glasses of water or its equivalent in other non-alcoholic fluids should be consumed per day.

Body weight should also be monitored to avoid unwanted weight loss.

ALKALINE URINE: Because brompheniramine maleate is alkaline, it is excreted at a normal rate only if your urine is acidic. However, if the quantity of alkaline foods in your diet is high, your urine will lose its acidity, and the excretion of this drug will be slowed. A hazardous buildup could conceivably result, increasing the potency of a given dose of this drug, leading to drowsiness, loss of concentration, ringing in the ears, headache, nausea, and slightly distorted vision.

Prevention and Treatment: Fruits, vegetables, and dairy products tend to be alkaline, and high-protein foods tend to be acidic. Foods causing the production of alkaline urine include milk, buttermilk, cream, almonds, chestnuts, coconuts, all vegetables except corn and lentils, and all fruits except cranberries, prunes, and plums.

Antacids that neutralize the acid in the stomach will also neutralize the acid in the urine, causing it to turn alkaline. Therefore, you should avoid antacids when taking this drug.

ALCOHOL INTERACTION: Alcohol heightens the danger of a loss of coordination. Dizziness, lassitude, fatigue, blurred vision, and double vision are likely to occur, as is an exacerbation of the gastric effects. Alcohol in any form should not be consumed concurrently with the drug.

BUSULFAN

DRUG FAMILY: Anti-cancer

BRAND NAME: Myleran

HOW TO TAKE BUSULFAN: As directed by your physician

FOODS TO AVOID: None

POSSIBLE SIDE EFFECTS: Deficiencies of niacin, riboflavin, folic acid, and vitamin B_6; poor appetite, nausea, and other gastrointestinal disturbances

ACTION OF BUSULFAN: This drug acts by preventing the tumor cells from dividing.

HIGH-RISK GROUPS: Anyone who uses this drug

NUTRITIONAL INTERACTIONS

NIACIN AND RIBOFLAVIN DEFICIENCIES: Use of busulfan is likely to lead to some nutritional deficiencies, especially of Vitamin B_6, niacin (vitamin B_3), and riboflavin (vitamin B_2).

The symptoms are most likely to be cheilosis, dry skin around the nose and lips and a cracking in the corners of the mouth, and glossitis, a smooth, sore tongue. Riboflavin and vitamin B_6 deficiencies cause cheilosis; vitamin B_6, niacin, and folacin deficiencies cause glossitis.

Busulfan functions as an anti-cancer agent by preventing the formation of new cells; it has the same effect on the healthy body systems, including those areas where cells are continuously wearing out and need to be replaced. These include the lining of the gastrointestinal tract, the surface of the lips, and the surface of the tongue.

The problem in the lining of the intestine will prevent the normal absorption of nutrients, including those required to replace old cells. Hence, the cheilosis and glossitis are the result of the combination of these two problems. Good nutrition cannot solve the problem of nutritional deficiencies, but it can at least limit it.

Prevention and Treatment: Good sources of riboflavin, niacin, vitamin B_6, and folic acid should be included in the diet while taking busulfan. Riboflavin is a key factor in the conversion of all food substances to energy, and in maintaining body tissues in a healthy state, especially the eyes and skin.

Milk usually contributes about 50 percent of our riboflavin intake, meat about 25 percent, and dark green leafy vegetables and enriched cereals and breads the remainder. The need for riboflavin provides a major reason for including milk in some form in every day's meals; no other food that is commonly eaten can make such a substantial contribution to our daily needs. People who don't use milk products can substitute a generous serving of dark green leafy vegetables, because a cup of greens such as collards provides about the same amount of riboflavin as a cup of milk.

Among the meats, liver is the richest source, but all lean meats, as well as eggs, can provide some riboflavin. Riboflavin is light-sensitive; it can be destroyed by the ultraviolet rays of the sun and by fluorescent lamps. For this reason, milk is seldom sold, and should not be stored, in transparent glass containers. Cardboard or plastic containers protect the riboflavin in the milk from ultraviolet rays.

Niacin is found in many foods. Milk, eggs, meat, poultry, and fish contribute about half the niacin consumed by most people, and about one fourth comes from enriched breads and cereals. Niacin permits all the tissues in the body to derive energy from the food we eat. It comes in two forms, nicotinic acid and nicotinamide (sometimes called niacinamide). Niacin is unique among the B vitamins in that can be made from protein. Tryptophan, one of the amino acids (the constituent building blocks of protein), can be converted to niacin in the body. Every 6 grams of protein in the diet contains 60 mg of tryptophan, which is sufficient to make 1 mg of niacin. Thus, a food containing, for example, 1 mg niacin and 60 mg tryptophan contains the equivalent of 2 mg niacin. However, not all the tryptophan in the diet is available to be made into niacin, since the tryptophan is also needed to build body proteins. The need for niacin is proportional to the energy intake.

Vegetarians are well advised to emphasize nuts and legumes in their diets, since these are good sources of niacin and protein.

VITAMIN B_6 DEFICIENCY: Vitamin B_6 is a key factor in the body's breakdown of protein, and dietary needs are roughly proportional to protein intakes. Common symptoms of vitamin B_6 deficiency are a sore mouth and tongue, cracks in the lips and corners of the mouth, and patches of itching, scaling skin. A severe vitamin B_6 deficiency may cause depression and confusion.

Vitamin B_6 deficiencies are common among the elderly. Alcoholics, as well, often experience this deficiency, since alcohol interferes with the body's ability to use B_6. Smokers also tend to have low body levels of this vitamin. It is estimated that one of every two Americans consumes less than 70 percent of the Recommended Dietary Allowance of B_6.

Prevention and Treatment: To avoid a B_6 deficiency, you should consume a diet featuring food sources of vitamin B_6 such as liver (beef, calf, and pork), herring, salmon, walnuts, peanuts, wheat germ, carrots, peas, potatoes, grapes, bananas, and yeast. (See table of Vitamin B_6(Pyridoxine)-Rich Foods, page 311.) The vitamin is present in significant amounts in meats, fish, fruits, cereals, and vegetables, and to a lesser extent in milk and other dairy products.

Since vitamin B_6 is decomposed at high temperatures, modern food processing often diminishes dietary sources of the vitamin. Consequently, the more processed foods you eat, the more susceptible you will be to a deficiency of this vitamin. The same losses also occur in cooking: meat loses as much as 45 to 80 percent, vegetables 20 to 30 percent.

FOLIC ACID DEFICIENCY: Folacin is required for any form of cell multiplication. For example, the cells on the surface of the tongue are continuously being replaced, but with-

out folacin this cannot occur. Thus, a sore tongue is one symptom of folic acid deficiency. Folacin is also needed for the manufacture of new blood cells.

Frequently, the first symptom of a folic acid or folacin deficiency is inflamed and bleeding gums. The symptoms that follow are a sore, smooth tongue; diarrhea; forgetfulness; apathy; irritability; and anemia. Despite the fact that folacin is found in a variety of foods, folacin deficiency is still the most common vitamin deficiency in the United States.

Folacin is not stored by the body in any appreciable amounts, so an adequate supply must be consumed on a daily basis. In adults, deficiencies are limited almost exclusively to the elderly and women, 30 percent of whom have intakes below the recommended daily allowance and 5 to 7 percent of whom also have severe anemia. There are several factors that account for this bias, but one of the most obvious reasons is that oral contraceptive use decreases the absorption of folic acid. Constant dieting also limits folacin intake, and alcohol interferes with the body's use of folic acid, as well.

Folic acid is also crucial to the normal metabolism of proteins.

Prevention and Treatment: To counteract a deficiency in folic acid, your diet should contain liver, yeast, and leafy vegetables such as spinach, kale, parsley, cauliflower, brussels sprouts, and broccoli. The fruits that are highest in folic acid are oranges and cantaloupes. To a lesser degree, folacin is found in almonds and lima beans, corn, parsnips, green peas, pumpkins, sweet potatoes, bran, peanuts, rye, and whole grain wheat. (See table of Folacin-Rich Foods, page 297.) Approximately one half of the folic acid you consume is absorbed by your body.

Normal cooking temperatures (110 to 120 degrees for 10 minutes) destroy 65 percent of your dietary folacin. Your daily diet, therefore, should include some raw vegetables and fruits. Cooking utensils made out of copper speed up folacin's destruction.

The recommended daily consumption of folacin is 400 mcg.

Cancer patients usually have poor appetites, and chemotherapy with its associated nausea tends to make the situation worse. Therefore, if you cannot eat a well-balanced diet while taking busulfan, or if the glossitis and cheilosis persist despite a good diet, you should take a supplement containing 5 mg riboflavin, 15 to 25 mg niacin, 5 mg vitamin B$_6$, and .4 to .8 mg of folacin.

OTHER ADVICE: Busulfan can also cause gastrointestinal distress and weight loss.

CAFFEINE

DRUG FAMILY: Stimulant

BRAND NAMES: A.P.C. with Codeine; Amaphen; Amaphen with Codeine; Anacin Analgesic; Anacin Maximum Strength Analgesic; Anoquan; Buff-A Comp; Buff-A Comp No. 3; Cafergot; Cafergot P-B; Cafetrate-PB; Compal; Dexatrim 18 Hour; Di-Gesic; Dihydrocodeine Compound; Efed II; Esgic; Excedrin Extra-Strength; Fiorinal; Fiorinal w/Codeine; G-1; Korigesic; Migralam; No Doz; Pacaps; Propoxyphene Compound 65; Repan; SK-65 Compound; Soma Compound; Soma Compound w/Codeine; Synalgos-DC; Two-Dyne; Vanquish

HOW TO TAKE CAFFEINE: Just after meals

FOODS TO AVOID: None

POSSIBLE SIDE EFFECTS: Iron deficiency

ACTION OF CAFFEINE: Caffeine constricts cerebral blood vessels and may contribute to relief of headaches caused by high blood pressure. It also elevates mood, reduces fatigue, and improves your intellectual performance.

HIGH-RISK GROUPS: Premenopausal women, especially those who menstruate heavily, the elderly, teenagers, children, vegetarians

NUTRITIONAL INTERACTIONS

IRON DEFICIENCY: Caffeine impairs the absorption of iron in the diet. Particularly in the risk groups cited above, a deficiency could conceivably result. Iron is especially important to the oxygen-carrying cells of the blood and muscles, which consume two thirds of the iron your body requires. As a result, an iron shortage reduces the blood's oxygen-carrying capacity, and the upshot can be an anemia signaled by such symptoms as tiredness, general feelings of malaise, irritability, decreased attention span, pale complexion, rapid heart rhythm, headaches, loss of concentration, and breathlessness on exertion. A mild iron deficiency will also impair the functioning of your immune system.

In order for iron to be absorbed from any vegetable source, it must be converted to another form by the action of the hydrochloric acid produced in the stomach. Many elderly people secrete less hydrochloric acid than normal, so they absorb iron poorly under even normal circumstances. The diets of many Americans lack adequate quantities of this mineral for their normal needs. For example, 10 percent of American women suffer from an iron deficiency, and up to 30 percent have inadequate iron stores. Other people who are at significant risk of an iron deficiency are women who have had several pregnancies and those whose menstrual periods are heavy.

The lack of sufficient iron in many diets is due not only to the choice of foods that are poor sources of iron, but also to the switch from cast-iron cookware to aluminum, stainless steel, and nonstick surfaces. Iron used to be leached from the surface of iron pots and pans, and became available as dietary iron.

Prevention and Treatment: To counteract an iron deficiency, iron-rich foods should be included in your diet: liver, whole grain products, oysters, dried apricots, prunes, peaches, leafy green vegetables, and lean red meats. (See table of Iron-Rich Foods, page 299.)

Remember that a variety of other foods and drugs has an impact on the way your body absorbs (or does not absorb) iron. There are two kinds of iron in food sources: heme iron in meat and ionic iron in vegetables. Up to 30 percent of the iron from meat, fish, and poultry is absorbed, but less than 10 percent is absorbed from eggs, whole grains, nuts, and dried beans. Only 10 percent of ionic iron is absorbed from vegetable sources, with as little as 2 percent being absorbed from spinach. Antacids will interfere with iron absorption in vegetables, as will commercial black and pekoe tea, taken in substantial quantities, because of its tannin content. Coffee also seems to decrease iron absorption, but not to the same degree as tea. Vitamin C supplements or citrus juices increase the absorption of iron from vegetable sources by two to three times if taken simultaneously.

You will have impaired iron absorption if your diet is rich in high-fiber foods, because the fiber will bind with the iron and pass it out in the stool. This is the same action that contributes to the low absorption of iron from vegetable sources. Foods high in phosphorus (e.g. meat) interfere with iron absorption, which explains why only 30 percent of the iron in meat is captured. (However, meat and fish facilitate iron absorption from vegetables.) For that matter, any use of large quantities of mineral supplements, such as zinc, will impair iron absorption. Because iron can be leached from vegetables if they are cooked in large amounts of water, it is preferable to steam them.

Iron supplements should not be taken without a physician's recommendation, because an accumulation of too much iron can lead in extreme cases to such serious problems as anemia, malfunctioning of the pancreas and the heart, cirrhosis of the liver, a brown cast to the skin, and depression.

CALCIUM CARBONATE

DRUG FAMILY: Antacids

BRAND NAMES: Calcet; Cal-Sup; Camalox; Fosfree; Iromin-G; Mission Prenatal; Mission Prenatal F.A.; Mission Prenatal H.P.; Natacomp-FA; Natalins Rx; Natalins; Nu-Iron-V; Os-Cal; Pramet FA; Pramilet FA; Prenate 90; Zenate

HOW TO TAKE CALCIUM CARBONATE: For hyperacidity, it should be taken as needed. As a supplement, it should be taken between meals with water and at bedtime. One half of the daily dose should always be taken at bedtime.

FOODS TO AVOID: Fatty foods; people with hyperacidity should also avoid very acidic foods such as fruit juice, soda pop, and wine, and large of amounts of foods and beverages rich in caffeine, such as tea, coffee, cola, and chocolate.

POSSIBLE SIDE EFFECTS: Deficiencies of phosphate, folacin, iron, and thiamin and, in rare instances, magnesium; constipation

ACTION OF CALCIUM CARBONATE: This drug is used as a therapy for stomach hyperacidity and as a preventive measure against the development and in the treatment of osteoporosis.

HIGH-RISK GROUPS: Heavy drinkers, the elderly, young women, lactating women, pregnant women, oral contraceptive users, vegetarians, teenagers

NUTRITIONAL INTERACTIONS

PHOSPHATE AND OTHER NUTRIENT DEFICIENCIES: Calcium carbonate decreases the absorption of magnesium in all users, but deficiencies are highly unlikely and extremely rare, the exception being with alcoholics. It also decreases the absorption of folacin and iron, and is instrumental in destroying thiamin. Consumption of too much calcium carbonate (more than 2 grams of calcium per day for prolonged periods) can lead to loss of appetite, nausea, vomiting, headache, and general feelings of weakness

owing to a phosphate deficiency. It can also lead to deposition of calcium in the cornea, resulting in impaired vision. The elderly, particularly those with kidney problems, are especially at risk.

Prevention and Treatment: To counteract the possibility of any difficulties due to low phosphate levels, your diet should contain liver, peas, beans, whole grain cereals, eggs, milk, green vegetables, fish and nuts (almonds and cashews, in particular) on a regular basis. (See table of Phosphorus-Rich Foods, page 302.)

Take a one-a-day vitamin containing the Recommended Dietary Allowances if you are using calcium carbonate on a regular basis.

OTHER ADVICE: Calcium carbonate is a potent drug. By increasing its dosage beyond recommended levels, you are more likely to increase your discomfort than to lessen it. Your stomach reacts to more of this drug by producing even more acid than before, with the result that the hyperacidity worsens.

It is conceivable that you will experience malnutrition as a result of excessive self-medication with antacids, as a result of malabsorption of nutrients. It should be emphasized that nutrient depletion from antacid use is gradual, and evidence of malnutrition does not make its appearance until nutrient stores are exhausted.

People taking antacids therapeutically should avoid large amounts of acidic foods, such as fruit juices and foods containing caffeine, that irritate the stomach wall.

This kind of antacid also leads to constipation in some individuals and, in rare instances, malabsorption of fat. The appearance of either constipation or greasy stools should provide you with the stimulus to switch to a different antacid.

CALCIUM FENOPROFEN

DRUG FAMILY: Anti-inflammatory

BRAND NAME: Nalfon

HOW TO TAKE CALCIUM FENOPROFEN: At least half an hour before a meal

FOODS TO AVOID: None

POSSIBLE SIDE EFFECTS: Gastrointestinal disturbances

ACTION OF CALCIUM FENOPROFEN: This anti-inflammatory drug is used as an anti-arthritic agent. It reduces joint swelling, pain, and the duration of morning stiffness.

HIGH-RISK GROUPS: People with a history of abdominal distress

NUTRITIONAL INTERACTIONS

GASTROINTESTINAL DISTRESS: Calcium fenoprofen can cause gastrointestinal disturbances.

Prevention and Treatment: The absorption and the effectiveness of the drug are impaired if it is taken with meals, so in order to prevent gastrointestinal discomfort you should take antacids with the drug. Calcium fenoprofen should always be taken at least half an hour before a meal.

CALCIUM SUPPLEMENTS

DRUG FAMILY: Mineral supplements

BRAND NAMES: [GENERIC/Brand] CALCIUM CARBONATE/Calcet; Cal-Sup; Camalox; Fosfree; Iromin-G; Mission Prenatal; Mission Prenatal F.A.; Mission Prenatal H.P.; Natacomp-FA; Natalins Rx; Natalins; Nu-Iron-V; Os-Cal 250; Os-Cal 500; Pramet FA; Pramilet FA; Prenate 90; Zenate (see also separate entry for Calcium Carbonate). CALCIUM GLUCONATE/Calcet; Fosfree; Iromin-G; Mission Prenatal; Mission Prenatal F.A.; Mission Prenatal H.P.; CALCIUM LACTATE/Calcet; Calphosan; Calphosan B-12; Fosfree; Iromin-G; Mevanin-C; Mission Prenatal; Mission Prenatal F.A.; Mission Prenatal H.P.; CALCIUM (OYSTER SHELL)/Os-Cal 250; Os-Cal 500; Os-Cal Forte; Os-Cal Plus; Os-Cal-Gesic

HOW TO TAKE CALCIUM SUPPLEMENTS: Half the daily dose should be taken at bedtime, half between meals.

FOOD TO AVOID: None

POSSIBLE SIDE EFFECTS: An overdose can result in loss of appetite, headaches, excessive thirst, and irritability.

ACTION OF CALCIUM COMPOUNDS: These drugs are used to supplement dietary sources of calcium, as a preventive measure to protect you from osteoporosis.

HIGH-RISK GROUPS: Anyone who takes this drug

NUTRITIONAL INTERACTIONS

CALCIUM ABSORPTION: The absorption of calcium is decreased by oxalate, phytic acid, and phosphorus. Corticosteroid drugs too decrease its absorption. On the other hand, too much calcium absorption can result in hypercalcemia (high blood calcium levels), particularly when large doses of vitamin D are also being consumed. Hypercalcemia is characterized by a loss of appetite, headache, excessive thirst, and irritability.

Prevention and Treatment: Within a period of 2 hours before and 2 hours after taking the calcium supplement, you should not consume foods rich in oxalate (spinach, beet greens, rhubarb, celery, and peanuts; see also table of Oxalate-Rich Foods, page 301); phytic acid (oatmeal and other whole grain cereals); or phosphorus (chocolate, cocoa, dried beans and peas, dried fruit, canned fish, game, nuts, organ meats, peanut butter, and whole grains). In practice, then, calcium supplements should not be taken at meals, and half the supplement should be taken before bedtime, since this helps to limit the loss of calcium from your bones while you sleep.

No more than 500 to 800 IU of vitamin D should be taken along with a calcium supplement unless specifically prescribed by your doctor.

CAPTOPRIL

DRUG FAMILY: Anti-hypertensive

BRAND NAME: Capoten

HOW TO TAKE CAPTOPRIL: One hour before meals

FOODS TO AVOID: None

POSSIBLE SIDE EFFECTS: Sodium deficiency

ACTION OF CAPTOPRIL: This drug blocks the production of angiotensin II, which is a natural hormone produced by the kidneys that elevates blood pressure. It is used in patients who do not respond to other therapy or who develop side effects taking other types of anti-hypertensive medications.

HIGH-RISK GROUPS: Heart patients, hypertensives

NUTRITIONAL INTERACTIONS

SODIUM DEFICIENCY: Captopril can cause sodium depletion in its users by increasing its rate of excretion. Under these circumstances, blood sodium levels will be extremely low (hyponatremia). Common symptoms include anorexia, nausea, vomiting, and muscle weakness.

Prevention and Treatment: If you are taking captopril, you should not be on a diet that restricts your sodium intake to less than 2 grams per day.

CARAMIPHEN EDISYLATE

DRUG FAMILY: Cough medicine

BRAND NAMES: Rescaps-D T.D.; Tuss-Ade; Tuss-Ornade

HOW TO TAKE CARAMIPHEN EDISYLATE: With meals or milk

FOODS TO AVOID: All alcoholic beverages

POSSIBLE SIDE EFFECTS: Stomach upset

ACTION OF CARAMIPHEN EDISYLATE: This drug is used to relieve coughing and nasal congestion associated with the common cold.

HIGH-RISK GROUPS: Heavy drinkers

NUTRITIONAL INTERACTIONS

GASTROINTESTINAL DISTRESS: Caramiphen edisylate tends to irritate the gastrointestinal tract.

Prevention and Treatment: This drug should be taken with meals or milk to avoid a possible upset stomach.

OTHER ADVICE: Caramiphen edisylate enhances the depressive effects of alcohol, so alcohol should not be consumed concurrently with it.

CARBAMAZEPINE

DRUG FAMILY: Anti-epileptic; analgesic

BRAND NAME: Tegretol

HOW TO TAKE CARBAMAZEPINE: With meals or milk

FOODS TO AVOID: None

POSSIBLE SIDE EFFECTS: Sodium deficiency; constipation; loss of appetite

ACTION OF CARBAMAZEPINE: This drug is used in treating seizures in patients who do not respond well to other seizure-preventing drugs. Carbamazepine is also used in treating neuralgia (nerve pain).

HIGH-RISK GROUPS: The elderly, children, heart patients, hypertensives

NUTRITIONAL INTERACTIONS

SODIUM DEFICIENCY: This drug tends to encourage water retention. This can lead to the dilution of the blood sodium levels to lower than normal levels (hyponatremia). Such symptoms as loss of appetite, nausea, vomiting, and muscle weakness may occur. If the blood sodium levels drop extremely low, the senses are impaired, and the low sodium levels can cause seizures.

Prevention and Treatment: Fluid intake should be limited to no more than 6 glasses per day, to reduce the risk of hyponatremia. Your consumption of salt, however, should not be increased.

GASTROINTESTINAL DISTRESS: Carbamazepine is likely to cause gastrointestinal disturbances, including constipation, and can cause the loss of appetite.

Prevention and Treatment: This drug should be taken with meals or milk to minimize these problems. Weight should be carefully monitored to avoid unwanted weight loss.

If constipation does occur, it is usually safely remedied by an increase in the bulk in the diet. This means consuming larger servings of any of the following: dried or fresh fruits, salad vegetables, radishes, oatmeal, and whole grain foods (brown rice, whole wheat breads, and cereals). It is not necessary to purchase products that claim "extra fiber" has been added to them. (See table of Dietary Fiber-Rich Foods, page 293.)

OTHER ADVICE: Oral contraceptive users should note that this drug is likely to accelerate the rate at which their contraceptive pills are broken down, and that will make them less effective.

CEPHALOSPORINS

DRUG FAMILY: Antibiotic

BRAND NAMES: [GENERIC/Brand] CEPHAL-EXIN/Keflex; CEPHRADINE/Anspor; Velosef; CEFACLOR/Ceclor; CEFADROXIL/Duricef; Ultracef

HOW TO TAKE CEPHALOSPORINS: Between meals, on an empty stomach

FOODS TO AVOID: None

POSSIBLE SIDE EFFECTS: Diarrhea and, rarely, nausea and vomiting

ACTION OF CEPHALOSPORINS: These anti-bacterial agents are used to treat infections of the respiratory tract, skin and soft tissues, bones and joints, urinary tract, and bloodstream.

NUTRITIONAL INTERACTIONS

GENERAL ADVICE: The absorption of cephalosporins is delayed by the presence of food in the gastrointestinal tract, so they should be taken on an empty stomach. However, these drugs do sometimes cause diarrhea, nausea, and vomiting.

CHLORAL HYDRATE

DRUG FAMILY: Anti-anxiety

BRAND NAMES: SK-Chloral Hydrate; Noctec

HOW TO TAKE CHLORAL HYDRATE: Immediately after meals with a full glass of a beverage

FOODS TO AVOID: Carbonated beverages, beans, peas, cabbage, and large amounts of salad vegetables and fruit; all alcoholic beverages

POSSIBLE SIDE EFFECTS: Stomachache, nausea, vomiting, flatulence, and decreased appetite

ACTION OF CHLORAL HYDRATE: This drug is prescribed as a sedative, an anti-anxiety agent, and often to combat insomnia.

HIGH-RISK GROUPS: Heavy drinkers

NUTRITIONAL INTERACTIONS

GASTROINTESTINAL IRRITATION: Chloral compounds are gastric irritants, and their consumption can lead to abdominal pain, nausea, occasional vomiting, and flatulence. Chloral hydrate is bad tasting. Consequently, this drug may decrease appetite and food intake.

Prevention and Treatment: This drug should be well diluted in water or milk to reduce its unpleasant gastric side effects. It should be taken after meals, when the stomach is full. In this way, the unpleasant taste will not reduce the appetite, and the drug will least upset the stomach. Foods that cause gas, such as carbonated beverages, beans, peas, vegetables in the cabbage family, bran in excessive amounts, salad vegetables, and fruit, should be limited to prevent flatulence.

ALCOHOL INTERACTION: Alcohol prolongs the activity of the drug, which will increase sleeping time. By the same token, chloral hydrate decreases the rate of metabolism of alcohol and so prolongs its effects.

Prevention and Treatment: The drug should never be taken with alcohol.

CHLORAMBUCIL

DRUG FAMILY: Anti-leukemia

BRAND NAME: Leukeran

HOW TO TAKE CHLORAMBUCIL: With milk or meals

FOODS TO AVOID: None

POSSIBLE SIDE EFFECTS: Reduced appetite, minor gastrointestinal discomfort

ACTION OF CHLORAMBUCIL: This anti-cancer drug is used in the treatment of chronic, lymphocytic leukemia and in treating Hodgkin's disease. Chlorambucil is also the treatment of choice for primary macroglobulinemia.

HIGH-RISK GROUPS: Anyone who takes this drug

NUTRITIONAL INTERACTIONS

GASTROINTESTINAL DISTRESS: Chlorambucil reduces appetite and consequently food consumption in many who use it. It also causes minor gastrointestinal discomfort.

Prevention and Treatment: Food intake should be carefully monitored to prevent unwanted weight loss. To minimize the gastrointestinal side effects, this drug should always be taken with milk or food.

CHLORAMPHENICOL

DRUG FAMILY: Antibiotic

BRAND NAME: Chloromycetin

HOW TO TAKE CHLORAMPHENICOL: With meals or milk

FOODS TO AVOID: None

POSSIBLE SIDE EFFECTS: Deficiencies of riboflavin, and vitamins B_6 and B_{12}; occasionally, nausea, vomiting, and diarrhea

ACTION OF CHLORAMPHENICOL: This antibiotic is usually reserved for use against serious infections.

HIGH-RISK GROUPS: Infants, children, anyone who consumes alcohol, vegetarians, young women, users of oral contraceptives, teenagers, the elderly

NUTRITIONAL INTERACTIONS

RIBOFLAVIN DEFICIENCY: A deficiency in riboflavin is likely since this drug increases your requirements for riboflavin.

The symptoms of a deficiency of riboflavin (vitamin B_2) most likely to appear are dermatitis around the nose and lips, cracking at the corners of the mouth, and a soreness in the lips, mouth, or tongue. Discomfort in eating and swallowing may result. The eyes may burn, itch, be more sensitive than usual to light, and tend to be bloodshot. However, be aware that any B vitamin deficiency can cause similar symptoms.

Riboflavin helps the body transform protein, fats, and carbohydrates into the energy needed to maintain body tissues and to protect the body against common skin and eye disorders.

Prevention and Treatment: Good sources of riboflavin should be included in the diet. Milk usually contributes about 50 percent of our riboflavin intake, meat about 25 percent, and dark green leafy vegetables and enriched cereals and breads the rest. The need for riboflavin provides a major reason for including milk in some form in every day's meals; no other food that is commonly eaten can make such a substantial contribution to meeting our daily riboflavin needs. People who don't use milk products can substitute a generous serving of dark green leafy vegetables, because a cup of greens such as collards provides about the same amount of riboflavin as a cup of milk. (See table of vitamin B_2(Riboflavin)-Rich Foods, page 310.)

Among the meats, liver is the richest source, but all lean meats, as well as eggs, can provide some riboflavin. Riboflavin is light-sensitive; it can be destroyed by the ultraviolet rays of the sun or fluorescent lamps. For this reason, milk is seldom sold, and should not be stored, in transparent glass containers. Cardboard or plastic containers protect the riboflavin in the milk from ultraviolet rays.

A 5 mg supplement of riboflavin should be taken daily by people on this drug. This is especially important in oral contraceptive users, who have a great need for this vitamin.

VITAMIN B_6 DEFICIENCY: A deficiency of this vitamin is also likely, since chloramphenicol increases your body's requirements for vitamin B_6. Common symptoms of this deficiency are a sore mouth and tongue, cracks in the lips and corners of the mouth, and patches of itching, scaling skin. A severe vitamin B_6 deficiency may cause depression and confusion.

Vitamin B_6 deficiencies are common among the elderly. Alcoholics, as well, often experience this deficiency, since alcohol interferes with the body's ability to use B_6. In addition, smokers tend to have less than optimal body levels of this vitamin. It is estimated that one of every two Americans consumes less than 70 percent of the Recommended Dietary Allowance of B_6.

Prevention and Treatment: To avoid a B_6 deficiency, you should consume a diet featuring food sources of vitamin B_6 such as liver (beef, calf, and pork), herring, salmon, walnuts, peanuts, wheat germ, carrots, peas, potatoes, grapes, bananas, and yeast. (See table of Vitamin B_6(Pyridoxine)-Rich Foods, page 311.) While the vitamin is present in significant amounts in meats, fish, fruits, cereals, and vegetables, it is present to a lesser extent in milk and other dairy products.

Since vitamin B_6 is decomposed at high temperatures, modern food processing often diminishes dietary sources of the vitamin. Consequently, the more processed foods you eat, the more susceptible you will be to a deficiency of this vitamin. The same losses also occur in cooking: meat loses as much as 45 to 80 percent, vegetables 20 to 30 percent.

It has been observed that 15 to 20 percent of oral contraceptive users show direct evidence of vitamin B_6 deficiency. If you are among these people, you should take 5 mg of vitamin B_6 per day. Other people should take a 2 mg supplement as a preventive measure. However, keep in mnd that you can take too much vitamin B_6; people taking over 1 gram per day have been reported to have developed nerve degeneration.

VITAMIN B_{12} DEFICIENCY: As in the case of riboflavin and vitamin B_6, chloramphenicol increases the body's need for vitamin B_{12}. A deficiency of this vitamin is therefore possible, though the chances are somewhat less. Vitamin B_{12} is needed for the normal development of red blood cells and for the healthy functioning of all cells, in particular those of the bone marrow, nervous system, and intestines.

The most common result of a B_{12} deficiency is pernicious anemia, which is characterized by listlessness, fatigue (especially following such physical exertion as climbing a flight of stairs), numbness and tingling in the fingers and toes, palpitations, angina, light-headedness, and a pale complexion. A vitamin B_{12} deficiency can also lead to an irreversible breakdown in the brain membranes, causing loss of coordination, confusion, memory loss, paranoia, apathy, tremors, and hallucinations. In extreme cases, degeneration of the spinal cord can also result.

Since vitamin B_{12} can be obtained only from animal food sources, strict vegetarians are at particular risk here. Oral contraceptive users too have a greater chance of experiencing this deficiency, since they often have a poor vitamin B_{12} status to begin with, as do many smokers. Heavy consumers of alcohol, as well, frequently lack B_{12} because alcohol impairs the absorption of the vitamin. Patients with bacterial or parasitic infections of the intestine also have difficulty in absorbing this vitamin, as do many elderly people. In any case, anyone who is likely to have a vitamin B_{12} absorption problem should be alert for signs of pernicious anemia while taking this drug.

Prevention and treatment: A balanced diet containing plenty of vitamin B_{12} sources is advised. Only animal products, including dairy foods and fish and shellfish, contain natural vitamin B_{12}. However, some vegetable products are supplemented with vitamin B_{12}; many soy products, for example, are enriched with vitamin B_{12} to safeguard vegetarians. (See table of Vitamin B_{12}-Rich Foods, page 312.)

Vitamin B_{12} is stored in the liver, so one meal that includes a B_{12}-rich source such as calf's liver will normally fulfill your body's need for this vitamin for 2 or 3 weeks. (One 3-ounce serving of calf's liver contains 100 mcg of vitamin B_{12}.) If none of these products figures prominently in your diet, you should take a 6 mcg supplement each day while you are on chloramphenicol.

People who use major amounts of vitamin C should be aware that vitamin C supplements of more than 500 mg per day can damage B_{12} and contribute to a B_{12} deficiency. However, anyone who eats red meat two times a week has a three- to five-year supply of B_{12} in his liver.

The presence of baking soda in cooking will destroy vitamin B_{12} and should be avoided whenever possible. B_{12} also degrades at high temperatures, as when meat is placed on a hot griddle. The pasteurization of milk and the sterilization in boiling water of a bottle of milk also cause the loss of some B_{12}.

OTHER ADVICE: Chloramphenicol inhibits the degradation of anti-coagulants such as warfarin, and makes them more potent. If you are taking an anti-coagulant, you should advise your physician so that he may adjust the dosage, if necessary.

Gastrointestinal discomfort occasionally occurs in users of this drug. This may be alleviated by taking the drug with meals or milk.

CHLORPHENIRAMINE MALEATE

DRUG FAMILY: Decongestant

BRAND NAMES: Allerest; Anafed; Anamine; Anatuss; Brexin; Chlorafed; Chlor-Trimeton; Citra Forte; Codimal; Colrex; Comhist; Comtrex; Contac; Co-Pyronil 2; Coricidin; Coryban-D; CoTylenol; Deconamine; Decongestant-AT; Dehist; Dristan, Advanced Formula; Dristan Ultra Colds Formula; Drize; Dura-Vent; E.N.T.; Extendryl; 4-Way Cold Tablets; Fedahist; Headway; Histalet; Histaspan; Histor-D; Hycomine; Iophen-C; Isoclor; Korigesic; Kronofed-A; Kronohist; Naldecon; Neotep; Nolamine; Novafed A; Novahistine DH; Ornade; P-V-Tussin; Pediacof; Pertussin Complex D; Phenate; Protid; Pyrroxate; Quelidrine; Resaid; Rescaps; Rhinolar; Ru-Tuss; Ryna; Ryna-C; Scot-Tussin; Sinarest; Sine-off; Singlet; Sinovan; Sinulin; Sinutab; Teldrin; Triaminic; Triaminicol; Trind; Tussar

HOW TO TAKE CHLORPHENIRAMINE MALEATE: With meals

FOODS TO AVOID: All alcoholic beverages

POSSIBLE SIDE EFFECTS: Nausea

ACTION OF CHLORPHENIRAMINE MALEATE: This drug is prescribed to relieve nasal congestion, catarrh, sinusitis, seasonal allergies, and acute upper-respiratory infections.

HIGH-RISK GROUPS: Anybody with a history of gastrointestinal distress

NUTRITIONAL INTERACTIONS

GASTROINTESTINAL DISTRESS: Chlorpheniramine maleate causes nausea in some people.

Prevention and Treatment: If this drug is taken with meals, the risk of nausea is much reduced.

OTHER ADVICE: This drug may cause an inability to concentrate, dizziness, drowsiness, and impaired coordination. Alcohol exacerbates these effects and should not be consumed while you are taking this drug.

CHLORPROMAZINE HYDRO-CHLORIDE

DRUG FAMILY: Anti-psychotic

BRAND NAME: Thorazine

HOW TO TAKE CHLORPROMAZINE HYDROCHLORIDE: With meals

FOODS TO AVOID: All alcoholic beverages; large amounts of alkaline foods such as milk, buttermilk, cream, almonds, chestnuts, coconuts, all vegetables except corn and lentils, and all fruits except cranberries, prunes, and plums; foods rich in cholesterol

POSSIBLE SIDE EFFECTS: High blood cholesterol levels, gastrointestinal distress, and riboflavin deficiency

ACTION OF CHLORPROMAZINE HYDROCHLORIDE: This drug is used to treat psychiatric disorders and, in low doses, to control nausea and vomiting.

HIGH-RISK GROUPS: Heart patients, anyone who consumes alcohol, users of oral contraceptives, people taking anti-coagulants, the elderly, vegetarians

NUTRITIONAL INTERACTIONS

ALCOHOL INTERACTION: The effect of chlorpromazine hydrochloride is likely to be enhanced by alcohol. Central nervous system depression may be increased, in some cases with severe respiratory failure resulting. Chlorpromazine hydrochloride can also enhance the effects of alcohol in inhibiting motor driving skills, with a consequent increase in the chance of accident.

Prevention and Treatment: Alcohol should not be consumed concurrently with this drug.

ALKALINE URINE: Because chlorpromazine hydrochloride is alkaline, it is excreted at a normal rate only if your urine is acidic. However, if the quantity of alkaline foods in your diet is high, your urine will lose its acidity, and the excretion of this drug will be slowed. A hazardous buildup is likely to result. The symptoms of such a buildup or overdose are drowsiness, dizziness, rapid heart rate, low blood pressure (especially on standing), momentary fainting, muscle spasms, and jitteriness.

Prevention and Treatment: Fruits, vegetables, and dairy products tend to be alkaline, and high-protein foods tend to be acidic. Foods causing the production of alkaline urine include milk, buttermilk, cream, almonds, chestnuts, coconuts, all vegetables except corn and lentils, and all fruits except cranberries, prunes, and plums.

Antacids that neutralize the acid in the stomach will also neutralize the acid in the urine, causing it to turn alkaline. Therefore, you should avoid taking antacids while on this drug.

CHOLESTEROL BUILDUP: Thorazine is likely to induce high blood cholesterol, and so will increase the risk of heart attack in susceptible individuals.

Prevention and Treatment: Elevated blood cholesterol levels have been shown to be associated with an increased risk of heart attack. Thorazine elevates cholesterol levels and hence the risk of heart disease. As a rule of thumb, everybody should limit his cholesterol intake to less than 300 mg per day, which means being careful about such high-cholesterol foods as red meat, eggs, and liver. (See table of Cholesterol-Rich Foods, page 290.)

A reduction in the fat content of your diet to less than 30 percent of your food consumption will also tend to lower blood cholesterol levels. This 30 percent should be comprised of equal amounts of so-called polyunsaturated, monounsaturated, and saturated fats. Saturated fats are found in meat, fish, and avocados; monounsaturated fats, in fish and some vegetable oils; including olive oil; and polyunsaturated fats, mainly in vegetables.

A diet based on the four food groups will help give you the right balance of fats.

GASTROINTESTINAL DISTRESS: Chlorpromazine hydrochloride could conceivably cause you to experience gastric irritation and should not be taken on an empty stomach. However, this drug also increases appetite and leads to weight gain in some people.

Prevention and Treatment: This drug should always be taken with a meal to prevent stomach irritation. You should also carefully monitor your weight, to ensure that the drug does not cause an obesity problem with its associated health risks.

RIBOFLAVIN DEFICIENCY: Chlorpromazine increases your body's need for riboflavin (vitamin B$_2$), and is likely to lead to a deficiency.

The symptoms most likely to appear will be dry skin around the nose and lips, cracks in the corners of the mouth, and a sore and shiny tongue. Discomfort in eating and swallowing may result. The eyes may burn, itch, be more sensitive than usual to light, and tend to be bloodshot.

Riboflavin helps the body transform protein, fats, and carbohydrates into the energy needed to maintain body tissues and to protect the body against common skin and eye disorders.

Prevention and Treatment: Good sources of riboflavin should be included in the diet. Milk usually contributes about 50 percent of our riboflavin intake, meat about 25 percent, and dark green leafy vegetables and enriched cereals and breads the rest. The need for riboflavin provides a major reason for including milk in some form in every day's meals; no other food that is commonly eaten can make such a substantial contribution to meeting our daily riboflavin needs. People who don't use milk products can substitute a generous serving of dark green leafy vegetables, because a cup of greens such as collards provides about the same amount of riboflavin as a cup of milk. (See table of Vitamin B$_2$(Riboflavin)-Rich Foods, page 310.)

Among the meats, liver is the richest source, but all lean meats, as well as eggs, can provide some riboflavin. Riboflavin is light-sensitive; it can be destroyed by the ultraviolet rays of the sun or fluorescent lamps. For this reason, milk is seldom sold, and should not be stored, in transparent glass containers. Cardboard or plastic containers protect the riboflavin in the milk from ultraviolet rays.

OTHER ADVICE: Chlorpromazine diminishes the effectiveness of anti-coagulants such as warfarin.

CHLORPROPAMIDE

DRUG FAMILY: Anti-diabetic

BRAND NAME: Diabinese

HOW TO TAKE CHLORPROPAMIDE: With milk or immediately after eating

FOODS TO AVOID: All alcoholic beverages and foods containing alcohol; large quantities of salty foods such as anchovies, dill pickles, sardines, green olives, canned soups and vegetables, TV dinners, soy sauce, processed cheeses, salty snack foods, cold cuts, and catsup

POSSIBLE SIDE EFFECTS: Hypoglycemia, hyperglycemia, edema, flatulence, loose stools, and diarrhea

ACTION OF CHLORPROPAMIDE: This drug is a member of the sulfonylurea family and is prescribed to reduce blood glucose levels by stimulating the pancreas to produce insulin.

HIGH-RISK GROUPS: The elderly, heavy drinkers

NUTRITIONAL INTERACTION

HYPOGLYCEMIA AND HYPERGLYCEMIA: Hypoglycemia or hyperglycemia, respectively, could conceivably be caused by too high or too low a dose of chlorpropamide. Hypoglycemia is a condition in which there is too little sugar (glucose) in the blood. If your blood sugar levels drop to below 30 mg/100 ml of blood (a normal level is 100 mg/100 ml of blood), you may become mentally confused due to a lack of glucose reaching the brain. Other early symptoms are headaches, hunger, and a general sensation resembling mild drunkenness. Below 10 mg/100 ml, you could go into a diabetic coma. If the situation is not corrected within a few minutes, permanent brain damage may occur.

If too little chlorpropamide is taken, you will experience the opposite problem, hyperglycemia, from too much sugar in the blood. This condition results when the drug causes the pancreas to release amounts of insulin insufficient to allow the cells in the body to absorb glucose, which starves the cells of the energy they need. In this instance, as well, coma can result.

Alcohol and aspirin enhance the blood-glucose-lowering activity of this drug and can cause the glucose levels to drop so low that the brain is starved of glucose and energy, and you can go into a coma.

Prevention and treatment: If you are diabetic, you must carefully monitor your food intake and avoid an excess of carbohydrates in the form of simple sugars, such as cookies, candies, sodas, honey, and table sugar. These foods are absorbed very rapidly and will increase your blood sugar to very high levels. Such blood sugar levels are dangerous to diabetics, because the limited amount of insulin produced by the pancreas may not be sufficient to bring the levels back into the normal range. A preferred diet is low in fats, but with plenty of complex carbohydrates such as starches, cereals, and vegetables. (See tables of Simple and Complex Carbohydrate Foods, page 305.)

Some studies suggest that a high-fiber diet may cause a slower and more sustained release of glucose from the gastrointestinal tract into the bloodstream, preventing the wide swings in blood sugar levels. It also helps the body to absorb glucose. For the diabetic, it is recommended that you remain physically active and exercise daily, because by doing so the cells are made more susceptible to the insulin available. Finally, a change in eating schedule from the standard three meals per day to five or six smaller meals a day will also help keep blood sugar levels within normal range.

PARKINSON'S DISEASE: Chlorpropamide is sometimes prescribed for nondiabetics suffering from Parkinson's disease, a nervous disorder involving a rhythmic tremor, rigidity of muscle action, and slowing of body motion. The elderly seem to be sensitive to this drug; in some cases, elderly patients taking this and other sulfonylurea drugs have developed hypoglycemia and in rare cases a few have succumbed to coma.

Prevention and Treatment: If you are an elderly patient, you should carry sugar cubes or candy just in case you experience hypoglycemia.

EDEMA: It is conceivable that use of this drug could lead to water and salt retention, which will tend to cause swelling (called edema) in your legs, ankles, feet, and breasts, and around your eyes. A rise in sodium and water retention may also increase the volume of blood in the body, which places an added strain on the heart and tends to elevate blood pressure.

Prevention and Treatment: While you are taking this drug, you should restrict your consumption of salt. In particular, those foods listed in the table of Sodium-Rich Foods (see page 306) should be avoided, or consumed in small quantities. You should not add salt at the table or in cooking, and should consume 6 to 8 glasses of water per day, as water is a natural diuretic.

The average American consumes some 15 pounds of salt a year, or 3 to 4 teaspoons a day. Even if you do not salt your food while preparing or eating it, you consume large quantities of salt in such foods as anchovies, dill pickles, sardines, green olives, canned soups and vegetables, so-called TV dinners, soy sauce, processed cheeses, many snack foods, cold cuts, and catsup. Sodium is consumed as a result of additives, such as baking soda and baking powder, that are widely used in the preparation of processed foods.

On average, one third of the salt we consume comes naturally in the food we eat, one third is added as table salt, and one third is added in processing.

ALCOHOL INTERACTION: Chlorpropamide inhibits the breakdown of acetaldehyde, which is produced when alcohol is broken down in the body. This causes a number of unpleasant symptoms. If alcohol is consumed after this drug is taken, severe headache, flushing, nausea, vomiting, hypertension, weakness, vertigo, blurred vision, and convulsions may occur. The reaction begins within 5 to 10 minutes of drinking the alcohol, and in sensitive people it may be caused by the intake of as little as a few sips.

The same reaction will occur when patients take such foods as wine vinegar, sauces containing wine, or desserts containing liquor. Alcohol may also cause the blood glucose level to drop below normal, leading to light-headedness and fatigue. Aspirin use with chlorpropamide further lowers blood glucose.

It is urged that you not take this drug with alcohol.

GASTROINTESTINAL DISTRESS: Chlorpropamide is likely to irritate your gastrointestinal tract, causing flatulence and loose stools or diarrhea. It is recommended that this drug be taken with milk or immediately after eating, to minimize gastric irritation.

CHOLESTYRAMINE

DRUG FAMILY: Cholesterol reducer

BRAND NAME: Questran

HOW TO TAKE CHOLESTYRAMINE: Before or during meals and at bedtime, mixed with pulpy fruit, such as applesauce, or liquids

FOODS TO AVOID: None

POSSIBLE SIDE EFFECTS: Deficiencies of vitamins D and A, and possibly vitamins K, E, and B_{12}, and folic acid; constipation

ACTION OF CHOLESTYRAMINE: This drug is prescribed to lower blood cholesterol levels in patients with arteriosclerosis.

HIGH-RISK GROUPS: The elderly, vegetarians, smokers, anyone who consumes alcohol

NUTRITIONAL INTERACTION

VITAMIN D DEFICIENCY: By causing fat malabsorption and hence malabsorption of the fat-soluble vitamins A, D, E, and K, cholestyramine could cause vitamin deficiencies if used over a prolonged period of time.

Vitamin D is needed for the body to absorb calcium and phosphorus, to promote the development of strong teeth and bones. Whenever calcium blood levels are low, the body will liberate the calcium it needs from the bones, where it is stored. The result will be a condition called osteomalacia, in which the bones are weakened, in severe cases to the degree that they will fracture easily. Prominent symptoms are bone pain in the back, thighs, shoulder region, or ribs; difficulty in walking; and weakness in the muscles of the legs. Osteomalacia is reversible once calcium blood levels are raised.

An extended calcium deficiency can also lead to a condition called osteoporosis, one fairly common among postmenopausal women. In osteoporosis, the bones are weakened and made brittle by an unexplained and rapid loss of calcium. Unlike those of osteomalacia, the effects of osteoporosis are irreversible. The common symptoms are backache, a gradual loss of height, and periodontal disease. Fractures of the vertebrae, hip, and wrist occur, sometimes spontaneously.

Prevention and Treatment: To avoid a vitamin D deficiency while taking cholestyramine, you should take 400 to 800 IU of vitamin D per day as a supplement and include in your diet foods rich in vitamin D, such as fortified milk, butter, liver, egg yolks, salmon, tuna, and sardines. (See table of Vitamin D-Rich Foods, page 313.)

Vitamin D is initially formed in the skin on exposure to sunlight, and activated in the liver and kidneys. The production of vitamin D is dependent upon climatic conditions, air pollution, skin pigmentation (the darker the skin, the lower the production), the area of skin exposed, the duration of exposure to the sun, and the use of sun screens. Adults who are not often exposed to sunlight (e.g. those who are housebound or by custom heavily clothed), require dietary sources of vitamin D to prevent osteomalacia.

This vitamin is also indispensable to infants, children, and to pregnant or lactating women, whose requirements are high due to bone growth or skeletal mineral replacement. Supplementation for pregnant women is crucial, since vitamin D deficiencies can cause fetal abnormalities. However, no more than 800 IU of the vitamin should be taken by pregnant women, because excessive consumption can cause kidney damage. In nonpregnant adults, 2,000 IU of the vitamin should be taken if osteomalacia is indicated.

If your intake of vitamin D exceeds 4,000 IU per day, vitamin D poisoning can occur. The symptoms are loss of appetite, headache, excessive thirst, irritability, and kidney stones.

In all of these cases, foods rich in calcium

should be included in the diet, especially dairy products. (See table of Calcium-Rich Foods, page 289.) If these foods must be avoided because of an intolerance to lactose, the sugar found in dairy products (some 30 million Americans have such a problem digesting dairy products), a 1,200 to 1,500 mg daily supplement of calcium should be taken. (See Calcium Supplements entry, page 51.)

VITAMIN A DEFICIENCY: Cholestyramine could conceivably induce a deficiency of vitamin A. Among the symptoms of vitamin A deficiency are night blindness, rough skin, drying of the eyes, and infection of the mucous membrane (the inner linings of the body).

Prevention and Treatment: A small dosage of vitamin A, such as the 5,000 IUs found in a multivitamin tablet, should counteract this deficiency. Vitamin A is another of the fat-soluble vitamins, and it is stored in the liver. Fat-soluble vitamins do not have to be consumed everyday, but because they are stored, it is advisable not to take large doses (over 10,000 IU per day). Over extended periods, such doses can be toxic and can lead to diarrhea, nausea, hair loss, and extreme fatigue.

Vitamin A can be found in foods such as fish oils, liver, whole milk, whole milk products, egg yolks, fortified margarine, green vegetables (spinach), and yellow fruit (cantaloupe). (See table for Vitamin A-Rich Foods, page 308.) Unlike most vitamins, cooking or exposure to high temperatures will not easily destroy vitamin A, but long exposure to sunlight will. Therefore, you should keep milk stored in opaque containers and cover vegetables.

VITAMIN E DEFICIENCY: Though it is highly unlikely, it is possible that a vitamin E deficiency could result from long-term use of cholestyramine. Vitamin E deficiencies have no clearly observable symptoms, but in the event of a severe vitamin E deficiency the blood cells wear out in a shorter period than normal, and this can result in anemia.

Prevention and Treatment: If cholestyramine is used frequently, a supplement of vitamin E is advised, approximately 2 to 2.5 mg daily. Note, however, the interaction of vitamins K and E described below.

VITAMIN K DEFICIENCY: People with abnormally low dietary intakes of vitamin K could conceivably experience a deficiency of this vitamin while taking cholestyramine. In that event the risk is of hemorrhage, since vitamin K is needed to promote blood clotting.

Normally vitamin K helps produce blood-clotting substances in the liver. Without sufficient levels of this vitamin in the diet, however, bleeding may take place in the gastrointestinal tract (causing black or blood-stained stools), in the urinary tract (causing blood in the urine), and in the uterus (causing blood loss at times other than the normal menstrual periods). Excessive blood loss may occur from an injury or surgery. Another sign of a deficiency of this vitamin is more frequent and more visible bruising than normal.

Many elderly people are at risk of a vitamin K deficiency because they have a problem of poor fat absorption, and vitamin K, a fat-soluble vitamin, must be accompanied by sufficient dietary fat to be properly absorbed. Finally, anyone who suffers from a kidney disease or cancer, or who is under prolonged antibiotic therapy, may be at risk.

Prevention and Treatment: A vitamin K deficiency can be countered by a vitamin K supplement of 100 mcg per day, plus a diet that includes such foods as kale, spinach, cabbage, cauliflower, leafy green vegetables, liver (especially pork liver), and fish. (See table of Vitamin K-Rich Foods, page 315.)

Vitamin E supplements should not be taken when there is risk of a vitamin K shortage, because vitamin E impairs the absorption of K.

VITAMIN B_{12} DEFICIENCY: It is conceivable that a vitamin B_{12} deficiency will occur while you are taking cholestyramine. This vitamin is needed for the normal development of red blood cells and for the healthy functioning of all cells in the body, in particular those of the bone marrow and nervous system.

The most common result of a B_{12} deficiency is pernicious anemia, which is characterized by listlessness, fatigue (especially following heavy physical exertion such as climbing a flight of stairs), numbness and tingling in the fingers and toes, palpitations, angina, light-headedness, and a pale complexion. A vitamin B_{12} deficiency can also lead to an irreversible breakdown in the brain membranes, causing a loss of coordination, confusion, memory loss, paranoia, apathy, tremors, and hallucinations. In extreme cases, degeneration of the spinal cord can also result.

Since vitamin B_{12} can be obtained only from animal food sources, strict vegetarians are at particular risk here. Oral contraceptive users too have a greater chance of experiencing this deficiency, since they often have a poor vitamin B_{12} status to begin with, as is sometimes the case with smokers. Heavy consumers of alcohol, as well, frequently lack B_{12} because alcohol impairs the absorption of the vitamin. Some elderly people do not absorb vitamin B_{12} very well. In any case, everyone who is likely to have a vitamin B_{12} absorption problem should be alert for signs of pernicious anemia while taking cholestyramine.

Prevention and Treatment: A balanced diet containing plenty of vitamin B_{12} sources is advised. Only animal products, including dairy foods and fish and shellfish, contain the natural vitamin. However, some vegetable matter is supplemented with vitamin B_{12}; many soy products, for example, are enriched with the vitamin to safeguard vegetarians. (See table of Vitamin B_{12}-Rich Foods, page 312.)

Vitamin B_{12} is stored in the liver, so one meal that includes a B_{12}-rich source, such as calf's liver, will normally fulfill your body's need for this vitamin for 2 to 3 weeks. (One 3-ounce serving of calf's liver contains 100 mcg of vitamin B_{12}.) If none of these products figures prominently in your diet, you should take a 6 mcg supplement each day while on this drug.

People who use major amounts of vitamin C should be aware that vitamin C supplements of more than 500 mg per day can destroy B_{12} and contribute to a B_{12} deficiency. However, anyone who eats red meat two times a week has a three- to five-year supply of B_{12} in his liver.

The presence of baking soda in cooking will destroy this vitamin and should be avoided whenever possible. B_{12} also breaks down at high temperatures, as when meat is placed on a hot griddle. The pasteurization of milk and the sterilization in boiling water of a bottle of milk also cause the loss of some B_{12}.

FOLIC ACID DEFICIENCY: A folic acid or folacin deficiency is also conceivable while you are taking cholestyramine. Often the first sign of a folic acid or folacin deficiency is inflamed or bleeding gums. The symptoms that follow are a sore, smooth tongue; diarrhea; forgetfulness; apathy; irritability; anemia; and a reduced resistance to infection.

Although folacin is found in a variety of foods, folacin deficiency is still the most common vitamin deficiency in the United States. In adults, deficiencies are limited almost exclusively to the elderly and women, 30 percent of whom have intakes below the Recommended Dietary Allowance, and 5 to 7 percent of whom also have severe anemia. There are several factors that account for this bias, but among the most obvious are that oral contraceptive use decreases the absorption of folic acid and that constant dieting limits folacin intake. Alcohol interferes with the body's absorption and utilization of folic acid, as well.

Folic acid is crucial to the normal metabolism of proteins. Since folacin is also required for cell growth, a deficiency of this vitamin during pregnancy can lead to birth defects. Folacin is not stored by the body in any appreciable amounts, so an adequate supply must be consumed on a daily basis.

Prevention and Treatment: To counteract a deficiency in folic acid, your diet should contain liver, yeast, and leafy vegetables such as spinach, kale, parsley, cauliflower, brussels sprouts, and broccoli. The fruits that are highest in folic acid are oranges and cantaloupes. To a lesser degree, folacin is found in almonds and lima beans, corn, parsnips, green peas, pumpkins, sweet potatoes, bran, peanuts, rye, and whole grain wheat. (See table of Folacin-Rich Foods, page 297.) Approximately one half of the folic acid you consume is absorbed by your body.

Normal cooking temperatures (110 to 120 degrees for 10 minutes) destroy as much as 65 percent of the folacin in your food. Your daily diet, therefore, should include some raw vegetables and fruits. Cooking utensils made out of copper speed up folacin's destruction.

The recommended daily consumption of folacin is 400 mcg. Lactating women should assume a daily need of 1,200 mcg. Pregnant women and oral contraceptive users should consume 800 mcg daily.

CONSTIPATION AND OTHER SIDE EFFECTS: Cholestyramine is likely to cause constipation, especially in elderly patients. Many people experiencing constipation will self-medicate with laxatives. As a consequence, they are more likely to experience the vitamin deficiencies described above (particularly vitamin D), because laxatives interfere with the body's ability to absorb vitamins and minerals.

The drug also has an unpleasant, chalky texture, and can cause nausea and abdominal discomfort.

Prevention and Treatment: Constipation is usually safely remedied by an increase in the bulk in the diet. This means increasing the servings of any of the following: dried or fresh fruits (especially unpeeled apples or pears), salad vegetables, radishes, oatmeal, and whole grain foods (brown rice, whole wheat breads, and cereals). It is not necessary to purchase products that claim "extra fiber" has been added to them.

Persistent constipation may also be relieved by doubling the amount of fluid consumed each day. Bran, if used, should be added to the diet gradually, and fluid should be increased by at least ¾ cup per teaspoon of bran. (See table of Dietary Fiber-Rich Foods, page 293.)

The unpleasant, chalky texture of cholestyramine may be masked with pulpy fruit, such as applesauce, or liquids. Nausea and abdominal pains can be alleviated by taking the drug just before or during meals.

OTHER ADVICE: Cholestyramine binds to the following drugs, and it is likely that it will interfere with their absorption: digitalis, glycosides, phenobarbital, iron supplements, sodium warfarin, thyroid preparations, tetracycline, and thiazide diuretics. These drugs should be taken at least 1 hour before cholestyramine to prevent this from happening.

CIMETIDINE

DRUG FAMILY: Histamine H2 receptor antagonist

BRAND NAME: Tagamet

HOW TO TAKE CIMETIDINE: With food or milk

FOODS TO AVOID: Pepper, chili powder, cocoa, cola beverages, tea, caffeinated and decaffeinated coffee, and alcohol

POSSIBLE SIDE EFFECTS: Iron deficiency and diarrhea

ACTION OF CIMETIDINE: This drug inhibits the secretion of gastric acid and is used in the treatment of duodenal and gastric ulcers, and other kinds of stomach hyperacidity.

Histamine is released by cells in the wall of the stomach when food enters. By binding to receptors (H2) in the acid-secreting cells in the stomach, the histamine causes them to secrete hydrochloric acid. Cimetidine binds to the H2 receptors, and blocks the binding of histamine and acid secretion.

An ulcer is the wearing away of the lining of the stomach or intestines. Eventually, it involves small blood vessels within the wall of the gastrointestinal tract, causing bleeding, which may be fatal. If a hole is worn all the way through the wall, a major infection called peritonitis quickly develops, which can also be fatal.

Under normal circumstances, the inside wall of the gastrointestinal tract is protected by a covering of mucus. If this covering becomes thin or is destroyed, an ulcer develops, causing a burning pain. Stress, which brings on excess acid secretion, can exacerbate or cause ulcers, as can cigarette smoking, poor nutrition, insufficient sleep, excess caffeine, and the use of drugs (like aspirin) that irritate the stomach wall.

HIGH-RISK GROUPS: The elderly, premenopausal women, vegetarians

NUTRITIONAL INTERACTIONS

IRON DEFICIENCY: Cimetidine decreases the absorption of iron, especially from vegetable products. Since it is usually only taken for periods of up to 8 weeks, a person in good iron status, eating a diet including red meat on a regular basis, should not develop a deficiency. However, it is conceivable that people with low iron stores could develop a deficiency while on cimetidine.

Iron is especially important to the oxygen-carrying cells of the blood and muscles, which consume two thirds of the iron your body requires. As a result, an iron shortage reduces the blood's oxygen-carrying capacity, leading to an anemia signaled by such symptoms as tiredness, general feelings of malaise, irritability, decreased attention span, pale complexion, rapid heart rhythm, headaches, loss of concentration, and breathlessness on exertion. A mild iron deficiency will also impair the functioning of your immune system.

In order to absorb iron from any vegetable source, the iron must be coverted to another form by the action of the hydrochloric acid produced in the stomach. Some elderly people secrete less hydrochloric acid than normal, so they absorb iron poorly even under normal circumstances. The diets of many Americans lack adequate quantities of this mineral for their normal needs. For example, 10 percent of American women suffer from an iron deficiency, and up to 30 percent have inadequate iron stores. Other people who are at significant risk of an iron deficiency are women who have had several pregnancies and those whose menstrual periods are heavy.

The shortage of iron in many diets is due not only to the selection of foods that are poor sources of iron, but also to the switch from cast-iron cookware to aluminum, stainless steel, and nonstick surfaces. Acids in the food used to leach iron from iron pots and pans, and made it available as dietary iron.

Prevention and Treatment: To counteract an iron deficiency, iron-rich foods should be included in your diet: liver, whole grain products, oysters, dried apricots, prunes, peaches, leafy green vegetables, and, occasionally, lean red meat. (See table of Iron-Rich Foods, page 299.)

Other foods and drugs have a considerable impact on the way your body absorbs (or does not absorb) iron. There are two kinds of iron in food sources: heme iron in meat and ionic iron in vegetables. Up to 30 percent of the iron from meat, fish, and poultry is absorbed, but less than 10 percent is absorbed from eggs, whole grains, nuts, and dried beans. Only 10 percent of ionic iron is absorbed from vegetable sources, with as little as 2 percent being absorbed from spinach. Antacids will interfere with iron absorption in vegetables, as will commercial black and pekoe tea, taken in substantial quantities, because of its tannin content. Coffee also seems to decrease iron absorption, but not to the same degree as tea. Vitamin C supplements or citrus fruit juices increase the absorption of iron from vegetable sources by two to three times if taken simultaneously.

If your diet is rich in high-fiber foods, you will have impaired iron absorption because the fiber will bind to the iron and pass it out in the stool. This same action contributes to the poor absorption of iron from vegetable sources. Foods high in phosphorus (e.g. meat) interfere with iron absorption, which explains why only 30 percent of the iron in meat is captured. (However, meat and fish facilitate iron absorption from vegetables.) For that matter, any use of large quantities of mineral supplements, such as zinc, will impair iron absorption. Because iron can be leached from vegetables if they are cooked in large amounts of water, it is preferable to steam them.

Iron supplements should not be taken without a physician's recommendation, because an accumulation of too much iron can lead in extreme cases to such serious problems as anemia, malfunctioning of the pancreas and the heart, cirrhosis of the liver, a brown cast to the skin, and depression.

OTHER ADVICE: Antacids impair the absorption of cimetidine and should not be taken within 1 hour of taking the drug, unless otherwise indicated by a physician.

Most often this drug is given along with a specific dietary plan from your doctor. That diet too is a crucial part of the treatment and should be followed carefully. This usually involves eliminating foods that cause indigestion or pain, avoiding pepper, chili powder, cocoa, cola beverages, tea, caffeinated and decaffeinated coffee, and alcohol.

Cimetidine finds its way into breast milk and therefore should not be taken by breast-feeding mothers.

Cimetidine and iron both can cause diarrhea and should be taken with meals to reduce the risk of this interaction—they should not, however, be taken at the same time.

CISPLATIN

DRUG FAMILY: Anti-cancer

BRAND NAME: Platinol

HOW TO TAKE CISPLATIN: Given intravenously

FOODS TO AVOID: None

POSSIBLE SIDE EFFECTS: Deficiencies of magnesium, potassium, and zinc; nausea, vomiting, impaired taste, and lack of appetite

ACTION OF CISPLATIN: This anti-cancer agent is particularly effective in treating testicular tumors. It is also used in the treatment of cancer of the ovary, bladder, and endometrium, as well as for chemotherapy of lymphomas and some cancers of children.

HIGH-RISK GROUPS: Anyone who takes this drug

NUTRITIONAL INTERACTIONS

MAGNESIUM DEFICIENCY: Cisplatin increases magnesium, potassium, and zinc excretion. Magnesium deficiencies are not common, because the average American diet contains appreciable amounts of magnesium. However, the high level of magnesium excretion resulting from the interaction with this drug makes such a deficiency conceivable.

Clinical signs of magnesium deficiency include muscle weakness, tremors, depression, instability, and irrational behavior. Alcohol also depletes magnesium.

Prevention and Treatment: A diet containing the four food groups provides the normal amount of magnesium. However, if possible, your diet while taking this drug should feature foods such as nuts (almonds and cashews are highest), meat, fish, milk, whole grains, and fresh greens, since cooking can wash away some magnesium. (See table of Magnesium-Rich Foods, page 300.) Alcohol provokes magnesium excretion, so its intake should be restricted to no more than two drinks per day while you are on this drug.

Because of the nausea and vomiting associated with the use of cisplatin, it may be impractical to acquire magnesium in adequate quantities in the diet. Supplements should not be taken without the advice of your physician, but he or she is likely to prescribe them at the level of the Recommended Dietary Allowance, or approximately 350 mg per day.

POTASSIUM DEFICIENCY: It is also conceivable that cisplatin will cause you to experience a potassium deficiency. Potassium regulates the amount of water in the cells of the body and is essential for the proper functioning of the kidneys and the heart muscle, and the secretion of stomach juices. The most alarming symptom of a potassium deficiency is an irregular heartbeat, which can lead to heart failure. Other symptoms of low blood levels of potassium are weakness, loss of appetite, nausea, vomiting, dryness of the mouth, increased thirst, listlessness, apprehension, and diffuse pain that comes and goes.

Prevention and Treatment: Potassium depletion can be avoided by including such potassium-rich foods in your diet as tomato juice, lentils, dried apricots, asparagus, bananas, peanut butter, chicken, almonds, and milk. (See table of Potassium-Rich Foods, page 302.)

Potassium supplements should never be taken unless prescribed by a physician. They can cause anemia by interfering with the absorption of vitamin B_{12}. Just a few grams can also drastically increase the risk of heart failure. If you experience difficulty in swallowing while taking potassium supplements, consult your physician immediately. If supplements are prescribed, be aware that the absorption of the supplements potassium iodide and potassium chloride is decreased by dairy products, and that both are gastric irritants and should be taken with meals.

Once again, the nausea and vomiting that often accompany the use of cisplatin may make acquiring sufficient potassium in your diet impractical. Your doctor may well elect to prescribe a supplement at the recommended daily allowance level of approximately 3,000 mg.

Diuretics, commonly prescribed for people with heart disease, decrease the level of body potassium. Therefore, the risk of a deficiency is significantly increased if they are taken concurrently with this drug. Laxatives may have the same effect.

Too much salt in your diet can also compromise your body's supply of potassium.

ZINC DEFICIENCY: The third mineral that could conceivably be excreted at a rate sufficient to cause a deficiency is zinc. A shortage of zinc in your system may result in impaired healing of wounds and ulcers, scaly dermatitis of the face and limbs, and anorexia associated with the loss of taste.

Prevention and Treatment: Patients using this drug should be sure to get the Recommended Dietary Allowance of zinc. Animal foods are good sources, with the richest being oysters, herring, milk, and egg yolks. Among plant foods, whole grains are richest in zinc, but it is not as well absorbed from them as from meat. Fiber and phytic acid in the cereal grains hinder its absorption.

The recommended intake of 15 mg a day for adults is usually easily met by the diet of the average middle-class person, but deficiencies are more likely if animal protein is underemphasized. As a rule of thumb, two small servings of animal protein a day will provide sufficient zinc.

Again, however, it may be impractical to acquire zinc from dietary sources, given the nausea and vomiting that often accompany this drug. Supplements should not be taken without the advice of your physician, but he may elect to prescribe them at the level of the Recommended Dietary Allowance for zinc.

GASTROINTESTINAL DISTRESS: As mentioned above, cisplatin is likely to cause nausea, vomiting, impaired taste, mouth sores, and anorexia.

Prevention and Treatment: Nausea and vomiting may be controlled by taking several basic steps. First, you should eat smaller meals and limit your intake of high-fat foods. Second, when you experience nausea, you should slowly sip clear beverages such as ginger ale. Sucking a Popsicle may also alleviate the condition. You should loosen your clothes and lie down in a well-ventilated room.

If you find that you vomit frequently, you should take plenty of liquids to prevent dehydration.

CLINDAMYCIN

DRUG FAMILY: Antibiotic

BRAND NAMES: Cleocin Hydrochloride; Cleocin Pediatric; Cleocin Phosphate

HOW TO TAKE CLINDAMYCIN: One hour before or 3 hours after meals

FOODS TO AVOID: None

POSSIBLE SIDE EFFECTS: Diarrhea and impaired sense of taste

ACTION OF CLINDAMYCIN: This anti-bacterial agent is most often prescribed for abdominal and pelvic abscesses, bacteremia, pneumonia, lung abscesses, emphysema, soft tissue infections, and bedsores.

HIGH-RISK GROUPS: Patients with a history of abdominal distress

NUTRITIONAL INTERACTIONS

GENERAL ADVICE: Clindamycin impairs the sense of taste and can therefore reduce the pleasure of eating. A more worrisome problem, however, is that in 8 percent of all patients given clindamycin, serious diarrhea is experienced.

Prevention and Treatment: In order to minimize the affects of this drug on the appetite, you should take it 1 hour before or 3 hours after meals. The absorption of clindamycin is delayed when it is taken with food.

If you experience severe diarrhea upon consuming this drug, you should discontinue the use of it and consult your physician about a substitute medication.

CLOFIBRATE

DRUG FAMILY: Cholesterol reducer

BRAND NAME: Atromid-S

HOW TO TAKE CLOFIBRATE: Before or during meals and at bedtime

FOODS TO AVOID: None

POSSIBLE SIDE EFFECTS: Deficiencies of vitamin B_{12} and iron; loss of appetite, nausea, diarrhea, and a decreased sense of taste

ACTION OF CLOFIBRATE: This drug reduces the blood levels of cholesterol and triglycerides.

HIGH-RISK GROUPS: The elderly, vegetarians, smokers, premenopausal women

NUTRITIONAL INTERACTIONS

VITAMIN B_{12} DEFICIENCY: Clofibrate may cause malabsorption of vitamin B_{12}, and it is conceivable that you will develop a vitamin B_{12} deficiency over a period of years. Vitamin B_{12} is needed for the normal development of red blood cells and for the healthy functioning of all cells, in particular those of the bone marrow, nervous system, and intestines.

Pernicious anemia is the most common result of a B_{12} deficiency. It is characterized by listlessness, fatigue (especially following such physical exertion as climbing a flight of stairs), a numbness and tingling in the fingers and toes, palpitations, angina, light-headedness, and a pale complexion. A vitamin B_{12} deficiency can also lead to an irreversible breakdown in the brain membranes (called myelin), causing loss of coordination, confusion, memory loss, paranoia, apathy, tremors, and hallucinations. In extreme cases, degeneration of the spinal cord can also result.

Strict vegetarians are at particular risk of this deficiency, since vitamin B_{12} can be obtained only from animal food sources. Oral contraceptive users also have a greater chance of experiencing this deficiency since they often have a poor vitamin B_{12} status to begin with, as do some smokers. Heavy consumers of alcohol, as well, frequently lack B_{12} because alcohol impairs the absorption of the vitamin. Older people sometimes have a reduced ability to absorb the vitamin. This is because vitamin B_{12} must be combined in the stomach with a substance known as intrinsic factor in order to be properly absorbed in the intestine. This substance is lacking in some elderly people. In any case, anyone who is likely to have a vitamin B_{12} absorption problem should be alert for signs of pernicious anemia while taking this drug.

Prevention and Treatment: A balanced diet containing plenty of vitamin B_{12} sources is advised. Only animal products, including dairy foods and fish and shellfish, contain the natural vitamin. However, some vegetable matter is supplemented with vitamin B_{12}; many soy products, for example, are enriched with vitamin B_{12} to safeguard vegetarians. (See table of Vitamin B_{12}-Rich Foods, page 312.)

Vitamin B_{12} is stored in the liver, so one meal that includes a B_{12}-rich source such as calf's liver will normally fulfill your body's need for this vitamin for 2 to 3 weeks. (One 3-ounce serving of calf's liver contains 100 mcg of vitamin B_{12}.) If none of these products figures prominently in your diet, you should take a 6 mcg supplement each day while on clofibrate.

People who use major amounts of vitamin C should be aware that vitamin C supplements of more than 500 mg per day can destroy B_{12} and contribute to a B_{12} deficiency. Anyone who eats red meat two times a week has a three- to five-year supply of B_{12} in his liver.

The presence of baking soda in cooking will destroy vitamin B_{12} and should be avoided whenever possible. B_{12} also degrades at high temperatures, as when meat is placed on a hot griddle or, in the case of liver, when it is boiled for 5 minutes. The pasteurization of milk and the sterilization in boiling water of a bottle of milk also cause the loss of some B_{12}.

IRON DEFICIENCY: As was the case with vitamin B_{12}, iron may conceivably become deficient in your system while you are taking clofibrate. Iron is crucial to the oxygen-carrying cells of the blood and muscles, since they use two thirds of the iron your body requires. Consequently, an iron shortage reduces the blood's oxygen-carrying capacity.

The result of an iron deficiency is anemia, signaled by such symptoms as tiredness, general feelings of malaise, irritability, decreased attention span, pale complexion, rapid heart rhythm, headaches, loss of concentration, and breathlessness on exertion. A mild iron deficiency will also impair the functioning of your immune system.

To be absorbed from any vegetable source, iron must be converted to another form by the action of the hydrochloric acid produced in the stomach. Many elderly people secrete less hydrochloric acid than normal, so they absorb iron poorly even under normal circumstances. The diets of many Americans lack adequate quantities of this mineral for their normal needs. For example, 10 percent of American women suffer from an iron deficiency, and up to 30 percent have inadequate iron stores. Other people who

are at significant risk of an iron deficiency are women who have had several pregnancies and those whose menstrual periods are heavy.

The shortage of iron in many diets is due not only to the selection of foods that are poor sources of iron, but also to the switch away from cast-iron cookware to aluminum, stainless steel, and nonstick surfaces. Iron used to be leached from iron pots and pans by the acids in the foods being cooked, and became available as dietary iron.

Prevention and Treatment: To counteract an iron deficiency, iron-rich foods should be included in your diet: liver, whole grain products, oysters, dried apricots, prunes, peaches, leafy green vegetables, and lean red meat. (See table of Iron-Rich Foods, page 299.)

Other foods and drugs impact upon on the way your body absorbs (or does not absorb) iron. There are two kinds of iron in food sources: heme iron in meat and ionic iron in vegetables. Up to 30 percent of the iron from meat, fish, and poultry is absorbed, but less than 10 percent is absorbed from eggs, whole grains, nuts, and dried beans. Only 10 percent of ionic iron is absorbed from vegetable sources, with as little as 2 percent being absorbed from spinach. Antacids will interfere with iron absorption from vegetables, as will commercial black and pekoe tea, taken in substantial quantities, because of its tannin content.

Coffee also seems to decrease iron absorption, but not to the same degree as tea. Vitamin C supplements or citrus fruit juices increase the absorption of iron from vegetable sources by two to three times if taken simultaneously. If your diet is rich in high-fiber foods, you will have impaired iron absorption, because the indigestible fiber will bind to the iron and pass it out in the stool. This same action contributes to the poor absorption of iron from vegetable sources. Foods high in phosphorus (e.g. meat) interfere with iron absorption, which explains why only 30 percent of the iron in meat is captured. (However, meat and fish facilitate iron absorption from vegetables.) The use of large quantities of mineral supplements, such as zinc, will impair iron absorption. Because iron can be leached from vegetables if they are cooked in large amounts of water, it is preferable to steam them.

Iron supplements should not be taken without a physician's recommendation, because an accumulation of too much iron can lead in extreme cases to such serious problems as anemia, malfunctioning of the pancreas and the heart, cirrhosis of the liver, a brown cast to the skin, and depression.

APPETITE LOSS: The drug is also likely to cause nausea, diarrhea, and a decreased sense of taste that may result in a loss of appetite and unwanted weight loss.

Prevention and Treatment: A balanced dietary regimen that includes all four food groups should be followed (see table of Recommended Dietary Allowances, page 317), with a caloric intake appropriate for your weight and body type. Usually, no vitamin supplements are required if you eat a balanced diet, but you should monitor your weight carefully.

OTHER ADVICE: Note that this drug may decrease the effectiveness of oral contraceptives.

CLONIDINE HYDROCHLORIDE

DRUG FAMILY: Anti-hypertensive

BRAND NAMES: Catapres; Combipres

HOW TO TAKE CLONIDINE HYDROCHLORIDE: At noon and at bedtime, with a nonalcoholic beverage

FOODS TO AVOID: Salty foods such as anchovies, dill pickles, sardines, green olives, canned soups and vegetables, TV dinners, soy sauce, processed cheeses, salty snack foods, cold cuts, and catsup; tyramine- and dopamine-rich foods such as aged cheeses, raisins, avocados, liver, bananas, eggplant, sour cream, alcoholic beverages, salami, meat tenderizers, chocolate, yeast, and soy sauce; licorice candy made from natural extract

POSSIBLE SIDE EFFECTS: Edema; constipation

ACTION OF CLONIDINE HYDROCHLORIDE: This drug is used primarily as an anti-hypertensive agent. It is also used for the treatment of migraine headaches.

HIGH-RISK GROUPS: Anyone who takes this drug

NUTRITIONAL INTERACTIONS

EDEMA: This drug is likely to lead to water and salt retention, which will tend to cause swelling (called edema) in your legs, ankles, feet, and breasts, and around your eyes. An increase in sodium and water retention may also increase the volume of blood in the body, which places an added strain on the heart and tends to elevate blood pressure.

Hence, this drug is usually given along with a diuretic to avoid these potential problems.

High sodium retention causes some women to experience irritability, depression, and headaches, in particular before the onset of their menstrual periods.

Prevention and Treatment: While taking clonidine hydrochloride, you should restrict your consumption of salt. In particular, those foods listed in the table of Sodium-Rich Foods (see page 306) should be avoided, or consumed in small quantities. You should not add salt at the table or in cooking.

Many people are unaware of how much salt their diet contains. The average American, in fact, consumes some 15 pounds of salt a year. Even if you do not salt your food while preparing or eating it, you consume quantities of salt in such foods as anchovies, dill pickles, sardines, green olives, canned soups and vegetables, so-called TV dinners, soy sauce, processed cheeses, salty snack foods, cold cuts, and catsup. Many additives, such as baking soda and baking powder, widely used in the preparation of processed foods, contain sodium as well.

CONSTIPATION: Clonidine hydrochloride could conceivably cause you to become constipated.

Prevention and Treatment: Often constipation is safely remedied by an increase in the bulk in the diet. This means consuming larger servings of any of the following: dried or fresh fruits (especially unpeeled apples or pears), salad vegetables, radishes, oatmeal, and whole grain foods (brown rice, whole wheat breads, and cereals). It is not necessary to purchase products that claim "extra fiber" has been added to them.

Persistent constipation may also be relieved by doubling the amount of fluid consumed each day. Bran, if used, should be added to the diet gradually, and fluid should be increased by at least ¾ cup per teaspoon of bran. (See table of Dietary Fiber-Rich Foods, page 293.)

Exercise will also help, for not only does exercise tone up muscle in the arms and legs, it also strengthens the muscles lining the gastrointestinal tract, which propel the food through the intestines. However, if you have hypertension, check with your doctor before beginning an exercise program.

TYRAMINE-RICH FOODS: Tyramine, a food substance, may decrease the effectiveness of this drug by causing an increase in blood pressure.

Prevention and Treatment: It is advisable to restrict tyramine-containing foods while you are being treated with clonidine. Tyramine is common in many foods, but it is found in the greatest amounts in high-protein foods that have undergone some decomposition, like aged cheese. Tyramine is also found in chicken and beef livers, bananas, eggplant, sour cream, alcoholic beverages, salami, meat tenderizers, chocolate, yeast, and soy sauce. (See table of Tyramine-Rich Foods, page 307.) Raisins and avocados should also be avoided, because they contain dopamine, which has the same effect as tyramine.

Licorice candy that is made with natural extract contains glycyrrhizic acid, which also can elevate blood pressure by causing sodium and water retention. As little as 3 ounces is enough to induce such a reaction, so it is best to avoid eating licorice when taking this drug.

ALCOHOL: If taken along with clonidine, alcohol can cause drowsiness and an enhanced drop in blood pressure.

Prevention and Treatment: Avoid alcoholic beverages as much as possible.

CODEINE

DRUG FAMILY: Analgesic

BRAND NAMES: A.P.C. with Codeine; Acetaco; Acetaminophen with Codeine Phosphate; Actifed with Codeine Cough Syrup; Amaphen with Codeine; Ambenyl Cough Syrup; Anacin-3 with Codeine; Anatuss with Codeine; Ascriptin with Codeine; Aspirin w/Codeine; Bancap c̄ Codeine; Bromanyl; Bromphen DC; Buff-A Comp No. 3; Calcidrine; Capital with Codeine; Codalan; Codeine Phosphate; Codeine Sulfate; Codimal PH; Colrex; Conex with Codeine; Decongestant Expectorant; Decongestant-AT; Deproist; Empirin with Codeine; Empracet with Codeine Phosphate; Fiorinal w/Codeine; G-2; G-3; Guiatuss A-C; Iophen-C; Naldecon-CX; Novahistine DH; Novahistine; Nucofed; Pediacof; Phenaphen w/Codeine; Phenaphen-650; Phenergan with Codeine; Phenergan VC with Codeine; Poly-Histine Expectorant with Codeine; Robitussin A-C; Robitussin-DAC; Ru-Tuss; Ryna-C; Ryna-CX; SK-APAP; Soma Compound w/Codeine; Stopayne; Terpin Hydrate & Codeine Elixir; Triafed-C; Triaminic Expectorant w/Codeine; Tussi-Organidin; Tussar SF; Tussar-2; Tylenol w/Codeine

HOW TO TAKE CODEINE: At meals or with milk

FOODS TO AVOID: All alcoholic beverages

POSSIBLE SIDE EFFECTS: Constipation, nausea, vomiting

ACTION OF CODEINE: This analgesic is prescribed for the relief of mild to moderately severe pain and as a cough suppressant.

HIGH-RISK GROUPS: The elderly, anyone who consumes alcohol

NUTRITIONAL INTERACTIONS

GASTROINTESTINAL DISCOMFORT: Codeine could conceivably cause you to become constipated. This reaction is seen most often among elderly users of the drug. Codeine may also cause nausea and vomiting.

Prevention and Treatment: Constipation is usually safely remedied by an increase in the bulk in the diet. This means consuming larger servings of any of the following: dried or fresh fruits (especially unpeeled apples or pears), salad vegetables (especially unpeeled carrots), radishes, oatmeal, and whole grain foods (brown rice, whole wheat breads, and cereals). It is not necessary to purchase products that claim "extra fiber" has been added to them.

Persistent constipation may also be relieved by doubling the amount of fluid consumed each day. Bran, if used, should be added to the diet gradually, and fluid should be increased by at least ¾ cup per teaspoon of bran. (See table of Dietary Fiber-Rich Foods, page 293.)

Codeine should be taken with milk or meals, to reduce the likelihood of nausea or vomiting.

SERIOUS RISKS: Alcohol enhances the effects of codeine in suppressing the activity of the brain, and the combination can cause coma. The drug is also addictive and should be used with caution by patients also taking anti-depressants.

Prevention and Treatment: Alcohol should never be consumed concurrently with codeine.

COLCHICINE

DRUG FAMILY: Anti-gout

BRAND NAMES: ColBENEMID; Col-Probenecid; Probenecid w/Colchicine

HOW TO TAKE COLCHICINE: Immediately after meals

FOODS TO AVOID: Coffee, tea, cola beverages, herbal teas, alcoholic beverages, dairy products; large amounts of foods rich in purines, such as sweetbreads, anchovies, sardines, liver, kidney, and meat extracts

POSSIBLE SIDE EFFECTS: Malabsorption of all nutrients; diarrhea.

ACTION OF COLCHICINE: This strong, anti-inflammatory drug is prescribed for patients with gout, where extreme pain is felt, and in some instances as a chemical agent in cancer therapy.

Colchicine helps the body excrete uric acid, which causes gout. Gout is an arthritis-type disease that occurs as a result of deposits of uric acid crystals in the joints. It usually occurs in single joints, most often the big toe, in painful episodes that last only a few days but are likely to recur. Middle-aged men are most often afflicted. This drug is not usually taken over long periods of time.

Your doctor is likely to recommend a special diet low in purine-rich foods in addition to prescribing this or another of the anti-gout medications. That diet is a crucial part of the treatment, because the purines in foods are broken down by your body to produce uric acid. (See table of Purine-Rich Foods, page 303.)

HIGH-RISK GROUPS: Anyone who takes this drug

NUTRITIONAL INTERACTION

NUTRITIONAL DEFICIENCIES: This drug destroys parts of the lining of the intestines, where the enzymes that digest your food are located. Consequences of this are likely to be the malabsorption of all nutrients and invariably diarrhea. Malabsorption of sugars, fats (and hence the fat-soluble vitamins A, D, E, and K), protein, iron, vitamin B_{12}, and folacin usually result. The diarrhea will also lead to the loss of minerals, including calcium, magnesium, and potassium, and a lot of water will be lost from the body.

Prevention and Treatment: Since colchicine is taken for very short periods of time, no nutritional deficiencies should occur. However, while you are using the drug, you should safeguard your nutritional status by taking a one-a-day vitamin containing the recommended daily allowances for vitamins and iron. This is especially true of elderly people and vegetarians, since both groups often have a poor vitamin B_{12} and iron status.

A low-fat, high-protein diet is recommended. This means cutting down on meats and processed foods, and increasing the consumption of vegetables, fruits, and cereals. The body's ability to digest milk sugar is decreased by as much as 85 percent while you are using colchicine, so milk should never be taken with this drug; otherwise diarrhea will result.

BILE SALT BUILDUP: The liver secretes bile to help digest fatty foods. The bile, along with the dietary fats, passes into the upper portion of the small intestine, where the fats are broken down into small globules that the fat-digesting enzymes can digest.

After they have done their work, one of the constituents of the bile, the bile salts, is reabsorbed in the lower regions of the small intestine and recycled. This lower region, called the jejunum, is also damaged by colchicine, and it is conceivable that, as a result, it will not be able to reabsorb the salts, so more of the bile salts end up in the colon. Studies have shown that bacteria in the colon convert bile salts to chemicals, and these chemicals have been implicated as a causal factor in colon cancer. Hence, patients regularly using colchicine should ensure that these salts are flushed out of the system as quickly as possible; eating a high-fiber diet is the best way to do that.

OTHER ADVICE: It is not wise to consume large quantities of coffee, tea, or cola beverages while you are taking colchicine, because they may reduce the effectiveness of the drug. Also avoid herbal teas, since these contain phenylbutazone, which raises blood uric acid levels.

Colchicine should be taken after eating to reduce stomach irritation. It should not be used at all if you have a history of peptic ulcers.

You should also avoid alcohol, especially beer, and simple sugars (see table of Simple and Complex Carbohydrates, page 305), because they can raise the blood level of uric acid and impair the drug's ability to manage chronic gout.

If obese, the gout sufferer should also achieve ideal body weight by gradual weight reduction (1 to 2 pounds per week). All sufferers should decrease their animal fat intake and increase their complex carbohydrate intake.

COLESTIPOL HYDROCHLORIDE

DRUG FAMILY: Cholesterol reducer

BRAND NAME: Colestid

HOW TO TAKE COLESTIPOL HYDROCHLORIDE: Just before or during meals and at bedtime, mixed with pulpy fruit, such as applesauce, or a liquid

FOODS TO AVOID: None

POSSIBLE SIDE EFFECTS: Folic acid deficiency, constipation, nausea, and stomachache, and, though less likely, possible deficiencies of vitamins A, D, E, and K

ACTION OF COLESTIPOL HYDROCHLORIDE: This drug lowers blood cholesterol and triglyceride levels.

HIGH-RISK GROUPS: The elderly, people taking anti-convulsants, chronic users of aspirin, heavy drinkers

NUTRITIONAL INTERACTIONS

FAT-SOLUBLE VITAMIN DEFICIENCIES: Although it is highly unlikely, there is a chance that while taking colestipol you will experience a slight malabsorption of the fat-soluble vitamins A, D, E, and K. Under normal circumstances, no symptoms of a deficiency of these vitamins will be evident.

Prevention and Treatment: To avoid fat-soluble vitamin deficiencies while taking colestipol, you should eat a balanced diet that includes all four food groups at the appropriate caloric intake for your weight and body type. (See table of Recommended Dietary Allowances, page 317.) In addition, if the drug is taken over extended periods, supplements are advised at the following levels: 2,000 to 5,000 IU of vitamin A; 200 to 800 IU of vitamin D; 10 to 15 IU of vitamin E.

FOLIC ACID DEFICIENCY: Conceivably, you could develop a folic acid deficiency while taking colestipol, since the drug impairs the absorption of this nutrient. Often the first sign of a folic acid or folacin deficiency is inflamed and bleeding gums. The symptoms that follow are a sore, smooth tongue; diarrhea; forgetfulness; apathy; irritability; anemia; and a reduced resistance to infection. Despite the fact that folacin is found in a variety of foods, folacin deficiency is still the most common vitamin deficiency in the United States.

In adults, deficiencies are limited almost exclusively to the elderly and women, 30 percent of whom have intakes below the recommended daily allowance, and 5 to 7 percent of whom also have severe anemia. There are several factors that account for this bias, but one of the most obvious reasons is that oral contraceptive use decreases the absorption of folic acid. Constant dieting also limits folacin intake, and alcohol interferes with the body's use of folic acid, as well.

Folic acid is crucial to the normal metabolism of proteins. As folacin is also required for cell growth, a deficiency of this vitamin during pregnancy can lead to birth defects. Folacin is not stored by the body in any appreciable amounts, so an adequate supply must be consumed on a daily basis.

Prevention and Treatment: To counteract a deficiency of folic acid, your diet should contain liver, yeast, and leafy vegetables such as spinach, kale, parsley, cauliflower, brussels sprouts, and broccoli. The fruits that are highest in folic acid are oranges and cantaloupes. To a lesser degree, folacin is found in almonds and lima beans, corn, parsnips, green peas, pumpkins, sweet potatoes, bran, peanuts, rye, and whole grain wheat. (See table of Folacin-Rich Foods, page 297.) Approximately one half of the folic acid you consume is absorbed by your body.

Normal cooking temperatures (110 to 120 degrees for 10 minutes) destroy up to 65 percent of the folacin in your food. Your daily diet, therefore, should include some raw vegetables and fruits. Cooking utensils made out of copper speed up folacin's destruction.

The Recommended Dietary Allowance of folacin is 400 mcg.

CONSTIPATION AND OTHER PROBLEMS: Colestipol is likely to cause constipation, especially in the elderly, and can provoke nausea and abdominal discomfort. It also has an unpleasant chalky texture.

Prevention and Treatment: Constipation is usually safely remedied by an increase in the bulk in the diet. This means consuming larger servings of any of the following: dried or fresh fruits, salad vegetables (especially unpeeled carrots), radishes, oatmeal, and whole grain foods (brown rice, whole wheat breads, and cereals). It is not necessary to purchase products that claim "extra fiber" has been added to them.

Persistent constipation may also be relieved by doubling the amount of fluid consumed each day. Bran, if used, should be added to the diet gradually, and fluid should be increased by at least ¾ cup per teaspoon of bran. (See table of Dietary Fiber-Rich Foods, page 293.)

The unpleasant texture of colestipol may be made more palatable by taking it with pulpy fruit, such as applesauce, or a liquid. To minimize the nausea and abdominal problems, take the drug just before or during meals.

OTHER ADVICE: Colestipol is also likely to decrease the absorption and effectiveness of acidic compounds such as iron supplements, sodium warfarin, thyroid preparations, tetracycline, and thiazide diuretics. These medications should be taken at least one hour before the colestipol.

CORTICOSTEROIDS

DRUG FAMILY: Anti-inflammatory

BRAND NAMES: [GENERIC/Brand] HYDRO-CORTISONE/Aeroseb-HC; Allersone; Alphaderm; Carmol HC; Cort-Dome; Cort-enema; Corticaine; Cortisporin; Cortixin; Cortril; Dermacort; Derma-Sone; Eldecort; F-E-P; Hill Cortac; Hytone; Otic-HC; Otobiotic Otic; Pedi-Cort V; Pricort; Pro-Cort; Proctocort; Pyocidin-Otic; Synacort; Terra-Cortril; Texacort; Vanoxide-HC; Vioform-Hydrocortisone; VōSol HC; Vytone; Anusol-HC; Coly-Mycin S Otic w/Neomycin & Hydrocortisone; Cortifoam; Derma Medicone; Epifoam; Hedal H-C; Hydrocortone Acetate; Komed HC; Mantadil; Ophthocort; Orabase HCA; Pramosone; Proctofoam-HC; Rectal Medicone-HC; Wyanoids HC; Barseb HC; Barseb Thera; A-hydroCort; Hydrocortisone Sodium Succinate; Solu-Cortef; Westcort; DEXAMETHASONE/Aeroseb-Dex; Decadron; Decaspray; Dexone; Hexadrol; SK-Dexamethasone; Dalalone D.P.; Dalalone I.L.; Dalalone L.A.; Decadron-LA; Dexasone; Neodecadron; Decadron Phosphate; Hexadrol Phosphate; METHYL-PREDNISOLONE/Medrol; DepMedalone "40"; DepMedalone "80"; Depo-Medrol; Medrol; Depo-Predate 40; Depo-Predate 80; Medrol Acetate; A-methaPred; Methylprednisolone Sodium Succinate; Solu-Medrol; PREDNISOLONE/Delta-Cortef; Metimyd; Predate 50; Metreton; Predate S; Hydeltra-T.B.A.; Predate TBA; PREDNISONE/Deltasone; Liquid Pred; SK-Prednisone; Sterapred Uni-Pak.

HOW TO TAKE CORTISONE DRUGS: With meals or milk

FOODS TO AVOID: Fatty foods; large amounts of those rich in sodium, such as anchovies, green olives, dill pickles, sardines, canned soups and vegetables, TV dinners, processed cheeses, cold cuts

POSSIBLE SIDE EFFECTS: Edema; hyperglycemia; loss of body calcium and protein; deficiencies of potassium, zinc, and vitamins B_6 and C; increased risk of heart disease; dehydration; increased appetite

ACTION OF CORTISONE DRUGS: These anti-inflammatory agents are used in treating arthritis, many skin diseases, severe allergic conditions, insufficiency of the adrenal glands, collagen diseases, thyroiditis, and hypercalcemia associated with cancer.

HIGH-RISK GROUPS: Anyone who takes this drug by mouth or injection

NUTRITIONAL INTERACTIONS

EDEMA: Corticosteroids tend to increase sodium and water retention, which can lead to a swelling (called edema) in your legs, ankles, feet, and breasts, and around your eyes. Water and sodium retention also increase the volume of blood, which can lead to high blood pressure.

High sodium retention can also cause some women to experience irritability, depression, and headaches, particularly prior to the onset of the menstrual period.

Prevention and Treatment: You should restrict your intake of dietary sodium, when you are taking corticosteroids, to no more than 2 to 3 grams per day, which is equivalent to 1 to 2 teaspoons of salt.

Most people are not aware of how much salt their diet contains. The average American consumes 15 pounds of salt annually, or 3 to 4 teaspoons a day. Do not salt your food at the table or add more than 1 teaspoon of salt during cooking. Foods rich in sodium, such as anchovies, green olives, dill pickles, sardines, canned soups and vegetables, so-called TV dinners, processed cheeses, cold cuts, many snack foods, soy sauce, and catsup, should be limited. (See table of Sodium-Rich Foods, page 306.) Salt comes into your diet through additives such as monosodium glutamate, which is widely used in the preparation of processed foods. Beware of foods in which sodium is placed high on the list of ingredients shown on the package. The higher it appears, the greater the amount of sodium present.

DIABETES REACTION: Corticosteroids can decrease your body's ability to absorb sugar, which can result in a diabeteslike state in susceptible individuals due to damage to the pancreas. Diabetes occurs when the pancreas fails to produce adequate amounts of insulin to clear the blood of excess glucose or sugar. A diet high in sugar increases the likelihood of a diabetic condition with this drug.

Symptoms of a glucose buildup in your blood are headaches, excessive hunger and thirst, and a need to urinate frequently.

Prevention and Treatment: Recent studies have demonstrated that a high-fiber diet may cause a slower and more sustained release of glucose from the gastrointestinal tract into the bloodstream, preventing the wide swings in blood sugar levels. If you are taking a corticosteroid, it is recommended that you remain physically active and exercise daily, because by this means the cells are made more susceptible to the insulin, and you absorb glucose more readily. Finally, a change in eating schedule from the standard three meals per day to five or six smaller meals will also help keep blood sugar levels within normal range.

CALCIUM LOSS: Extended use of corticosteroids can create a loss of calcium, since these drugs decrease calcium absorption and increase losses from the bones. The decrease in absorption is due to an inability to produce active vitamin D, which is essential to calcium absorption. These drugs also decrease the absorption of the mineral phosphorus, which may further exacerbate the loss of body calcium.

Whenever calcium blood levels are low, the body will liberate the necessary amounts of calcium from the bones, where it is stored, weakening them. This condition is called osteomalacia. Prominent symptoms are pain in the bones of the thighs, back, shoulder region, or ribs; difficulty in walking; and weakness in the muscles of the legs. This disease affects millions of older Americans, but also many younger people. One out of every four postmenopausal women suffers from this problem; it has been estimated that the average woman over forty-five consumes only 450 mg of calcium per day, when the Recommended Dietary Allowance is 800 to 1,200. The condition is reversible once calcium blood levels are corrected.

After a number of years without correction, however, osteomalacia may lead to osteoporosis, another condition in which the bones are made weak and brittle. However, osteoporosis, an unexplained and rapid loss of calcium from the bones, is irreversible and uneven. The early signs of the disease are backache, a gradual loss of height, and periodontal disease. Often the first sign of the disorder is a fracture, usually of a vertebra, the hip, or a wrist.

If this drug is given to children, a condition known as rickets can occur. Again, the effect is on the bones, which become bent or malformed. Children under four years of age may develop pigeon breast, bowlegs, a protruding abdomen due to a weakness of stomach muscles, and poorly formed teeth which tend to decay. (However, drugs that are known to induce rickets are rarely given to the very young.)

PREVENTION AND TREATMENT: While taking this drug, you should take 400 to 800 IU of vitamin D per day as a supplement to a diet of foods rich in vitamin D, such as cod-liver oil, fortified milk, butter, liver, egg yolks, salmon, tuna, and sardines. (See table of Vitamin D-Rich Foods, page 313.)

If demineralization of the bones is indicated, nonpregnant adults should take 2,000 IU per day of vitamin D.

A calcium depletion can be prevented by eating foods rich in calcium, particularly milk and dairy products, including yogurt and hard cheeses. (See table of Calcium-Rich Foods, page 289.) If dairy foods must be avoided because of an intolerance to lactose, the sugar found in dairy products, a 1,000 mg daily supplement of calcium should be taken. (See Calcium Supplements entry, page 51.) Since vitamin C assists calcium absorption, foods rich in that vitamin should also be consumed.

Foods that can decrease the absorption of calcium should be temporarily restricted, such as spinach, cocoa, chocolate, beet greens, and tea. A deficiency might arise also if the ratio of phosphorus to calcium in your diet is very high. The ideal ratio is essentially 1 to 1, as in dairy products; when the ratio is 15 or 20 to 1, as in meat, very little calcium is absorbed. Processed foods are particularly bad in this respect, with carbonated beverages having perhaps the highest phosphorus content. High-fiber foods may contribute to a calcium deficiency, because fiber binds to calcium and passes it out in the stool.

Since there is little calcium in strict vegetarian diets (those that avoid dairy products as well as meat), vegetarians are at greater risk of a deficiency when taking corticosteroids. Those who use diuretics, or magnesium- or aluminum-based antacids, are also more prone to calcium deficiencies, because both impair calcium absorption.

To safeguard women against osteoporosis and osteomalacia, many experts believe that their calcium intake should be increased to 1,200 to 1,500 mg per day. Besides a change in dietary habits and the use of calcium supplements, it is recommended that you adopt an exercise regimen that will strengthen the bones by supporting the weight of the body. A regular walking or jogging program, for example, can help prevent the bone degeneration of the spine, hips, and legs. Note, however, that swimming, though good for the heart as an aerobic exercise, is not especially beneficial for bone buildup.

PROTEIN LOSS: Corticosteroids can also contribute to the breakdown of body protein, which may lead to a loss of muscle, muscle weakness, and slowed wound healing. Protein is also lost from the bones, which leads to their breakdown and consequent loss of bone calcium.

Prevention and Treatment: To avoid a temporary protein deficiency while you are taking this drug, you should eat a diet rich in protein, including such foods as fish, soy products, beans, and peas. Protein, however, should not represent more than 20 percent of dietary calories, since more than this could accelerate bone loss. (See table of Protein-Rich Foods, page 304.)

POTASSIUM DEFICIENCY: Corticosteroids increase the rate of excretion of potassium, which is likely to lead to a deficiency of this important mineral. Potassium regulates the amount of water in the cells of the body, and is essential for the proper functioning of the kidneys and the heart muscle, and the secretion of stomach juices. The most alarming symptom of a potassium deficiency is an irregular heartbeat, which can lead to heart failure.

Low blood serum levels of potassium, called hypokalemia, are associated with laxative abuse, because many laxatives promote an increased loss of potassium in the gastrointestinal tract. This risk is especially high in elderly patients who consume diets not only low in potassium but also low in dietary fiber (which may, in fact, have played a part in the development of their constipation in the first place).

People who take the laxatives phenolphthalein, bisacodyl, and senna on a daily basis have been reported to have a much greater chance of experiencing serious hypokalemia. These people, and others with a potassium deficiency, may have such symptoms as weakness, loss of appetite, nausea, vomiting, dryness of the mouth, increased thirst, listlessness, apprehension, and diffuse pain that comes and goes.

Prevention and Treatment: Potassium depletion can be avoided by including such potassium-rich foods in your diet as tomato juice, lentils, dried apricots, asparagus, bananas, peanut butter, chicken, almonds, and milk. (See table of Potassium-Rich Foods, page 302.)

Diuretics, commonly prescribed for people with heart disease, decrease the level of body potassium. Therefore, the risk of a deficiency is significantly greater if they are taken concurrently with this drug.

Potassium supplements should never be used unless prescribed by a physician. They can cause anemia by interfering with the absorption of vitamin B_{12}. Just a few grams can also drastically increase the risk of heart failure. If you experience difficulty in swallowing while taking potassium supplements, consult your physician immediately. If supplements are prescribed, be aware that the absorption of the supplements potassium iodide and potassium chloride is decreased by dairy products, and that both are gastric irritants and should be taken with meals.

Too much salt in your diet can also compromise your body's supply of potassium, as can 1 to 3 ounces per day of natural licorice. Only imported licorice usually contains natural licorice.

ZINC DEFICIENCY: Since the excretion of zinc is increased by the corticosteroids, it is conceivable that you will experience a deficiency while taking a corticosteroid. A shortage of zinc in your system may result in impaired healing of wounds and ulcers, scaly dermatitis of the face and limbs, and anorexia associated with the loss of taste.

Prevention and Treatment: Patients using this drug should be sure to get the Recommended Dietary Allowance of zinc. An-

imal foods are good sources, with the richest being oysters, herring, milk, and egg yolks. Among plant foods, whole grains are richest in zinc, but it is not as well absorbed from them as from meat. Fiber and phytic acid in the cereal grains hinder its absorption. The recommended intake of 15 mg a day for adults is usually met easily by the diet of the average middle-class person, but deficiencies are more likely if animal protein is underemphasized. As a rule of thumb, two small servings of animal protein a day will provide sufficient zinc.

VITAMIN B_6 DEFICIENCY: These drugs speed up the reactions in the body that require vitamin B_6, and consequently a deficiency of this vitamin is conceivable.

Common symptoms of this deficiency are a sore mouth and tongue, cracks in the lips and corners of the mouth, and patches of itching, scaling skin. A severe vitamin B_6 deficiency may cause depression and confusion.

Vitamin B_6 deficiencies are common among the elderly. Alcoholics, as well, often experience this deficiency, since alcohol interferes with the body's ability to use B_6. It is estimated that one of every two Americans consumes less than 70 percent of the Recommended Dietary Allowance of B_6.

Prevention and Treatment: To avoid a B_6 deficiency, you should consume a diet featuring such food sources of vitamin B_6 as liver (beef, calf, and pork), herring, salmon, walnuts, peanuts, wheat germ, carrots, peas, potatoes, grapes, bananas, and yeast. (See table of Vitamin B_6-Rich Foods, page 311.) The vitamin is present in significant amounts in meats, fish, fruits, cereals, and vegetables, and to a lesser extent in milk and other dairy products.

Since vitamin B_6 is decomposed at high temperatures, modern food processing often diminishes dietary sources of the vitamin. Consequently, the more processed foods you eat, the more susceptible you will be to a deficiency of this vitamin. The same losses also occur in cooking: meat loses as much as 45 to 80 percent, vegetables 20 to 30 percent. As vitamin B_6 is light-sensitive, the amount of the vitamin in a container of milk left in the sunlight will gradually decrease.

It has been observed that 15 to 20 percent of oral contraceptive users show direct evidence of vitamin B_6 deficiency. If you are among these people, you should take a 5 mg supplement of vitamin B_6 per day. However, keep in mind that you can take too much vitamin B_6; people taking over 500 mg per day have been reported to experience a toxic reaction.

VITAMIN C DEFICIENCY: Corticosteroid drugs cause an increase in the excretion of vitamin C, as well as an increase in the rate of various reactions in the body that use vitamin C. Consequently, while you are on corticosteroids, your system has an added need for the vitamin; thus, unless your intake keeps pace with your needs, a deficiency is conceivable.

With an adequate vitamin C intake, the body normally maintains a fixed pool of the vitamin, and rapidly excretes any excess in the urine. Ordinarily, 60 to 100 mg of vitamin C per day will fulfill the body's needs. However, with an inadequate intake, the reservoir becomes depleted at the rate of up to 3 percent per day, and even more

quickly in users of this drug. Obvious symptoms of a vitamin C deficiency do not appear until the available vitamin C has been reduced to about one fifth of its optimal level, and this may take two months to occur.

The earliest signs of a deficiency are spongy or bleeding gums, slightly swollen wrists and ankles, and capillaries that break under the skin, producing pinpoint hemorrhages around the hair follicles on the arms and legs.

Vitamin C is important to the functioning of your bodily systems in a number of ways. When your body is deficient in Vitamin C, your white blood cells are less able to detect and destroy invading bacteria. On the other hand, megadoses of the vitamin (over 2 grams daily) can also impair this ability. Vitamin C also helps your body guard itself against such pollutants as known cancer-causing agents nitrites and nitrosamines, and protects vitamins A and E from degradation. In addition, it aids in iron absorption, speeds up wound healing, and strengthens blood vessels. Other well-known effects are that, in some people, vitamin C reduces the symptoms of a cold by one third and is important in preventing plaque formation on the teeth, which reduces the likelihood of gum disease and tooth decay.

Prevention and Treatment: Patients taking corticosteroids should be sure to get 100 mg per day of vitamin C. Vitamin C-rich foods include citrus fruits, broccoli, spinach, cabbage, and bananas. (See table of Vitamin C-Rich Foods, page 313.) In preparing foods rich in vitamin C, you should keep in mind that it is readily oxidized (during both food processing and storage, when exposed to the air), and that copper and iron cooking utensils will speed up the oxidization. Also, the longer the food is cooked and the higher the temperature, the greater the vitamin loss. Large amounts of water used in cooking will wash out the vitamin.

Supplements can be taken, although the body tends to eliminate any surplus of the vitamin, so supplements of more than 100 mg a day are unnecessary. In fact, megadoses of the vitamin can cause nausea, abdominal cramps, and diarrhea, among other undesirable side effects.

OTHER ADVICE: Corticosteroids should always be taken with meals or milk since they can cause upset stomach.

These drugs raise blood cholesterol and triglyceride levels, increasing the risk of heart disease.

There is also some risk of dehydration, so make sure you drink about 8 glasses of fluid per day. You need at least 4 a day under normal circumstances to rid your system of the waste products that build up in the body, but the additional 4 glasses will make it easier for your body to carry out its day-to-day functions. In general, people tend not to drink enough fluids, which makes them tired and less strong, and taxes the kidneys.

Corticosteroids stimulate the appetite in some people, so you should watch your weight carefully to avoid unwanted weight gain.

CYCLOBENZAPRINE HYDRO-CHLORIDE

DRUG FAMILY: Anti-spasmodic

BRAND NAME: Flexeril

HOW TO TAKE CYCLOBENZAPRINE HYDROCHLORIDE: With meals or milk

FOODS TO AVOID: All alcoholic beverages

POSSIBLE SIDE EFFECTS: Gastrointestinal disturbances

ACTION OF CYCLOBENZAPRINE HYDROCHLORIDE: This drug relieves muscle spasms associated with the acute musculoskeletal pains characteristic of such conditions as osteoarthritis. This drug is only effective for periods of 2 to 3 weeks.

HIGH-RISK GROUPS: Anyone who consumes alcohol, people with a history of gastrointestinal distress

NUTRITIONAL INTERACTIONS

GASTROINTESTINAL DISTRESS: Cyclobenzaprine hydrochloride is likely to cause you gastrointestinal disturbances.

Prevention and Treatment: This drug should be taken at mealtimes or with milk, to avoid gastric disturbances.

ALCOHOL INTERACTION: Consumption of alcohol exacerbates the side effects of the drug, including drowsiness and blurred vision.

Prevention and Treatment: Alcohol should not be taken concurrently with this drug.

CYCLOPHOSPHAMIDE

DRUG FAMILY: Anti-cancer

BRAND NAMES: Cytoxan; Neosar

HOW TO TAKE CYCLOPHOSPHAMIDE: Injection

FOODS TO AVOID: None

POSSIBLE SIDE EFFECTS: Sodium deficiency, impaired taste, nausea, vomiting, mouth sores, poor appetite

ACTION OF CYCLOPHOSPHAMIDE: This drug is prescribed to prevent cancer cells from proliferating.

HIGH-RISK GROUPS: Anyone who takes this drug

NUTRITIONAL INTERACTIONS

SODIUM DEFICIENCY: Cyclophosphamide causes a loss of body sodium and may lead to hyponatremia, a sodium deficiency. Common symptoms of hyponatremia (abnormally low blood levels of sodium) include loss of appetite, nausea, vomiting, and muscle weakness. Hyponatremia can eventually lead to depression of the senses and grand mal seizures.

Prevention and Treatment: Hyponatremia requires stopping this drug therapy.

GASTROINTESTINAL DISTRESS: Cyclophosphamide causes impaired taste, nausea, vomiting, mouth sores, and anorexia.

Prevention and Treatment: Nausea and vomiting may be controlled by taking several basic steps. First, you should eat smaller meals and limit your intake of high-fat foods. Second, when you experience nausea, you should slowly sip clear beverages like ginger ale. Sucking a Popsicle may also alleviate the condition. You should lie down, loosen your clothes, and get fresh air as well.

If you find that you vomit frequently, you should take plenty of liquids to prevent dehydration.

CYCLOSERINE

DRUG FAMILY: Anti-tubercular

BRAND NAME: Seromycin

HOW TO MAKE CYCLOSERINE: As directed by your physician

FOODS TO AVOID: All alcoholic beverages

POSSIBLE SIDE EFFECTS: Deficiencies of vitamins B_6, B_{12}, and K, and of folic acid, magnesium, and calcium

ACTION OF CYCLOSERINE: This drug is used to treat tuberculosis.

HIGH-RISK GROUPS: Heavy drinkers, vegetarians, oral contraceptive users, the elderly, smokers

NUTRITIONAL INTERACTIONS

VITAMIN B_{12} DEFICIENCY: Cycloserine impairs the absorption of vitamin B_{12}, but usually not sufficiently to cause deficiencies in most people. However, vegetarians who take no animal products (including milk and eggs), and who are normally in a marginal vitamin B_{12} status, could be at risk for a deficiency of this vitamin. Some elderly people also tend to absorb vitamin B_{12} inefficiently, as do heavy drinkers, while smokers often have lower body levels of this vitamin.

Vitamin B_{12} is needed for the normal development of red blood cells and for the healthy functioning of all cells, in particular those of the bone marrow, nervous system, and intestines. The most common result of a B_{12} deficiency is pernicious anemia, which is characterized by listlessness, fatigue (especially following such physical exertion as climbing a flight of stairs), numbness and tingling in the fingers and toes, palpitations, angina, light-headedness, and a pale complexion.

Prevention and Treatment: A balanced diet containing plenty of vitamin B_{12} sources is advised. Only animal products, including dairy foods and fish and shellfish, contain natural vitamin B_{12}. However, some vegetable products are supplemented with the vitamin; many soy products, for example, are enriched with vitamin B_{12} to safeguard vegetarians. (See table for Vitamin B_{12}-Rich Foods, page 312.)

Vitamin B_{12} is stored in the liver, so one meal that includes a B_{12}-rich source such as calf's liver will normally fulfill your body's need for this vitamin for 2 to 3 weeks. (One 3-ounce serving of calf's liver contains 100 mcg of vitamin B_{12}.) If none of these products figures prominently in your diet, you should take a 6 mcg supplement each day while taking cycloserine.

MAGNESIUM DEFICIENCY: Cycloserine decreases magnesium absorption. Heavy drinkers, who excrete large amounts of magnesium, could become magnesium deficient, even though these mineral deficiencies are uncommon, because the average American diet contains appreciable amounts of the mineral.

Clinical signs of magnesium deficiency include muscle weakness, tremors, depression, emotional instability, and irrational behavior.

Prevention and Treatment: A diet containing the four food groups provides the normal amount of magnesium. However, if a magnesium depletion is suspected, your diet should feature foods such as nuts (almonds and cashews are highest), meat, fish, milk, whole grains, and fresh greens, since cooking can wash away some magnesium. (See table of Magnesium-Rich Foods, page 300.)

CALCIUM DEFICIENCY: This drug could also lead to deficiencies of calcium, folic acid, vitamins B_6 and K, though these deficiencies are quite unlikely.

In the case of calcium, any shortage of it that results from taking cycloserine is not likely to be severe enough to cause osteomalacia, a disease in which the bones are weakened.

Prevention and Treatment: Nevertheless, the consumption of foods rich in calcium, particularly milk and dairy products (including yogurt and hard cheeses) is recommended. (See table of Calcium-Rich Foods, page 289.)

If calcium foods are to be avoided because of an intolerance to lactose, the sugar present in dairy products, a 1,000 mg daily supplement of calcium should be taken, 500 mg before bedtime and 500 mg at midmorning.

FOLIC ACID DEFICIENCY: Cycloserine impairs the body's use of folacin and can cause a deficiency of this vitamin. The first sign of a folacin deficiency is inflamed or bleeding gums. The symptoms that follow are a sore, smooth tongue; diarrhea; forgetfulness; apathy; irritability; anemia; and a reduced resistance to infection. This is the most common vitamin deficiency in the United States.

Folacin is essential to the synthesis of new cells, so a deficiency in pregnant women may result in birth defects.

Prevention and Treatment: To avoid this deficiency, your diet should contain liver, yeast, and leafy vegetables such as spinach, kale, parsley, cauliflower, brussels sprouts, and broccoli. The fruits that are highest in folic acid are oranges and cantaloupes. To a lesser degree, folacin is found in almonds and lima beans, corn, parsnips, green peas, pumpkins, sweet potatoes, bran, peanuts, rye, and whole grain wheat. (See table of Folacin-Rich Foods, page 297.)

VITAMIN B$_6$ DEFICIENCY: Cycloserine is an antagonist of vitamin B$_6$; therefore, users of this drug may experience a vitamin B$_6$ deficiency. Symptoms of this deficiency are a sore mouth and tongue, cracks in the lips and corners of the mouth, and patches of itching, scaling skin. A severe vitamin B$_6$ deficiency may cause depression and confusion.

Vitamin B$_6$ deficiencies are common among the elderly. Alcoholics, as well, often experience this deficiency, since alcohol interferes with the body's ability to use B$_6$. It is estimated that one of every two Americans consumes less than 70 percent of the Recommended Dietary Allowance of B$_6$.

Prevention and Treatment: To avoid a B$_6$ deficiency, you should consume a diet featuring food sources of vitamin B$_6$ such as liver (beef, calf, and pork), herring, salmon, walnuts, peanuts, wheat germ, carrots, peas, potatoes, grapes, bananas, and yeast. (See table of Vitamin B$_6$(Pyridoxine)-Rich Foods, page 311.) The vitamin is present in significant amounts in meats, fish, fruits, cereals, and vegetables, and to a lesser extent in milk and other dairy products. Since vitamin B$_6$ is decomposed at high temperatures, modern food processing often diminishes dietary sources of the vitamin.

It has been observed that 15 to 20 percent of oral contraceptive users show direct evidence of vitamin B$_6$ deficiency. If you are among these people, you should take a 5 mg supplement of vitamin B$_6$ per day.

VITAMIN K DEFICIENCY: Since cycloserine also kills many of the bacteria in the large intestine that make vitamin K, a deficiency of this vitamin is also possible.

Prevention and Treatment: As long as dietary sources are consumed, this should not be a problem. Good sources are green, leafy vegetables, cabbage, and milk. (See table of Vitamin K-Rich Foods, page 315.)

SPECIAL WARNING: Concurrent alcohol consumption can lead to seizures. Consequently, while you are taking cycloserine, you should never drink alcohol.

CYPROHEPTADINE

DRUG FAMILY: Antihistamine and anti-serotonin

BRAND NAME: Periactin

HOW TO TAKE CYPROHEPTADINE: Directly after meals

FOODS TO AVOID: All alcoholic beverages

POSSIBLE SIDE EFFECTS: Nausea, vomiting, diarrhea, and constipation; increased appetite and weight gain

ACTION OF CYPROHEPTADINE: This drug is used in the treatment of hay fever and the skin reactions associated with seasonal and food allergies, such as itching, hives, and rashes. Cyproheptadine blocks the action of the excessive histamine released by the eyes, nose, and skin as a response to the allergy.

As an anti-serotonin drug, it slows down the rate of contraction of the muscles lining the intestine, so it is used in patients after stomach surgery, in patients with cancer, and sometimes in the treatment of asthma in children.

HIGH-RISK GROUPS: Heavy drinkers, children

NUTRITIONAL INTERACTIONS

GASTROINTESTINAL DISTURBANCES: This drug can cause stomach upset, nausea, vomiting, diarrhea, and constipation.

Prevention and Treatment: The drug should be taken after meals to reduce the gastrointestinal discomfort. If constipation is experienced, plenty of dietary fiber should be included in the diet: fruit, vegetables, and whole-grain cereal products. (See table of Dietary Fiber-Rich Foods, page 293.) Bran is also a good source of fiber, but must be accompanied by ¾ cup fluid per teaspoon if it is to be effective.

OTHER ADVICE: This drug improves appetite and can cause significant weight gain in anyone who takes it. Alcohol should be consumed only with extreme caution by users of cyproheptadine, since it increases drowsiness and lack of coordination, and makes tasks like driving extremely dangerous.

DACTINOMYCIN

DRUG FAMILY: Anti-cancer

BRAND NAME: Cosmegen

HOW TO TAKE DACTINOMYCIN: Injection

FOODS TO AVOID: Limit the intake of fatty foods

POSSIBLE SIDE EFFECTS: Reduced appetite, nausea, vomiting, and diarrhea

ACTION OF DACTINOMYCIN: This anti-neoplastic agent prevents the cancer cells from replicating, and hence the tumor is prevented from growing.

HIGH-RISK GROUPS: Anyone who takes this drug

NUTRITIONAL INTERACTIONS

GASTROINTESTINAL DISTURBANCE: Dactinomycin causes reduced appetite and gastrointestinal disturbances. Since it impairs the ability of the body to build new tissue, the membranes lining the gastrointestinal tract, which are normally replaced every three days, will become worn and sore, as will your lips and tongue. The malabsorption of several vitamins, and such minerals as iron and calcium, will result.

Prevention and Treatment: This drug is only taken for periods of 5 days, so the long-term effects of calcium and iron malabsorption (namely, osteoporosis and anemia, respectively) should not result directly from its use. However, users of this drug would do well to take a nutrient supplement throughout the whole period that the drug is being given. The drug is usually taken for periods of 5 days' duration at 2- to 4-week intervals. The supplement should be taken during rest periods also. The supplement should contain Recommended Dietary Allowances for calcium, iron and all the vitamins, to reduce any risk of nutritional deficiencies. (See tables of Vitamin and Mineral Supplements, page 321, and Recommended Dietary Allowances, page 317.)

Any nausea and vomiting resulting from the use of this drug may be controlled by taking several basic steps. First, you should eat smaller meals and limit your intake of high-fat foods. Second, when you experience nausea, you should slowly sip clear beverages like ginger ale. Sucking a Popsicle may also alleviate the condition. You should loosen your clothes and lie down near an open window so that you can get as much fresh air as possible.

If you find that you vomit frequently, you should take plenty of liquids to prevent dehydration.

DAUNORUBICIN HYDROCHLORIDE

DRUG FAMILY: Anti-leukemia

BRAND NAME: Cerubidine

HOW TO TAKE DAUNORUBICIN HYDROCHLORIDE: Injection

FOODS TO AVOID: None

POSSIBLE SIDE EFFECTS: Riboflavin deficiency

ACTION OF DAUNORUBICIN HYDROCHLORIDE: This potent anti-cancer drug is used in the treatment of leukemia.

HIGH-RISK GROUPS: Anyone who takes this drug

NUTRITIONAL INTERACTIONS

RIBOFLAVIN DEFICIENCY: Daunorubicin impairs the conversion of riboflavin to its active form; thus, the drug is likely to cause a riboflavin deficiency. This may lead to heart failure in severe cases.

The symptoms most likely to appear will be a dry skin around the nose and lips, a cracking in the corners of the mouth, and a soreness or burning sensation in the lips, mouth, or tongue. Discomfort in eating and swallowing may result. The eyes may burn, itch, be more sensitive than usual to light, and tend to be bloodshot. However, be aware that any B vitamin deficiency can cause similar symptoms.

Riboflavin helps the body transform protein, fats, and carbohydrates into the energy needed to maintain body tissues and to protect the body against common skin and eye disorders.

Prevention and Treatment: Good sources of riboflavin should be included in the diet. Milk usually contributes about 50 percent of our riboflavin intake, meat about 25 percent, and dark green leafy vegetables and enriched cereals and breads the rest. The need for riboflavin provides a major reason for including milk in some form in every day's meals; no other food that is commonly eaten can make such a substantial contribution to meeting our daily riboflavin needs. People who don't use milk products can substitute a generous serving of dark green leafy vegetables, because a cup of greens such as collards provides about the same amount of riboflavin as a cup of milk. (See table of Vitamin B_2(Riboflavin)-Rich Foods, page 310.)

Among the meats, liver is the richest source, but all lean meats, as well as eggs, can provide some riboflavin. Riboflavin is light-sensitive; it can be destroyed by the ultraviolet rays of the sun or fluorescent lamps. For this reason, milk is seldom sold, and should not be stored, in transparent glass containers. Cardboard or plastic containers protect the riboflavin in the milk from ultraviolet rays.

Note that riboflavin supplements in excess of the Recommended Dietary Allowance may make the drug less effective and should not be taken.

DEXBROMPHENIRAMINE MALEATE

DRUG FAMILY: Antihistamine

BRAND NAMES: Drixoral; Disobrom

HOW TO TAKE DEXBROMPHENIRAMINE MALEATE: With meals

FOODS TO AVOID: All alcoholic beverages; alkaline foods such as milk, buttermilk, cream, almonds, chestnuts, coconuts, all vegetables except corn and lentils, and all fruits except cranberries, prunes, and plums should be taken in moderation.

POSSIBLE SIDE EFFECTS: Loss of appetite, nausea, vomiting, stomach cramps, constipation, diarrhea, increased urination, dryness of the mouth, weight loss

ACTION OF DEXBROMPHENIRAMINE MALEATE: This antihistamine is used in the treatment of seasonal allergies and motion sickness.

HIGH-RISK GROUPS: People with a history of abdominal distress, anyone who consumes alcohol

NUTRITIONAL INTERACTIONS

GASTROINTESTINAL DISTRESS: One likely side effect of this drug is gastrointestinal distress, which may include a loss of appetite, nausea, vomiting, stomach cramps, constipation, diarrhea, increased urination, and dryness of the mouth.

Prevention and Treatment: This drug should be taken with meals to avoid the gastric symptoms. To prevent dehydration due to excess urination, at least 6 to 8 glasses of water or its equivalent in other non-alcoholic fluids should be consumed per day.

Body weight should also be monitored to avoid unwanted weight loss.

ALKALINE URINE: Because dexbrompheniramine maleate is alkaline, it is excreted at a normal rate only if your urine is acidic. However, if the quantity of alkaline foods in your diet is high, your urine will lose its acidity, and the excretion of this drug will be slowed. A hazardous buildup could conceivably result, leading to drowsiness, lack of coordination, vertigo, dizziness, headache, insomnia, anxiety, tension, weakness, and palpitations.

Prevention and Treatment: Fruits, vegetables, and dairy products tend to be alkaline, and high-protein foods tend to be acidic. Foods causing the production of alkaline urine include milk, buttermilk, cream, almonds, chestnuts, coconuts, all vegetables except corn and lentils, and all fruits except cranberries, prunes, and plums.

Antacids that neutralize the acid in the stomach will also neutralize the acid in the urine, causing it to turn alkaline. Therefore, you should avoid antacids when taking this drug.

ALCOHOL INTERACTION: Alcohol is likely to heighten the chance of a loss of coordination. Dizziness, lassitude, uncoordination, fatigue, blurred vision, nervousness, and insomnia, as well as an exacerbation of the gastric effects, may result.

Alcohol in any form should not be consumed concurrently with the drug.

DIAZOXIDE

DRUG FAMILY: Anti-hypertensive (used as injection); anti-hypoglycemic (as capsule)

BRAND NAMES: Hyperstat; Proglycem

HOW TO TAKE DIAZOXIDE: With meals or milk

FOODS TO AVOID: Sodium-rich foods, such as anchovies, dill pickles, sardines, green olives, canned soups and vegetables, TV dinners, soy sauce, processed cheeses, salty snack foods, cold cuts, and catsup; foods rich in purines, such as sweetbreads, anchovies, corn, lentils, cranberries, prunes, plums, sardines, and large amounts of meat and fish; coffee, strong tea, chocolate, and cola beverages

POSSIBLE SIDE EFFECTS: Edema; hyperglycemia; gastrointestinal distress; gout

ACTION OF DIAZOXIDE: In hospitals, Hyperstat is used as an injection to reduce blood pressure in times of a hypertensive emergency (when a patient's blood pressure suddenly shoots up to life-threatening levels). The drug relaxes the muscles in the blood vessels, causing them to dilate and the blood pressure to go down.

Used in the form of orally administered Proglycem capsules, diazoxide inhibits the release of insulin by the pancreas and so elevates blood glucose levels.

HIGH-RISK GROUPS: Heart patients, the elderly, people with a history of gout, kidney patients

NUTRITIONAL INTERACTIONS

EDEMA: Use of diazoxide leads to water and sodium retention, which could conceivably cause swelling (called edema) in your legs, ankles, feet, and breasts, and around your eyes. A diet high in sodium will make the condition more likely to occur.

Prevention and Treatment: While you are taking this drug, you should restrict your consumption of sodium. In particular, those foods listed in the table of Sodium-Rich Foods (see page 306) should be avoided, or consumed in small quantities. You should not add salt at the table or in cooking.

Many people are unaware of how much sodium their diet contains. Each teaspoon of salt in the diet contains 2 grams of sodium. The average American, in fact, consumes some 15 pounds of salt a year, or 3 to 4 teaspoons per day. Even if you do not salt your food while preparing or eating it, you consume quantities of salt in such foods as anchovies, dill pickles, sardines, green olives, canned soups and vegetables, so-called TV dinners, soy sauce, processed cheeses, many snack foods, cold cuts, and catsup.

To sharpen your awareness of the sodium content of food products, read the list of ingredients that appears on the label of all packaged foods. Sodium can be present in a food as either common salt or sodium chloride, or as any other sodium-containing compound, monosodium glutamate being a common one. If salt (or its equivalent) appears as one of the first ingredients on the label, then the product contains a significant amount of sodium. If, on the other hand, it appears very near the end of the list (as in bread), then it need not be a concern.

HYPERGLYCEMIA: An abnormally high blood glucose level, called hyperglycemia, may occur in users of diazoxide. It is unlikely in most patients, but the chances are greater in people with severe kidney disease.

Prevention and Treatment: Symptoms of high blood glucose levels are headaches, excessive hunger and thirst, and a need to urinate frequently. If this happens, you should seek the help of your physician immediately.

GASTROINTESTINAL DISTRESS: This drug is likely to lead to gastrointestinal distress, so Proglycem should be taken with meals or milk.

OTHER ADVICE: Use of diazoxide leads to the retention of uric acid, which can form deposits in the joints and cause gout, an interaction that has been reported in some patients. Nevertheless, it is highly unlikely. Gout is an arthritislike disease that affects single joints, often the big toe, in painful episodes that last only a few days but are likely to recur. Middle-aged men are most often afflicted.

While you are taking this drug, you should avoid high intakes of rich sources of purines, which are broken down into uric acid in your body. Such foods include sweetbreads, anchovies, corn, lentils, cranberries, prunes, plums, sardines, meat, and fish. Also avoid caffeine-containing beverages, which increase the retention of uric acid. (See table of Purine-Rich Foods, page 303.)

DICUMAROL

DRUG FAMILY: Anti-coagulant

HOW TO TAKE DICUMAROL: With milk or meals

FOODS TO AVOID: Excess amounts of vitamin K-rich foods, such as cabbage, broccoli, asparagus, spinach, and turnip greens

POSSIBLE SIDE EFFECTS: Vitamin K deficiency; gastrointestinal disturbances

ACTION OF DICUMAROL: Commonly referred to as a blood thinner, dicumarol decreases the rate at which blood clots. Dicumarol is taken by arteriosclerosis patients, whose blood tends to clot more readily than normal. Clotting can lead to the blockage of blood vessels, and if this happens in the brain or heart, a stroke or heart attack will occur.

HIGH-RISK GROUPS: The elderly; heavy drinkers

NUTRITIONAL INTERACTIONS

VITAMIN K DEFICIENCY: An improper balance of anti-coagulants and vitamin K in the body is likely to cause interrelated problems. These drugs can prevent vitamin K from producing blood-clotting substances in the liver, but a diet that features excess amounts of vitamin K-rich foods can actually reduce the effectiveness of the drug.

People with an abnormally low dietary intake of vitamin K are at risk of hemorrhaging with unusual ease if they use this drug. Bleeding may take place in the gastrointestinal tract (causing black or blood-stained stools), in the urinary tract (causing blood in the urine), and in the uterus (causing blood loss at times other than the normal menstrual periods). Excessive blood loss may occur from an injury or surgery. Another sign of a deficiency of this vitamin is more frequent and more visible bruising than normal.

Women who have had several pregnancies or whose menstrual periods are heavy are at high risk for a vitamin K deficiency. Many of the elderly should also be careful because they have a problem of poor fat absorption, and vitamin K, a fat-soluble vitamin, must be accompanied by sufficient dietary fat to be properly absorbed.

Prevention and Treatment: You should not consume large amounts of foods rich in vitamin K. In particular, you should avoid eating large quantities of such foods as kale, spinach, cabbage, cauliflower, leafy green vegetables, and liver (especially pork liver). However, one should not go to the other extreme and risk a hemorrhage by cutting out all such foods. Moderation is the key here.

Vitamin E supplements should not be taken along with dicumarol, since vitamin E impairs vitamin K absorption and may cause bleeding. Nor should a dicumarol user take vitamin K supplements, which make the drug less effective. Do not drink alcohol concurrently with this medication. Alcohol and drugs are broken down in the liver by the same mechanism. If there is a high level of alcohol present, less of the drug is broken down. Hence, higher levels of this anti-coagulant build up in the body and can be extremely dangerous.

OTHER ADVICE: The antacid magnesium hydroxide speeds up the absorption of dicumarol, so its use should be discontinued and another antacid substituted while you are on dicumarol. However, your physician may have taken this factor into account when the appropriate dosage was decided on, so follow your doctor's specific directions.

Dicumarol has a tendency to cause gastrointestinal disturbances and should be taken with milk or meals.

DICYCLOMINE

DRUG FAMILY: Anti-spasmodic; anti-muscarinic

BRAND NAME: Bentyl

HOW TO TAKE DICYCLOMINE: One-half hour to 1 hour before eating

FOODS TO AVOID: None

POSSIBLE SIDE EFFECTS: Constipation

ACTION OF DICYCLOMINE: This drug is used in the treatment of infant colic and irritable bowel syndrome in adults. It prevents violent contractions in the muscles of the gastrointestinal tract, which can cause extreme pain.

HIGH-RISK GROUPS: The elderly

NUTRITIONAL INTERACTIONS

CONSTIPATION: Dicyclomine could conceivably cause you to become constipated.

Prevention and Treatment: Constipation is usually safely remedied in adults by an increase in the bulk in the diet. This means consuming larger servings of any of the following: dried or fresh fruits, salad vegetables, radishes, oatmeal, and whole grain foods (brown rice, whole wheat breads, and cereals). It is not necessary to purchase products that claim "extra fiber" has been added to them.

Constipation that persists may also be relieved by doubling the amount of fluid consumed each day. If you use bran, it should be added to the diet gradually, and fluid should be increased by at least ¾ cup per teaspoon of bran. (See table of Dietary Fiber-Rich Foods, page 293.)

Do not attempt to treat constipation in a young child without consulting your doctor, since great harm can be done to the child.

DIETHYLPROPION HYDROCHLORIDE

DRUG FAMILY: Appetite suppressants

BRAND NAMES: Tenuate Dospan; Tenuate; Tepanil

HOW TO TAKE DIETHYLPROPION HYDROCHLORIDE: One hour before meals

FOODS TO AVOID: None

POSSIBLE SIDE EFFECTS: Constipation

ACTION OF DIETHYLPROPION HYDROCHLORIDE: This appetite suppressant is used as a short-term adjunct to a treatment program for obesity. This drug tends to be addictive.

HIGH-RISK GROUPS: The elderly

NUTRITIONAL INTERACTIONS

CONSTIPATION: Diethylpropion hydrochloride could conceivably cause you to become constipated.

PREVENTION AND TREATMENT: Usually a safe remedy for constipation is an increase in the bulk in the diet. This means consuming larger servings of any of the following: dried or fresh fruits (especially unpeeled apples or pears), salad vegetables (especially unpeeled carrots), radishes, oatmeal, and whole grain foods (brown rice, whole wheat breads, and cereals). It is not necessary to purchase products that claim "extra fiber" has been added to them.

Constipation that persists may also be relieved by doubling the amount of fluid consumed each day. Bran, if used, should be added to the diet gradually, and fluid should be increased by at least ¾ cup per teaspoon of bran. (See table of Dietary Fiber-Rich Foods, page 293.)

DIGITALIS PREPARATIONS

DRUG FAMILY: Heart drugs

BRAND NAMES: [GENERIC/Brand] DIGITALIS GLYCOSIDE/Crystodigin; DIGOXIN/Lanoxicaps; Lanoxin

HOW TO TAKE DIGITALIS PREPARATIONS: Between meals, with nonalcholic beverages other than milk

FOODS TO AVOID: Alcoholic beverages; very sweet foods such as candy, cookies, and cake

POSSIBLE SIDE EFFECTS: Vitamin B_1 and zinc deficiencies; gastrointestinal distress

ACTION OF DIGITALIS: These drugs are taken by patients who suffer from cardiac insufficiency—that is, their hearts do not pump blood at an adequate rate. The drugs increase the force with which the heart pumps.

HIGH-RISK GROUPS: People taking diuretics, anyone who consumes alcohol, the elderly, vegetarians

NUTRITIONAL INTERACTIONS

POTASSIUM AND MAGNESIUM DEFICIENCIES: Digoxin is the seventh most frequently prescribed drug in the United States, which is not surprising given the fact that heart disease is the most common serious health ailment in this country.

The prevalence of heart disease leads to the widespread and prolonged use not only of digitalis preparations but also of diuretics. Diuretics lead to a loss of body potassium and magnesium. Alcohol use also leads to the loss of magnesium. The result of a combined intake of alcohol and diuretics could conceivably be deficiencies of magnesium or potassium. Deficiencies of either of these minerals tend to cause the heart muscle to take up excess digitalis, which in turn causes the heart to beat irregularly.

Prevention and Treatment: To prevent this from happening, digitalis users should make sure that they consume adequate quantities of these minerals. Potassium depletion can be avoided by including such potassium-rich foods in the diet as tomato juice, lentils, dried apricots, asparagus, bananas, peanut butter, chicken, almonds, and milk. (See table of Potassium-Rich Foods, page 302.)

Potassium supplements should never be taken unless prescribed by a physician. They can cause anemia by interfering with the absorption of vitamin B_{12}. Just a few grams can also drastically increase the risk of heart failure. If you experience difficulty in swallowing while taking potassium supplements, consult your physician immediately. If supplements are prescribed, be aware that the absorption of the supplements potassium iodide and potassium chloride is decreased by dairy products, and that both are gastric irritants and should be taken with meals.

Too much salt in your diet can also compromise your body's supply of potassium.

In the case of magnesium, a diet containing the four food groups provides the normal amount of magnesium. However, if a magnesium depletion is suspected, your diet should feature foods such as nuts (almonds and cashews are highest), meat, fish, milk, whole grains, and fresh greens, since cooking can wash away some magnesium. (See table of Magnesium-Rich Foods, page 300.) Alcohol provokes magnesium excretion, so its intake should be severely restricted when taking this drug.

VITAMIN B_1 DEFICIENCY: Digitalis users need an increased amount of vitamin B_1 (thiamin), so a B_1 deficiency is conceivable. Vitamin B_1 is essential to the body's ability to metabolize carbohydrates, to muscle coordination, and to healthy nerves.

When vitamin B_1 is in short supply in your body, heart palpitations may result, along with mental confusion, moodiness, and tiredness. Other symptoms of a B_1 deficiency are difficulty in walking, weight loss, and water retention, especially at the ankles. Heavy consumers of alcohol tend to be deficient in this vitamin and therefore are at higher risk. Antacids taken at meals destroy dietary thiamin and can contribute to this deficiency.

Older Americans are also frequently found to be marginally deficient in this vitamin. A severe deficiency in this age group can be the cause of symptoms resembling senility, which is reversible when the supply of B_1 is replenished. This vitamin is also said to stimulate appetite.

Prevention and Treatment: To avoid a thiamin deficiency, at least 3 mg of the vitamin should be included in your daily diet. This means including rich dietary sources, such as whole grain cereals, oatmeal, nuts, peas, lima beans, oysters, liver, pork (especially ham), beef, lamb, poultry, and eggs. (See table of Vitamin-B_1(Thiamin)-Rich Foods, page 309.)

The presence of baking soda in cooking will destroy vitamin B_1, so it should be avoided when possible. High temperatures too are very destructive to B_1. Blackberries, brussels sprouts, beets, red cabbage, and spinach contain the enzyme thiaminase, which inactivates the vitamin. Large quantities of these foods should not be consumed raw. The consumption of chocolate should be avoided by digitalis users, since it will have the same effect.

GASTROINTESTINAL DISTRESS: Some of the digitalis glycosides damage the wall of the stomach. These drugs also decrease your ability to absorb sugar by as much as 50 percent; consequently, a high-sugar diet is likely to lead to diarrhea and the loss of essential minerals and vitamins.

Prevention and Treatment: Although digitalis preparations are more rapidly absorbed on an empty stomach, they should be taken with food if you experience severe gastrointestinal disturbances. These drugs should not, however, be taken with milk. Restrict sweet foods in your diet, such as candy, cookies, cake, honey, and table sugar.

ZINC DEFICIENCY: Digitalis increases the rate of zinc excretion and could conceivably lead to a zinc deficiency. A shortage of zinc in your system may result in impaired healing of wounds and ulcers, scaly dermatitis of the face and limbs, and anorexia associated with the loss of taste.

Prevention and Treatment: Patients using this drug should be sure to get the Recommended Dietary Allowance of zinc. Animal foods are good sources, with the richest being oysters, herring, milk, and egg yolks. Among plant foods, whole grains are richest in zinc, but it is not as well absorbed from them as from meat. Fiber and phytic acid in the cereal grains hinder its absorption. The recommended intake of 15 mg a day for adults is usually met easily by the diet of the average middle-class person, but deficiencies are more likely if animal protein is underemphasized. As a rule of thumb, two small servings of animal protein a day will provide sufficient zinc.

OTHER ADVICE: Anybody who takes calcium supplements, or whose diet contains many calcium-rich foods, may suffer from digitalis toxicity, which is evidenced by an irregular heart rhythm, gastrointestinal disturbances, headache, drowsiness, and blurred vision.

Cholestyramine, a drug taken to lower blood fat levels, interferes with the absorption of digitalis, and so cholestyramine should be used at least 1 to 2 hours after the digitalis.

DIHYDROCODEINE

DRUG FAMILY: Analgesic

BRAND NAMES: Synalgos-DC; Compal

HOW TO TAKE DIHYDROCODEINE: With meals or milk

FOODS TO AVOID: Alcoholic beverages

POSSIBLE SIDE EFFECTS: Constipation; nausea

ACTION OF DIHYDROCODEINE: This analgesic is prescribed to relieve moderate to moderately severe pain. It also acts as a mild sedative and is addictive.

HIGH-RISK GROUPS: The elderly, anyone who consumes alcohol

NUTRITIONAL INTERACTIONS

GASTROINTESTINAL DISTRESS: Dihydrocodeine could conceivably cause you to experience nausea and constipation.

Prevention and Treatment: In order to minimize the gastrointestinal distress that this drug can cause, it should be taken with meals or milk.

Constipation is usually safely remedied by an increase in the bulk in the diet. This means consuming larger servings of any of the following: dried or fresh fruits (especially unpeeled apples or pears), salad vegetables, radishes, oatmeal, and whole grain foods (brown rice, whole wheat breads, and cereals). It is not necessary to purchase products that claim "extra fiber" has been added to them.

Constipation may also be relieved by doubling the amount of fluid consumed each day. Bran, if used, should be added to the diet gradually, and fluid should be increased by at least ¾ cup per teaspoon of bran. (See table of Dietary Fiber-Rich Foods, page 293.)

ALCOHOL INTERACTION: Alcohol further depresses the central nervous system, and exacerbates the adverse side effects of drowsiness and dizziness associated with dihydrocodeine use. It also increases irritation to the gastrointestinal tract.

Prevention and Treatment: Alcohol should never be taken concurrently with this drug.

DIHYDROMORPHINONE OR HYDRO-MORPHONE HYDROCHLORIDE

DRUG FAMILY: Analgesic

BRAND NAME: Dilaudid

HOW TO TAKE HYDROMORPHONE HYDROCHLORIDE: As directed by your physician

FOODS TO AVOID: None

POSSIBLE SIDE EFFECTS: Constipation

ACTION OF HYDROMORPHONE HYDROCHLORIDE: This drug relieves moderate to severe pain especially in patients with cancer and following surgery of any kind. Hydromorphone hydrochloride is also in syrups used to control persistent coughs.

HIGH-RISK GROUPS: Anyone who takes this drug

NUTRITIONAL INTERACTIONS

CONSTIPATION: Long-term use of this drug could conceivably cause you to become constipated.

Prevention and Treatment: Constipation is usually safely remedied by an increase in the bulk in the diet. This means consuming larger servings of any of the following: dried or fresh fruits, salad vegetables, radishes, oatmeal, and whole grain foods (brown rice, whole wheat breads, and cereals). It is not necessary to purchase products that claim "extra fiber" has been added to them.

Persistent constipation may also be relieved by doubling the amount of fluid consumed each day. Bran, if used, should be added to the diet gradually, and fluid should be increased by at least ¾ cup per teaspoon of bran. (See table of Dietary Fiber-Rich Foods, page 293.)

DIOCTYL SODIUM SULFOSUCCINATE

DRUG FAMILY: Laxative

BRAND NAMES: Bilax; Colace; Disonate; Docusate Sodium; Ferro-Sequels; Geriplex-FS; Liqui-Doss; Materna 1.60; Modane Plus; Modane Soft; Neolax; Peri-Colace; Peritinic; Prenate 90; Senokot-S; Trilax

HOW TO TAKE DIOCTYL SODIUM SULFOSUCCINATE: In capsule or tablet form, this drug should be taken with meals. In liquid form, it should be mixed with half a glass of milk or fruit juice, to mask its bitter taste, and taken with or just after meals.

FOODS TO AVOID: None

POSSIBLE SIDE EFFECTS: Deficiencies of vitamins A and D if taken regularly; malabsorption of sodium and glucose

ACTION OF DIOCTYL SODIUM SULFOSUCCINATE: Although this drug is technically not a laxative, since it does not increase the rate at which the intestinal muscles contract, it is used to ensure easy and natural passage of the stool by softening it.

This drug is most often used in cases of constipation caused by hard stools. It decreases the absorption of water by the colon and thereby increases the quantity of water retained by the feces. The stools become softer and more bulky.

HIGH-RISK GROUPS: The elderly

NUTRITIONAL INTERACTIONS

VITAMIN AND MINERAL DEFICIENCIES: Dioctyl sodium sulfosuccinate will reduce your absorption of sodium and glucose but generally not to such levels that any symptoms will be apparent.

Prevention and Treatment: This drug should not be taken regularly except under the supervision of a physician. Furthermore, it should be accompanied by a daily vitamin supplement containing 500 to 1,000 IU of vitamin A per day and 400 to 800 IU of vitamin D.

MINERAL OIL INTERACTION: Dioctyl sodium sulfosuccinate may increase the absorption of mineral oil, as well as other fats and oils. In the case of mineral oil (a mixture of liquid hydrocarbons obtained from petroleum), there is cause for concern, because mineral oil is toxic to the system if absorbed—in large enough quantitites, it can increase your risk of cancer.

Prevention and Treatment: Dioctyl sodium sulfosuccinate should not be taken with mineral oil. If you are accustomed to taking mineral oil to soften the stool, this drug should substitute for it.

OTHER ADVICE: Dioctyl sodium sulfosuccinate can be taken with half a glass of milk or fruit juice, to mask its bitter taste.

DIPHENYLMETHANE CATHARTICS

DRUG FAMILY: Laxative

BRAND NAMES: [GENERIC/Brand] BISACODYL/Dulcolax; Evac-Q-Kwik; Fleet Bisacodyl; PHENOLPHTHALEIN/Agoral; Correctol Laxative; Evac-Q-Kit; Evac-U-Gen; Ex-Lax; Feen-A-Mint; Prulet; Trilax; Yellolax

HOW TO TAKE DIPHENYLMETHANE CATHARTICS: Swallow whole at bedtime without chewing or crushing, with a beverage that does not contain milk or milk products

FOODS TO AVOID: Do not take this drug within an hour of consuming milk or milk products or antacids

POSSIBLE SIDE EFFECTS: Deficiencies of potassium, calcium, and vitamin D

ACTION OF DIPHENYLMETHANE CATHARTICS: These laxatives function by increasing the action of the muscles lining the intestines and so reduce the time required for food to pass through the intestinal tract. They also cause a secretion of water into the large intestine and so increase the bulk of the stools. Oral doses take 6 to 8 hours to induce defecation.

HIGH-RISK GROUPS: Heart patients, the elderly

NUTRITIONAL INTERACTIONS

POTASSIUM DEFICIENCY: The frequent use of diphenylmethane cathartics could conceivably cause the malabsorption of a variety of nutrients by your body. The most crucial of these is potassium, since potassium regulates the amount of water in the cells of the body, and is essential for the proper functioning of the kidneys and the heart muscle, and the secretion of stomach juices. The most alarming symptom of a potassium deficiency is an irregular heartbeat, which can lead to heart failure.

This deficiency is especially likely if you also take any of the diuretics that cause potassium deficiencies.

People with a potassium deficiency may have such symptoms as weakness, loss of appetite, nausea, vomiting, dryness of the mouth, increased thirst, listlessness, apprehension, and diffuse pain that comes and goes.

Proper potassium levels in your body can also be threatened if diphenylmethane cathartics are taken concurrently with cortisone-containing drugs.

Prevention and Treatment: Potassium depletion can be avoided by including such potassium-rich foods in your diet as tomato juice, lentils, dried apricots, asparagus, bananas, peanut butter, chicken, almonds, and milk. (See table of Potassium-Rich Foods, page 302.)

Potassium supplements should never be taken unless prescribed by a physician. They can cause anemia by interfering with the absorption of vitamin B_{12}. Just a few grams can also drastically increase the risk of heart failure. If you experience difficulty in swallowing while taking potassium supplements, consult your physician immediately. If supplements are prescribed, be aware that the absorption of the supplements potassium iodide and potassium chloride is decreased by dairy products, and that both are gastric irritants and should be taken with meals.

Too much salt in your diet can also compromise your body's supply of potassium as can consuming large amounts daily (1 ounce or more) of licorice candy made from natural extract. Usually only imported licorice contains natural licorice extract; check the package.

VITAMIN D AND CALCIUM DEFICIENCY: The malabsorption of nutrients that results from the frequent use of these drugs also makes it conceivable that you will experience vitamin D and/or calcium deficiencies while taking these laxatives.

Vitamin D is needed for the body to absorb calcium and phosphorus, to promote the development of strong teeth and bones. Whenever calcium blood levels are low, which can result from a deficiency of either vitamin D or calcium itself, the body will liberate the calcium it needs from the bones, where it is stored. The bones thus become weakened, in severe cases so much so that they will fracture easily. Osteomalacia, as this condition is called, is more likely after middle age, since in older people the body uses dietary calcium less efficiently. Prominent symptoms are bone pain in the back, thighs, shoulder region, or ribs; difficulty in walking; and weakness in the muscles of the legs. Osteomalacia is reversible, however, once calcium blood levels are raised.

After prolonged periods of calcium deficiency, osteoporosis may develop. Osteoporosis is another condition where the bones are weakened and made brittle, but a much more serious one—an unexplained and rapid loss of calcium from the bones. Unlike osteomalacia, the effects of osteoporosis are irreversible. The common symptoms are backache, a gradual loss of height, and periodontal disease. Fractures of the vertebrae, hip, and wrist occur, sometimes spontaneously.

Approximately 7 percent of women fifty years of age and older have osteoporosis, and certain observers believe that the incidence of this disease is on the rise. Between 15 and 20 million Americans are said to have osteoporosis today. In some 30 percent of people over sixty-five, the disease is severe enough to result in fractures. By age eighty, virtually all women experience some degree of osteoporosis; early menopause is a strong predictor of the disease. One out of five cases of the disease is found in men, but generally men get it at a later age and less severely than women.

Prevention and Treatment: To avoid a vitamin D deficiency while you are on diphenylmethane, you should take 400 to 800 IU of vitamin D per day as a supplement to a diet of foods rich in vitamin D, such as fortified milk, butter, liver, egg yolks, salmon, tuna, and sardines. (See table of Vitamin D-Rich Foods, page 313.)

Vitamin D is initially formed in the skin on exposure to sunlight and activated in the liver and kidneys. The production of vitamin D is dependent upon climatic conditions, air pollution, skin pigmentation (the darker the skin, the lower the production), the area of skin exposed, the duration of exposure to the sun, and the use of sun screens. Adults who are not often exposed to sunlight (e.g. those who are housebound or are by custom heavily clothed), require dietary sources of vitamin D to prevent osteomalacia.

Vitamin D is indispensable to infants, children, and to pregnant or lactating women, whose requirements are high due to bone growth or skeletal mineral replacement. Supplementation for pregnant women is crucial since vitamin D deficiencies can cause fetal abnormalities. However, no more than 800 IU of the vitamin should be taken by pregnant women because excessive consumption can cause fetal kidney damage. In nonpregnant adults, 2,000 IU of the vitamin should be taken if osteomalacia is indicated. If your intake of vitamin D exceeds 4,000 IU per day, toxicity of vitamin D poisoning can occur. The symptoms are loss of appetite, headache, excessive thirst, emotional instability, and kidney stones.

In all of these cases, foods rich in calcium should be included in the diet, especially dairy products. (See table of Calcium-Rich Foods, page 289.) If these foods must be avoided, because of an intolerance of lactose, the sugar found in dairy products (some 30 million Americans have such a problem digesting dairy products), a 1,000 mg daily supplement of calcium should be taken. (See Calcium Supplement entry, page 51.)

The Recommended Dietary Allowance for calcium is 800 mg, and the latest evidence shows that all women should take in 1,200 mg of calcium per day. The average intake in the United States, however, is only 450 to 550 mg. For the elderly, and women who have already reached menopause or are about to, this should be increased to 1,500 mg by the consumption of foods rich in calcium, particularly milk and dairy products (including yogurt and hard cheeses) and, to a lesser extent, almonds. Three 8-ounce glasses of milk, for example, provide 1,500 mg of calcium. (See table of Calcium-Rich Foods, page 289.)

As most of the calcium lost from the body is leached from the bones at night, 500 mg of the supplement should be taken at bedtime. Calcium carbonate does have a tendency to cause constipation, so the supplements containing magnesium are to be preferred. Magnesium prevents the associated constipation and in small amounts improves calcium absorption.

Keep in mind that vitamin C assists calcium absorption, while cigarette smoking tends to reduce body calcium, as does excessive alcohol consumption. Diphenylmethane users should temporarily limit their consumption of foods that can decrease the absorption of calcium: kale, rhubarb, spinach, cocoa, chocolate, beet greens, tea, and caffeine. A deficiency might arise also if the ratio of phosphorus to calcium in your diet is very high; processed foods, especially carbonated beverages, are particularly high in phosphorus. The ideal ratio is 1 to 1, as in dairy products; when the ratio is 15 or 20 to 1, as in meat, very little calcium is absorbed. High-fiber foods may contribute to a calcium deficiency, since fiber binds to calcium and passes it out in the stool. Excess fat and protein in the diet also hinder absorption.

Since there is little calcium in strict vegetarian diets (those that avoid dairy products as well as meat), vegetarians are at greater risk of a calcium deficiency. People who take magnesium- or aluminum-based antacids are also more prone to calcium deficiencies, because both magnesium and aluminum in excess impair calcium absorption.

Besides a change in dietary habits and the use of calcium supplements, it is recommended that anyone at risk of this deficiency adopt an exercise regimen that causes the bones to support the weight of the body, to strengthen the bones and to counteract the loss of bone density. A regular walking or jogging program, for example, can help prevent the bone degeneration of the spine, hips, and legs. Note, however, that swimming, though good for the heart as an aerobic exercise, is not especially beneficial for bone buildup.

It has been observed that oral contraceptives seem to help calcium absorption, and that during pregnancy the body absorbs calcium more effectively, making the mother's bones actually stronger despite the calcium needs of the fetus.

OTHER ADVICE: Bisacodyl should not be taken for 1 hour before or after either antacids or milk. The coating of the tablet dissolves in an alkaline medium (such as milk, milk products, or antacids), and as a result will be released in the stomach rather than in the intestine, where it normally works. Gastric irritation may occur, with accompanying pain.

DIPYRIDAMOLE

DRUG FAMILY: Vasodilator

BRAND NAME: Persantine

HOW TO TAKE DIPYRIDAMOLE: One hour before or 3 hours after meals

FOODS TO AVOID: None

POSSIBLE SIDE EFFECTS: Allergic reactions

ACTION OF DIPYRIDAMOLE: This drug causes the coronary arteries to dilate and is used as a long-term treatment for angina pectoris.

HIGH-RISK GROUPS: Allergy sufferers

Nutritional Interactions

ALLERGIC REACTIONS: Persantine contains Federal Drug and Cosmetic (FD&C) Yellow Dye No. 5 (otherwise known as tartrazine), which may cause allergic reactions (including bronchial asthma) in susceptible individuals. Although the general incidence of sensitivity to the dyes is low, it is frequently seen in those patients who are hypersensitive to aspirin.

Tartrazine and other colorings made from coal tar, namely Red No. 3, Red No. 40, Blue No. 1, Orange B, and Citrus Red No. 2, are used as food colorings. A lot of controversy surrounds the use of these synthetic colorings in food. Natural colorings such as paprika, saffron, turmeric, fruit and vegetable juices, carrot oil, grape-skin extract, and beet powder have been safely used for centuries. However, any synthetic coloring added to food must be proved to be harmless. This means the Food and Drug Administration tests them out by doing long-term feeding studies in at least two species of animals before their use is permitted. Even with all these precautions, the odd person is found to be sensitive to one or more of the dyes, as is the case with tartrazine. Red Dye No. 3 is believed to be a factor in some cases of hyperactivity in children.

Prevention and Treatment: You should be alert for any signs of allergic reaction, including runny nose, congestion, and asthma. If you experience any of these, you should inform your doctor immediately.

OTHER ADVICE: Food decreases the absorption of the drug. Consequently, this drug should never be taken at mealtimes. The ideal time to take it is 1 hour before or 3 hours after meals, when the upper portion of the intestinal tract is free of food.

DISULFIRAM

DRUG FAMILY: Anti-alcoholism

BRAND NAME: Antabuse

HOW TO TAKE DISULFIRAM: Usually in the morning, but not within 12 hours of consuming any alcoholic beverage or food containing alcohol

FOODS TO AVOID: Any food, beverage, or medication (such as cough medicines) that contains alcohol

POSSIBLE SIDE EFFECTS: An interaction with alcohol causing such symptoms as headache, nausea, vertigo, and blurred vision

ACTION OF DISULFIRAM: This drug is prescribed for the treatment of chronic alcoholism.

HIGH-RISK GROUPS: Anyone who takes this drug

NUTRITIONAL INTERACTIONS

ALCOHOL INTERACTION: Disulfiram prevents the breakdown of acetaldehyde (a metabolite of alcohol) which, as a result, builds up rapidly in the blood. If alcohol is consumed after this drug is taken, it will cause symptoms such as severe headaches, flushing, nausea and vomiting, low blood pressure, weakness, vertigo, blurred vision, and possibly convulsions.

The reaction begins within 5 to 10 minutes of drinking the alcohol. In sensitive people, the reaction may result from consuming as little as a few sips. The same effects will occur if, after taking this drug, you consume such foods as sauces or casseroles containing wine, desserts containing liquor, or wine vinegar.

Prevention and Treatment: No alcohol, or any food or beverage containing alcohol, should be consumed while taking this drug.

DOXORUBICIN HYDROCHLORIDE

DRUG FAMILY: Anti-cancer

BRAND NAME: Adriamycin

HOW TO TAKE DOXORUBICIN HYDROCHLORIDE: Injection

FOODS TO AVOID: None

POSSIBLE SIDE EFFECTS: Riboflavin deficiency

ACTION OF DOXORUBICIN HYDROCHLORIDE: This potent drug is used against a wide range of human tumors.

HIGH-RISK GROUPS: Anyone who takes this drug

NUTRITIONAL INTERACTIONS

RIBOFLAVIN DEFICIENCY: Doxorubicin hydrochloride impairs the conversion of riboflavin to its active form; thus, the drug is likely to cause a riboflavin deficiency. This may lead to heart failure in severe cases.

The symptoms most likely to appear will be a dermatitis around the nose, cracks in the corners of the mouth, and a soreness or burning sensation in the lips, mouth, and tongue. Discomfort in eating and swallowing may result. The eyes may burn, itch, be more sensitive than usual to light, and tend to be bloodshot. However, be aware that any B vitamin deficiency can cause similar symptoms.

Riboflavin helps the body transform protein, fats, and carbohydrates into the energy needed to maintain body tissues and to protect the body against common skin and eye disorders.

Prevention and Treatment: Good sources of riboflavin should be included in the diet. Milk usually contributes about 50 percent of our riboflavin intake, meat about 25 percent, and dark green leafy vegetables and enriched cereals and breads the rest. The need for riboflavin provides a major reason for including milk in some form in every day's meals; no other food that is commonly eaten can make such a substantial contribution to meeting our daily riboflavin needs. People who don't use milk products can substitute a generous serving of dark green leafy vegetables, because a cup of greens such as collards provides about the same amount of riboflavin as a cup of milk. (See table of Vitamin B_2(Riboflavin)-Rich Foods, page 310.)

Among the meats, liver is the richest source, but all lean meats, as well as eggs, can provide some riboflavin. Riboflavin is light-sensitive; it can be destroyed by the ultraviolet rays of the sun or fluorescent lamps. For this reason, milk is seldom sold, and should not be stored, in transparent glass containers. Cardboard or plastic containers protect the riboflavin in the milk from ultraviolet rays.

Note that riboflavin supplements in excess of the Recommended Dietary Allowance may make the drug less effective and should not be taken.

ERYTHROMYCIN

DRUG FAMILY: Antibiotic

BRAND NAMES: A/T/S; E.E.S.; E-Mycin; E-Mycin E; ERYC; EryDerm; EryPed; Ery-Tab; Erythrocin Lactobionate-I.V.; Erythrocin Piggyback; Erythrocin Stearate; Erythromycin Base; Erythromycin Estolate; Erythromycin Ethylsuccinate; Erythromycin Stearate; Ilosone; Ilotycin; Ilotycin Gluceptate; Pediamycin; Pediazole; Robimycin; SK-Erythromycin; Wyamycin E

HOW TO TAKE ERYTHROMYCIN: With water, on an empty stomach 1 hour before or 3 hours after meals

FOODS TO AVOID: Acidic beverages such as fruit juices, colas, sodas, and wine should not be consumed within 1 hour of taking the drug

POSSIBLE SIDE EFFECTS: Deficiencies of folic acid; vitamins B_6, B_{12}, and K; calcium; and magnesium

ACTION OF ERYTHROMYCIN: This anti-bacterial agent is frequently prescribed for pneumonia, Legionnaire's disease, diphtheria, whooping cough, scarlet fever, syphilis, and gonorrhea, and to prevent the recurrences of rheumatic fever and a variety of other bacterial infections.

HIGH-RISK GROUPS: Oral contraceptive users, heavy drinkers, pregnant women, the elderly, vegetarians, children, smokers, teenagers, lactating women

NUTRITIONAL INTERACTIONS

FOLIC ACID DEFICIENCY: It is conceivable that while taking erythromycin you will develop a folic acid deficiency, since the drug impairs your body's ability to use this nutrient. Often, the first sign of a folic acid or folacin deficiency is inflamed and bleeding gums. The symptoms that follow are a sore, smooth tongue; diarrhea; forgetfulness; apathy; irritability; anemia; and a reduced resistance to infection. Despite the fact that folacin is found in a variety of foods, folacin deficiency is still the most common vitamin deficiency in the United States.

In adults, deficiencies are limited almost exclusively to the elderly and women, 30 percent of whom have intakes below the recommended daily allowance, and 5 to 7 percent of whom also have severe anemia. There are several factors that account for this bias, but one of the most obvious reasons is that oral contraceptive use decreases the absorption of folic acid. Constant dieting also limits folacin intake, and alcohol interferes with the body's use of folic acid, as well.

Folacin is not stored by the body in any appreciable amounts, so an adequate supply must be consumed on a daily basis. Folic acid is crucial to the normal metabolism of protein. Since this vitamin is also needed for the growth of all new cells, a deficiency during pregnancy can lead to birth defects.

Prevention and Treatment: To counteract a deficiency in folic acid, your diet should contain liver, yeast, and leafy vegetables such as spinach, kale, parsley, cauliflower, brussels sprouts, and broccoli. The fruits that are highest in folic acid are oranges and cantaloupes. To a lesser degree, folacin is found in almonds and lima beans, corn, parsnips, green peas, pumpkins, sweet potatoes, bran, peanuts, rye, and whole grain wheat. (See table of Folacin-Rich Foods, page 297.) Approximately one half of the folic acid you consume is absorbed by your body.

As much as 65 percent of dietary folacin is destroyed by normal cooking temperatures (110 to 120 degrees for 10 minutes). Your daily diet, therefore, should include some raw vegetables and fruits. Cooking utensils made out of copper speed up folacin's destruction.

The recommended daily consumption of folacin is 400 mcg. Lactating women should assume a daily need of 1,200 mcg. Pregnant women and oral contraceptive users should consume 800 mcg daily.

VITAMIN B_6 DEFICIENCY: A deficiency of vitamin B_6 is also conceivable in those taking erythromycin, since the drug is an antagonist of vitamin B_6. Common symptoms of this deficiency are a sore mouth and tongue, cracks in the lips and corners of the mouth, and patches of itching, scaling skin. A severe vitamin B_6 deficiency may cause depression and confusion.

A vitamin B_6 deficiency is often found in the elderly. Alcoholics, as well, often experience this deficiency, since alcohol interferes with the body's ability to use B_6. Smokers also seem to have lower than normal body levels. It is estimated that one of every two Americans consumes less than 70 percent of the Recommended Dietary Allowance of B_6.

Prevention and Treatment: To avoid a B_6 deficiency, you should consume a diet featuring such food sources of vitamin B_6 as liver (beef, calf, and pork), herring, salmon, walnuts, peanuts, wheat germ, carrots, peas, potatoes, grapes, bananas, and yeast. (See table of Vitamin B_6(Pyridoxine)-Rich Foods, page 311.) The vitamin is present in significant amounts in meats, fish, fruits, cereals, and vegetables, and to a lesser extent in milk and other dairy products.

Since vitamin B_6 is decomposed at high temperatures, modern food processing often diminishes dietary sources of the nutrient. Consequently, the more processed foods you eat, the more susceptible you will be to a deficiency of this vitamin. The same losses also occur in cooking: meat loses as much as 45 to 80 percent, vegetables 20 to 30 percent.

It has been observed that 15 to 20 percent of oral contraceptive users show direct evidence of vitamin B_6 deficiency. If you are among these people, you should take 5 mg of vitamin B_6 per day. However, keep in mind that you can take too much vitamin B_6; people taking over 1 gram per day have been reported to experience nerve degeneration.

VITAMIN K DEFICIENCY: Erythromycin decreases vitamin K synthesis by killing the bacteria in the large intestine that produce it; thus, a deficiency in this vitamin is conceivable. People with an abnormally low dietary intake of vitamin K are at risk of bleeding with unusual ease if they use erythromycin for a long period of time.

Normally, vitamin K helps produce blood-clotting substances in the liver. Without sufficient levels of vitamin K in the diet, however, bleeding may take place in the gastrointestinal tract (causing black or blood-stained stools), in the urinary tract (causing blood in the urine), and in the uterus (causing blood loss at times other than the normal menstrual periods). Excessive bleeding may occur from an injury or surgery. Another sign of a deficiency of this vitamin is more frequent and more visible bruising than normal.

Half the vitamin K in humans comes from dietary sources: predominantly green leafy vegetables, and to a lesser extent fruit, cereals, dairy products, and meat. The rest of the vitamin K in our bodies is synthesized by the bacteria in the intestines. The daily need for the vitamin is in the range of 70 to 140 mcg.

Pregnant women are at high risk because a vitamin K deficiency can lead to hemorrhaging in the fetus. A fetus is more susceptible than an adult, since it does not have a bacterial population in its large intestine to make vitamin K and does not develop the capacity to do so for the first week of life. Women who have had several pregnancies or whose menstrual periods are heavy should also be careful. Many of the elderly are at risk of a vitamin K deficiency because they have a problem of poor fat absorption, and vitamin K, a fat-soluble vitamin, must be accompanied by sufficient dietary fat to be properly absorbed.

Prevention and Treatment: A vitamin K deficiency can be countered by a vitamin K supplement of 100 mcg per day and a diet that includes foods rich in the vitamin, such as kale, spinach, cabbage, cauliflower, leafy green vegetables, liver (especially pork liver), and fish. (See table of Vitamin K-Rich Foods, page 315.) Pregnant women on this drug should take 5 mg of vitamin K per day for 3 days prior to anticipated delivery, but only under the guidance of a physician. A newborn baby whose mother is on erythromycin should be given 1 mg per day to avoid the risk of anemia caused by the destruction of red blood cells. Infant formulas are often fortified with vitamin K.

Vitamin E supplements should not be taken when at risk of a vitamin K shortage, because vitamin E impairs the absorption of K.

VITAMIN B_{12} DEFICIENCY: Erythromycin decreases vitamin B_{12} absorption as well, and it is conceivable that a deficiency will result. Vitamin B_{12} is needed for the normal development of red blood cells and for the healthy functioning of all cells, in particular those of the bone marrow, nervous system, and intestines.

The most common result of a B_{12} deficiency is pernicious anemia, which is characterized by listlessness, fatigue (especially following such physical exertion as climbing a flight of stairs), numbness and tingling in the fingers and toes, palpitations, angina, light-headedness, and a pale complexion. A vitamin B_{12} deficiency can also lead to an irreversible breakdown in the brain membranes, causing loss of coordination, confusion, memory loss, paranoia, apathy, tremors, and hallucinations. In extreme cases, degeneration of the spinal cord can also result.

Since vitamin B_{12} can be obtained only from animal food sources, strict vegetarians are at particular risk here. Oral contraceptive users too have a greater chance of experiencing this deficiency since they often have a poor vitamin B_{12} status to begin with, as do smokers in many cases. Heavy consumers of alcohol, as well, frequently lack B_{12} because alcohol impairs the absorption of the vitamin. Some elderly people and patients with bacterial or parasitic infections of the intestine also have difficulty in absorbing this vitamin. In any case, anyone who is likely to have a vitamin B_{12} absorption problem should be alert for signs of pernicious anemia while taking erythromycin.

Prevention and Treatment: A balanced diet containing plenty of vitamin B_{12} sources is advised. Only animal products, including dairy foods and fish and shellfish, contain natural vitamin B_{12}. However, some vegetable products are supplemented with vitamin B_{12}; many soy products, for example, are enriched with B_{12} to safeguard vegetarians. (See table of Vitamin B_{12}-Rich Foods, page 312.)

Vitamin B_{12} is stored in the liver, so one meal that includes a B_{12}-rich source such as calf's liver will normally fulfill your body's need for this vitamin for 2 to 3 weeks. (One 3-ounce serving of calf's liver contains 100 mcg of vitamin B_{12}.) If none of these products figures prominently in your diet, you should take a 6 mcg supplement each day while on erythromycin.

People who use major amounts of vitamin C should be aware that vitamin C supplements of more than 500 mg per day can damage B_{12} and contribute to a B_{12} deficiency. However, anyone who eats red meat two times a week has a three- to five-year supply of B_{12} in his liver.

The presence of baking soda in cooking will destroy vitamin B_{12} and should be avoided whenever possible. B_{12} also degrades at high temperatures, as when meat is placed on a hot griddle. The pasteurization of milk and the sterilization in boiling water of a bottle of milk also cause the loss of some B_{12}.

CALCIUM DEFICIENCY: Erythromycin also decreases calcium absorption, so a deficiency of calcium is conceivable if erythromycin is taken for long periods. Whenever calcium blood levels are low, the body will liberate the necessary amounts of calcium from the bones, where it is stored, thereby weakening them and making them more susceptible to fractures. A condition called osteomalacia can result. This is more likely after middle age, because in older people the body uses dietary calcium less efficiently.

Osteomalacia is a weakening of the bones as a consequence of uniform and steady calcium loss. This disease affects millions of older Americans, but also many younger people. In fact, one out of every four postmenopausal women suffers from this problem. Prominent symptoms are bone pain in the back, thighs, shoulder region, or ribs; difficulty in walking; and weakness in the muscles of the legs. The condition is reversible once blood calcium levels are raised.

If a calcium deficiency persists for several years, it can lead to osteoporosis, another condition in which the bones are made weak and brittle. However, osteoporosis, an unexplained and rapid loss of calcium from the bones, is irreversible. Here the first symptoms are backache, a gradual loss of height, and periodontal disease. In cases of osteoporosis, fractures of the vertebrae, hip, and wrist occur frequently, sometimes spontaneously.

Some 7 percent of women fifty years of age and older have osteoporosis, and certain observers believe that the incidence of this disease is on the rise; between 15 and 20 million Americans are said to have osteoporosis today. In some 30 percent of people over sixty-five, the disease is severe enough to result in fractures. By age eighty, virtually all women experience some degree of osteoporosis. Early menopause is a strong predictor of the disease. One out of five cases of the disease is found in men, but generally men get it at a later age and less severely than women.

Prevention and Treatment: The Recommended Dietary Allowance for calcium is 800 mg, and all women should consume at least 1,200 mg of calcium per day. The average intake in the United States, however, is only 450 to 550 mg. For the elderly, and women who have already reached menopause or are about to, this should be increased to 1,500 mg by the consumption of foods rich in calcium, particularly milk and dairy products (including yogurt and hard cheeses) and, to a lesser extent, almonds. Three 8-ounce glasses of milk, for example, provide 1,500 mg of calcium. (See table of Calcium-Rich Foods, page 289.)

If you are one of the 30 million Americans for whom digesting calcium foods is a problem because of an intolerance to lactose, the sugar found in dairy products, you should take a 1,000 mg daily supplement of calcium. The best-absorbed supplement is calcium carbonate. (See Calcium Supplements entry, page 51.) If magnesium is included in the supplement, the calcium is slightly better absorbed, and any tendency to constipation is reduced. The supplement should be taken in two 500 mg doses, one of which should be consumed before bedtime because most of the calcium loss from your body occurs while you sleep.

Vitamin C assists calcium absorption, while cigarette smoking leads to the loss of calcium from the body, as does excessive alcohol consumption. Users of erythromycin should temporarily avoid foods that can decrease the absorption of calcium, such as kale, rhubarb, spinach, cocoa and chocolate, beet greens, tea, and coffee. A deficiency might arise also if the ratio of phosphorus to calcium in your diet is very high; processed foods, especially carbonated beverages, are particularly high in phosphorus. The ideal ratio is essentially 1 to 1, as in dairy products; when the ratio is 15 or 20 to 1, as in meat, very little calcium is absorbed. High-fiber foods may contribute to a calcium deficiency, since fiber binds to calcium and passes it out in the stool. Excess

fat and protein in the diet also hinder absorption.

Since there is little calcium in strict vegetarian diets (those that avoid dairy products as well as meat), vegetarians are at greater risk of a calcium deficiency. People who take magnesium- or aluminum-based antacids are also more prone to calcium deficiencies, because both magnesium and aluminum in excess impair calcium absorption.

Besides a change in dietary habits and the use of calcium supplements, it is recommended that anyone at risk of this deficiency adopt an exercise regimen that causes the bones to support the weight of the body, to strengthen bones and to counteract the loss of bone density. A regular walking or jogging program, for example, can help prevent the bone degeneration of the spine, hips, and legs. Note, however, that swimming, though good for the heart as an aerobic exercise, is not especially beneficial for bone buildup.

It has been observed that oral contraceptives seem to help calcium absorption, and that during pregnancy the body absorbs calcium more effectively, making the mother's bones actually stronger, despite the calcium needs of the fetus.

OTHER ADVICE: Consumption of meals close to the time of administration of this drug delays its absorption except in cases of erythromycin estolate (Ilosone), where food aids absorption. Erythromycin is also destroyed by acidic beverages such as fruit juices and colas, so it is best taken with water, on an empty stomach, 1 hour before or 3 hours after a meal.

Erythromycin may decrease your magnesium absorption. A deficiency could occur, particularly if you are a heavy drinker, if you regularly use diuretics, or if you take oral contraceptives. It is unlikely that this will be a serious mineral deficiency, but foods rich in magnesium should be included in the diet, such as nuts (almonds and cashews are highest), meat, fish, milk, whole grains, and fresh greens, since cooking can wash away some magnesium. (See table of Magnesium-Rich Foods, page 300.)

ESTROGENS AND PROGESTINS

DRUG FAMILY: Oral contraceptives

BRAND NAMES: [GENERIC/Brand] ETHYNODIOL DIACETATE/Demulen 1/35-21; Ovulin-21; MESTRANOL/Enovid, Enovid-E; Norinyl 1+50; Norinyl 1+80; Norinyl 2 mg.; Ortho-Novum 1/50; Ortho-Novum 1/80; Ovulen-21; Ovulen-28; NORETHINDRONE/Aygestin; Norlutate; Brevicon; Loestrin 1/20; Loestrin 1.5/30; Micronor; Modicon; Norinyl 1+35; Norinyl 1+50; Norinyl 1+80; Norinyl 2 mg; Norlestrin 21; Norlestrin 1/50; Norlestrin 2.5/50; Norlutin; Nor-Q.D.; Ortho-Novum 1/35; Ortho-Novum 1/50; Ortho-Novum 1/80; Ortho-Novum 10/11; Ortho-Novum 2 mg; Ovcon-35; Ovcon-50; NORGESTREL/Lo/Ovral; Ovral; Ovrette

HOW TO TAKE ORAL CONTRACEPTIVES: At approximately the same time every day

FOODS TO AVOID: None

POSSIBLE SIDE EFFECTS: Deficiencies of riboflavin, folic acid, and vitamins B_6, B_{12}, and C

ACTION OF ORAL CONTRACEPTIVES: These drugs, which are a combination of the hormones estrogen and progestin, prevent pregnancy by suppressing ovulation.

HIGH-RISK GROUPS: Anyone who takes these drugs.

NUTRITIONAL INTERACTIONS

RIBOFLAVIN DEFICIENCY: Women who do not eat a balanced diet and therefore consume only very small amounts of riboflavin may suffer from a clinical deficiency. Estrogen stimulates many reactions in the body that require riboflavin, so riboflavin needs are increased. A woman with only a marginal intake of riboflavin to start with is likely to be pushed over the line into a deficiency state while taking oral contraceptives.

The symptoms most likely to appear will be a dermatitis around the lips and nostrils, a cracking in the corners of the mouth, and a sore tongue. Discomfort in eating and swallowing may result. The eyes may burn, itch, be more sensitive than usual to light, and tend to be bloodshot. However, be aware that any B vitamin deficiency can cause some of these same symptoms.

Riboflavin helps the body transform protein, fats, and carbohydrates into the energy needed to maintain body tissues and to protect the body against common skin and eye disorders.

Prevention and Treatment: Good sources of riboflavin should be included in the diet. About 50 percent of our riboflavin comes from milk, while meat contributes about 25 percent, and dark green leafy vegetables and enriched cereals and breads the rest. The need for riboflavin provides a major reason for including milk in some form in every day's meals; no other food that is commonly eaten can make such a substantial contribution to meeting our daily riboflavin needs. People who don't use milk products can substitute a generous serving of dark green leafy vegetables, because a cup of greens such as collards provides about the same amount of riboflavin as a cup of milk. (See table of Vitamin B₂(Riboflavin)-Rich Foods, page 310.)

Liver is the richest source of riboflavin among the meats, but all lean meats, as well as eggs, can provide some riboflavin. Riboflavin is light-sensitive; it can be destroyed by the ultraviolet rays of the sun or fluorescent lamps. For this reason, milk is seldom sold, and should not be stored, in transparent glass containers. Cardboard or plastic containers protect the riboflavin in the milk from ultraviolet rays.

FOLIC ACID DEFICIENCY: There is considerable evidence to show that people taking birth control pills have an increased need for folacin. They appear not to absorb it as efficiently as nonusers, and because of the increased protein synthesis caused by estrogen, they need more than usual and are likely to develop a deficiency.

Many women in America normally consume too little folacin in their diets, so this is a matter for real concern. Folacin is required for the production of all new cells in the body. Hence, any area of the body where rapid cell replacement occurs can become sore if the diet contains inadequate amounts of the vitamin. The tongue becomes smooth and sore. The lining of the gastrointestinal

tract becomes sore and less able to absorb food, resulting in diarrhea. The lining of the vagina may also become sore, and breakthrough bleeding may occur.

The end result of a folacin deficiency is anemia. Anemia is characterized by pallor, irritability, lassitude, and breathlessness on exertion. It should be emphasized that only a few women suffer from any of these more serious symptoms while taking birth control pills, with the anemia and vaginal soreness being very rare. However, many women do experience sore and bleeding gums, which is usually a distinct sign of a mild deficiency. You should keep in mind that the longer you are on the pill, the greater your risk of a folate deficiency. After 4 or 5 years on the pill, most people will suffer from some kind of deficiency.

Inflamed and bleeding gums are often the first sign of a folic acid or folacin deficiency. The symptoms that follow are a sore, smooth tongue; diarrhea; forgetfulness; apathy; irritability; and anemia. Despite the fact that folacin is found in a variety of foods, folacin deficiency is still the most common vitamin deficiency in the United States.

In adults, deficiencies are limited almost exclusively to the elderly and women, 30 percent of whom have intakes below the Recommended Dietary Allowance, and 5 to 7 percent of whom also have severe anemia due to the deficiency. There are several factors that account for this bias, but one of the most obvious reasons is the oral contraceptive use discussed above. Constant dieting also limits folacin intake, and alcohol interferes with the body's use and absorption of folic acid, as well. Folacin is not stored by the body in any appreciable amounts, so an adequate supply must be consumed on a daily basis.

Prevention and Treatment: To counteract a deficiency in folic acid, your diet should contain liver, yeast, and leafy vegetables such as spinach, kale, parsley, cauliflower, brussels sprouts, and broccoli. The fruits that are highest in folic acid are oranges and cantaloupes. To a lesser degree, folacin is found in almonds and lima beans, corn, parsnips, green peas, pumpkins, sweet potatoes, bran, peanuts, rye, and whole grain wheat. (See table of Folacin-Rich Foods, page 297.) Approximately one half of the folic acid you consume is absorbed by your body.

Normal cooking temperatures (110 to 120 degrees for 10 minutes) reduce the amount of useful folacin in your food by as much as 65 percent. Your daily diet, therefore, should include some raw vegetables and fruits. Cooking utensils made out of copper speed up folacin's destruction.

The recommended daily consumption of folacin is 400 mcg. Oral contraceptive users should consume 800 mcg daily.

A mild deficiency is not generally a major problem for the average woman. However, if you should become pregnant shortly after terminating contraceptive use, a serious problem could arise. Your developing fetus has a critical need for folacin for its rapidly dividing cells, and inadequate folacin at this time can lead to congenital malformations.

In any case, all women using any of the varieties of the birth control pill should take a .4 to 1.0 mg daily supplement of folacin.

VITAMIN B$_6$ DEFICIENCY: Oral contraceptives increase the need for vitamin B$_6$. Estrogen stimulates many reactions in the body that require vitamin B$_6$, including reactions involved in the breakdown of dietary protein. If you have a marginal intake of vitamin B$_6$, there may be insufficient quantities of the vitamin available in your system to keep all the reactions that require it working at their optimal rate, and it is conceivable that you will develop a B$_6$ deficiency. This is especially likely in smokers, who seem to have an increased need for the vitamin.

One reaction that relies upon B$_6$ is the production of serotonin. Serotonin is a substance in the brain that elevates mood. Many gynecologists believe that vitamin B$_6$ deficiencies in women taking the contraceptive pill account for much of the depression, and many of the emotional disturbances and headaches, experienced by these women. Common symptoms of this deficiency are a sore mouth and tongue, cracks in the lips and corners of the mouth, and patches of itching, scaling skin. A severe vitamin B$_6$ deficiency may cause depression and confusion. Alcohol interferes with the body's ability to use B$_6$, so consumers of alcohol are more likely to be subject to this deficiency. It is also estimated that one of every two Americans consumes less than 70 percent of the Recommended Dietary Allowance of B$_6$.

Prevention and Treatment: To avoid a B$_6$ deficiency, you should consume a diet featuring such food sources of vitamin B$_6$ as liver (beef, calf, and pork), herring, salmon, walnuts, peanuts, wheat germ, carrots, peas, potatoes, grapes, bananas, and yeast. (See table of Vitamin B$_6$(Pyridoxine)-Rich Foods, page 311.) The vitamin is present in significant amounts in meats, fish, fruits, cereals, and vegetables, and to a lesser extent in milk and other dairy products.

Since vitamin B_6 is decomposed at high temperatures, modern food processing often diminishes dietary sources of the vitamin. Consequently, the more processed foods you eat, the more susceptible you will be to a deficiency of this vitamin. The same losses also occur in cooking: meat loses as much as 45 to 80 percent, vegetables 20 to 30 percent. Since vitamin B_6 is light-sensitive, the amount of the vitamin in a container of milk left in the sunlight will gradually decrease.

It has been observed that 15 to 20 percent of oral contraceptive users show direct evidence of vitamin B_6 deficiency. You should take a supplement of 5 mg of B_6 per day while taking oral contraceptives. However, keep in mind that you can take too much vitamin B_6; people taking over 1 gram have been reported to experience a toxic reaction.

VITAMIN B_{12} DEFICIENCY: Women who have a very low intake of vitamin B_{12} may be at risk of a B_{12} deficiency. Estrogen reduces the net absorption of vitamin B_{12} but, under normal circumstances, only vegetarians who do not consume any animal products (or vegetable products supplemented with vitamin B_{12}, such as soy-supplemented products) need be concerned with a vitamin B_{12} deficiency. Smokers also seem to have an increased need for the vitamin.

Since they are at risk, vegetarians should be on the alert for pernicious anemia, which is characterized by listlessness, fatigue (especially following such physical exertion as climbing a flight of stairs), numbness and tingling in the fingers and toes, and a pale complexion. A vitamin B_{12} deficiency can also lead to an irreversible breakdown in the brain membranes, causing loss of coordination, confusion, memory loss, paranoia, apathy, tremors, and hallucinations. In extreme cases, degeneration of the spinal cord can also result.

Heavy consumers of alcohol, often lack B_{12} because alcohol impairs the absorption of the vitamin. Patients with bacterial or parasitic infections of the intestine also have difficulty in absorbing this vitamin. In any case, anyone who is likely to have a vitamin B_{12} absorption problem should be alert for signs of pernicious anemia while taking oral contraceptives.

Prevention and Treatment: A balanced diet containing plenty of vitamin B_{12} sources is advised. Only animal products, including dairy foods and fish and shellfish, contain natural vitamin B_{12}. Some vegetable matter is supplemented with B_{12}; many soy products, for example, are enriched with this nutrient to safeguard vegetarians. (See table of Vitamin B_{12}-Rich Foods, page 312.)

As vitamin B_{12} is stored in the liver, one meal that includes a B_{12}-rich source such as calf's liver will normally fulfill your body's need for this vitamin for 2 to 3 weeks. (One 3-ounce serving of calf's liver contains 100 mcg of vitamin B_{12}.) If none of these products figures prominently in your diet, you should take a 6 mcg supplement each day while using an oral contraceptive.

People who use major amounts of vitamin C should be aware that vitamin C supplements of more than 500 mg per day can damage B_{12} and contribute to a B_{12} deficiency. However, anyone who eats red meat two times a week has a three- to five-year supply of B_{12} in his liver.

The presence of baking soda in cooking will destroy vitamin B_{12} and should be avoided whenever possible. B_{12} also degrades at high temperatures, as when meat is placed on a hot griddle. The pasteurization of milk and the sterilization in boiling water of a bottle of milk also cause the loss of some B_{12}.

VITAMIN C DEFICIENCY: Contraceptive users break down vitamin C more rapidly than normal, so if you have a marginal intake, you could conceivably develop a deficiency. With an adequate vitamin C intake, the body normally maintains a fixed pool of the vitamin and rapidly excretes any excess in the urine. Ordinarily, 60 to 100 mg of vitamin C per day will fulfill the body's requirements, except in the case of some smokers who have an increased need for this vitamin.

With an inadequate intake, however, the reservoir becomes depleted at the rate of up to 3 percent per day, and even more quickly in users of this drug. Obvious symptoms of a vitamin C deficiency do not appear until the available vitamin C has been reduced to about one fifth of its optimal level, and this may take two months to occur.

Spongy or bleeding gums are the earliest sign of a deficiency, and this sign is often accompanied by slightly swollen wrists and ankles, and capillaries that break under the skin, producing pinpoint hemorrhages around the hair follicles on the arms and legs.

Vitamin C is important to the functioning of your bodily systems in a number of ways. When your body is deficient in Vitamin C, your white blood cells are less able to detect and destroy invading bacteria. On the other hand, megadoses of the vitamin (over 2 grams daily) can also impair this ability. Vitamin C also helps your body guard itself against such pollutants as known cancer-causing agents nitrites and nitrosamines and protects vitamins A and E from degradation. It also aids in iron absorption, speeds up wound healing, and strengthens blood vessels. Other well-known effects are that, in some people, vitamin C reduces the symptoms of a cold by one third, and that it is important in preventing plaque formation on the teeth, which reduces the likelihood of gum disease and tooth decay.

Prevention and Treatment: Patients taking this drug should be sure to get 100 mg per day of vitamin C. Vitamin C-rich foods include citrus fruits, broccoli, spinach, cabbage, and bananas. (See table of Vitamin-C Rich Foods, page 313.) In preparing foods rich in vitamin C, you should keep in mind that it is readily oxidized (when exposed to the air during both food processing and storage). Copper and iron cooking utensils will speed up the oxidization; also, the longer the food is cooked and the higher the temperature, the greater the vitamin loss. Large amounts of water used in cooking will wash out the vitamin. Vitamin C is also destroyed when fruit and vegetables are cut or bruised.

Supplements can be taken, although once again the body tends to eliminate any surplus of the vitamin, so supplements of more than 100 mg a day are unnecessary. The increased need for vitamin C while taking a birth control pill is small, and a large vitamin C supplement will be counterproductive, since it decreases the effectiveness of the pill. Never take more than 1,000 mg of vitamin C when on the birth control pill; a 100 mg daily supplement is recommended. In fact, megadoses of the vitamin can cause nausea, abdominal cramps, and diarrhea, among other undesirable side effects.

OTHER ADVICE: There is some evidence that suggests that the need for vitamin K is reduced in women taking oral contraceptives. Supplements of vitamin K should never be taken by such women since they will increase chances of blood clots. This risk is already elevated by the estrogen in the pill, although not to such a degree that one should be overly concerned.

There is also some indication that oral contraceptives increase the body's need for zinc and magnesium. However, it is unlikely that a deficiency of either will occur. To be sure, include in your diet foods rich in zinc (meat, oysters, herring, milk, and egg yolk) and magnesium (nuts, beans, peas, lentils, dark green vegetables, cereal grains, seafoods).

Some drugs decrease oral contraceptive effectiveness, such as anti-epileptic drugs and the anti-tubercular drug rifampin. If you are taking these medications, you should consult with both your regular physician and your gynecologist.

One last concern: Some people find that birth control pills stimulate their appetite. You should watch your weight carefully while taking oral contraceptives, since you could find yourself overeating.

Oral contraceptives also decrease the body's ability to metabolize caffeine. Hence, tea or coffee will have an enhanced effect.

ETHACRYNIC ACID AND SODIUM ETHACRYNATE

DRUG FAMILY: Diuretic

BRAND NAMES: [GENERIC/Brand] SODIUM ETHACRYNATE/Edecrin Sodium; ETHACRYNIC ACID/Edecrin

HOW TO TAKE ETHACRYNIC ACID: With meals

FOODS TO AVOID: Large amounts of sweetbreads, anchovies, corn, lentils, cranberries, prunes, plums, sardines, meat, and fish (see table of Purine-Rich Foods, page 303); cola beverages, strong tea, coffee, and chocolate; alcoholic beverages

POSSIBLE SIDE EFFECTS: Deficiencies of potassium, magnesium, and calcium; gout

ACTION OF ETHACRYNIC ACID: This drug is prescribed as a diuretic.

HIGH-RISK GROUPS: The elderly, heavy drinkers, users of oral contraceptives, smokers, vegetarians

NUTRITIONAL INTERACTIONS

POTASSIUM DEFICIENCY: Since this drug impairs the body's ability to absorb potassium and increases its rate of excretion, it is conceivable that, while taking sodium ethacrynate or ethacrynic acid, you will develop a potassium deficiency. Potassium regulates the amount of water in the cells of the body, and is essential for the proper functioning of the kidneys and the heart muscle, and the secretion of stomach juices. The most alarming symptom of a potassium deficiency is an irregular heartbeat, which can lead to heart failure.

Prevention and Treatment: Potassium depletion can be avoided by including such potassium-rich foods in your diet as tomato juice, lentils, dried apricots, asparagus, bananas, peanut butter, chicken, almonds, and milk. (See table of Potassium-Rich Foods, page 302.)

Potassium supplements should never be taken unless prescribed by a physician. They can cause anemia by interfering with the absorption of vitamin B_{12}. Just a few grams can also drastically increase the risk of heart failure. If you experience difficulty in swallowing while taking potassium supplements, consult your physician immediately. If supplements are prescribed, be aware that the absorption of the supplements potassium iodide and potassium chloride is decreased by dairy products, and that both are gastric irritants and should be taken with meals.

Too much salt in your diet can also compromise your body's supply of potassium, as can 1 to 3 ounces per day of licorice candy made from natural extract, which contains a substance called glycyrrhizic acid. This substance can also elevate blood pressure by causing sodium and water retention, so it is best to avoid eating licorice when taking this drug. Only imported licorice usually contains natural licorice extract; check the package.

MAGNESIUM DEFICIENCY: It is conceivable that, while taking this drug, you will experience a magnesium deficiency, although magnesium deficiencies are not common because the average American diet contains appre-

ciable amounts of the mineral. However, the high level of magnesium excretion resulting from the use of ethacrynic acid makes such a deficiency far more likely.

Clinical signs of magnesium deficiency include muscle weakness, tremors, depression, emotional instability, and irrational behavior.

Prevention and Treatment: A diet containing the four food groups provides the normal amount of magnesium. However, if a magnesium depletion is suspected, your diet should feature foods such as nuts (almonds and cashews are highest), meat, fish, milk, whole grains, and fresh greens, since cooking can wash away some magnesium. (See table of Magnesium-Rich Foods, page 300.) Alcohol provokes magnesium excretion, so its intake should be restricted to two drinks per day while you are on this drug.

CALCIUM DEFICIENCY: Because of increased excretion, it is conceivable that you will develop a calcium deficiency while taking this drug. Whenever calcium blood levels are low, the body liberates the necessary calcium from the bones, where it is stored. Over a prolonged period, the bones can become weakened and more susceptible to fractures, and a condition called osteomalacia can result. This is more likely after middle age, since in older people the body uses dietary calcium less efficiently.

Osteomalacia is a weakening of the bones as a consequence of uniform and steady calcium loss. This disease affects millions of older Americans, but also many younger people. In fact, one out of every four postmenopausal women suffers from this problem. Prominent symptoms are pain in the back, thighs, shoulder region, or ribs; difficulty in walking; and weakness in the leg muscles. The condition is reversible once calcium blood levels are raised.

A prolonged loss of bone calcium is believed to increase the risk of contracting the disease called osteoporosis, another condition in which the bones are made weak and brittle. However, osteoporosis, an unexplained and rapid loss of calcium from the bones, is irreversible. Here the first symptoms are backache, a gradual loss of height, and periodontal disease. In cases of osteoporosis, fractures of the vertebrae, hip, and wrist occur frequently, sometimes spontaneously.

Approximately 7 percent of women fifty years of age and older have osteoporosis, and certain observers believe that the incidence of this disease is on the rise; between 15 and 20 million Americans are said to have osteoporosis today. In some 30 percent of people over sixty-five, the disease is severe enough to result in fractures. By age eighty, virtually all women experience some degree of osteoporosis. Early menopause is a strong predictor of the disease. One out of five cases of the disease is found in men, but generally men get it at a later age and less severely than women.

Prevention and Treatment: The Recommended Dietary Allowance for calcium is 800 mg, and all women should consume at least 1,200 mg of calcium per day. The average intake in the United States, however, is only 450 to 550 mg. For women who have already reached menopause, or are about to, this should be increased to 1,500 mg by the consumption of foods rich in calcium, particularly milk and dairy products (including yogurt and hard cheeses) and, to a lesser extent, almonds. Three glasses of milk, for example, provide 800 mg of calcium. (See table of Calcium-Rich Foods, page 289.)

If calcium foods must be avoided because of an intolerance to lactose, the sugar found in dairy products (a problem for an estimated 30 million Americans), a 1,000 mg daily supplement of calcium should be taken. The best-absorbed supplement is calcium carbonate. (See Calcium Supplements entry page 51.) If magnesium is included in the supplement, the calcium is slightly better absorbed, and any tendency to constipation is reduced. The supplement should be taken in two 500 mg dosages, one of which should be consumed before bedtime because most of the calcium loss from your body occurs while you sleep.

Keep in mind that vitamin C assists calcium absorption, while cigarette smoking makes the body lose calcium, as does excessive alcohol consumption. Users of ethacrynic acid should temporarily avoid foods that can decrease the absorption of calcium, such as kale, rhubarb, spinach, cocoa, chocolate, beet greens, tea, and coffee. A deficiency might also arise if the ratio of phosphorus to calcium in your diet is very high; processed foods are particularly high in phosphorus. The ideal ratio is essentially 1 to 1, as in dairy products; when the ratio is 15 or 20 to 1, as in meat, very little calcium is absorbed. High-fiber foods may contribute to a calcium deficiency, since fiber binds to calcium and passes it out in the stool. Excess fat and protein in the diet also hinder absorption.

Since there is little calcium in strict vegetarian diets (those that avoid dairy products as well as meat), vegetarians are at greater risk of a calcium deficiency. People who take magnesium- or aluminum-based antacids are also more prone to calcium deficiencies, because both magnesium and aluminum in excess impair calcium absorption.

Besides a change in dietary habits and the use of calcium supplements, it is recommended that anyone at risk of this deficiency adopt an exercise regimen that causes the bones to support the weight of the body, to strengthen bones and to counteract the loss of bone calcium. A regular walking or jogging program, for example, can help prevent the bone degeneration of the spine, hips, and legs. Note, however, that swimming, though good for the heart as an aerobic exercise, is not especially beneficial for bone buildup.

It has been observed that oral contraceptives seem to help calcium absorption, and that during pregnancy the body absorbs calcium more effectively, making the mother's bones actually stronger despite the calcium needs of the fetus.

GOUT COMPLICATION: This drug may also cause gout in susceptible people. Gout is an arthritis-like disease that affects single joints, often the big toe, in painful episodes that last only a few days but are likely to recur. Middle-aged men are most often afflicted.

Gout is caused by deposits in the joints of uric acid crystals. When purines are taken in the diet, they are normally excreted as uric acid; however, ethacrynic acid causes a buildup of uric acid, which can result in gout. Caffeine can increase this tendency, as can alcohol.

Prevention and Treatment: If you have a predisposition to gout, you should avoid high intakes of rich sources of purines, such as sweetbreads, anchovies, corn, lentils, cranberries, prunes, plums, sardines, meat, fish, and caffeine- and alcohol-containing beverages. (See table of Purine-Rich Foods, page 303.)

OTHER ADVICE: The drug also irritates the stomach wall. The gastric effects are minimized when the drug is given with food, so the drug should never be taken on an empty stomach.

ETHAMBUTOL HYDROCHLORIDE

DRUG FAMILY: Anti-tubercular

BRAND NAME: Myambutol

HOW TO TAKE ETHAMBUTOL HYDROCHLORIDE: One hour before or 2 to 3 hours after meals

FOODS TO AVOID: Large amounts of sweet breads, anchovies, corn, lentils, cranberries, prunes, plums, sardines; coffee, strong tea, cola, and chocolate; alcoholic beverages

POSSIBLE SIDE EFFECTS: Gout; zinc deficiency

ACTION OF ETHAMBUTOL HYDROCHLORIDE: This drug kills tuberculosis-causing bacteria that are resistant to other anti-tubercular agents. It is used in combination with isoniazid.

HIGH-RISK GROUPS: Vegetarians, anyone who consumes alcohol regularly, oral contraceptive users, teenagers, pregnant women, the elderly

NUTRITIONAL INTERACTIONS

GOUT COMPLICATION: This drug may cause gout in susceptible people. Gout is an arthritis-like disease that affects single joints, often the big toe, in painful episodes that last only a few days but are likely to recur. Middle-aged men are most often afflicted.

Gout is caused by deposits in the joints of uric acid crystals. When purines are taken in the diet, they are normally secreted as uric acid; however, ethambutol causes a buildup of uric acid in the body, which can result in gout. This effect is exacerbated by vitamin B_6 supplements, which should not be taken to excess (more than 50 mg); by caffeine; and by alcohol.

Prevention and Treatment: If you have a predisposition to gout, you should avoid high intakes of rich sources of purines: sweet-breads, anchovies, corn, lentils, cranberries, prunes, plums, sardines, meat, fish; and caffeine- and alcohol-containing beverages. (See table of Purine-Rich Foods, page 303.)

ZINC DEFICIENCY: Ethambutol causes the excretion of large amounts of body zinc. A consequent deficiency is unlikely, but for heavy drinkers, pregnant women (in whom a deficiency can lead to fetal-growth retardation), and users of oral contraceptives, the chances are somewhat higher. A shortage of zinc in your system may result in impaired healing of wounds and ulcers, scaly dermatitis of the face and limbs, and anorexia associated with the loss of taste.

Prevention and Treatment: Patients using ethambutol should be sure to get the Recommended Dietary Allowance of zinc. Animal foods are good sources, with the richest being oysters, herring, milk, and egg yolks. Among plant foods, whole grains are richest in zinc, but it is not as well absorbed from them as from meat. Fiber and phytic acid in the cereal grains hinder its absorption.

The recommended intake of 15 mg a day for adults is usually easily met by the diet of the average middle-class person, but deficiencies are more likely if animal protein is underemphasized. As a rule of thumb, two small servings of animal protein a day will provide sufficient zinc. Supplements should not be necessary, providing good sources of the nutrients are included in the diet.

OTHER INTERACTIONS: The presence of food in the stomach impairs the absorption of this drug, so the daily dose should be taken 1 hour before or 2 to 3 hours after meals.

ETHIONAMIDE

DRUG FAMILY: Antibiotic

BRAND NAMES: Trecator-SC

HOW TO TAKE ETHIONAMIDE: With meals or milk

FOODS TO AVOID: None

POSSIBLE SIDE EFFECTS: Vitamin B_6 deficiency; gastrointestinal distress

ACTION OF ETHIONAMIDE: This drug is used to treat tuberculosis if the more usual drugs (such as isoniazid, streptomycin, and aminosalicylic acid) fail to achieve the desired improvement. Ethionamide is only given in conjunction with these anti-tubercular agents.

HIGH-RISK GROUPS: Anyone who takes this drug

NUTRITIONAL INTERACTIONS

VITAMIN B6 DEFICIENCY: Since ethionamide is an antagonist of vitamin B_6, users of this drug are likely to experience a vitamin B_6 deficiency. Common symptoms of this deficiency are a sore mouth and tongue, cracks in the lips and corners of the mouth, and patches of itching, scaling skin. A severe vitamin B_6 deficiency may cause depression and confusion.

Vitamin B_6 deficiencies are common among the elderly and sometimes occur in smokers. Alcoholics, as well, often experience this deficiency, since alcohol interferes with the body's ability to use B_6. It is estimated that one of every two Americans consumes less than 70 percent of the Recommended Dietary Allowance of B_6.

Prevention and Treatment: To avoid a B_6 deficiency, you should consume a diet featuring such food sources of vitamin B_6 as liver (beef, calf, and pork), herring, salmon, walnuts, peanuts, wheat germ, carrots, peas, potatoes, grapes, bananas, and yeast. (See table of Vitamin B_6(Pyridoxine)-Rich Foods, page 311.) The vitamin is present in significant amounts in meats, fish, fruits, cereals, and vegetables, and to a lesser extent in milk and other dairy products.

Since vitamin B_6 is decomposed at high temperatures, modern food processing often diminishes dietary sources of the vitamin. Consequently, the more processed foods you eat, the more susceptible you will be to a deficiency of this vitamin. The same losses also occur in cooking: meat loses as much as 45 to 80 percent, vegetables 20 to 30 percent.

It has been observed that 15 to 20 percent of oral contraceptive users show direct evidence of vitamin B_6 deficiency. If you are among these people, you should take a supplement of 5 mg of vitamin B_6 per day. However, keep in mind that you can take too much vitamin B_6; people taking over 500 mg have been reported to experience a toxic reaction.

GASTROINTESTINAL DISTRESS: Ethionamide also causes severe gastrointestinal disturbances, so it should always be taken with meals or milk.

ETHYLENEDIAMINETETRAACETIC ACID (EDTA)

DRUG FAMILY: Chelating agents

BRAND NAMES: [GENERIC/Brand] CALCIUM DISODIUM EDETATE; Calcium Disodium Versenate

HOW TO TAKE EDTA: Usually injected

FOODS TO AVOID: None

POSSIBLE SIDE EFFECTS: Vitamin B_6 deficiency, and loss of body calcium, zinc, manganese, iron, and copper

ACTION OF EDTA: These compounds bind to metals in the body and carry them out via the urine. Used in the treatment of lead poisoning, the emergency treatment of hypercalcemia (abnormally high blood calcium levels, which can cause heart failure), and occasionally to treat the irregular heart rate accompanying an overdosage of digitalis.

HIGH-RISK GROUPS: The elderly, children, anyone who consumes alcohol, premenopausal women, smokers, teenagers

NUTRITIONAL INTERACTIONS

CALCIUM DEFICIENCY: Use of this drug leads to a decrease in the absorption of a variety of metals, including calcium, zinc, manganese, iron, and copper. However, as the normal course of treatment with EDTA is five days, mineral deficiencies should not develop.

Prevention and Treatment: Taking a mineral supplement containing the Recommended Dietary Allowances for these minerals both during the treatment and for a month afterward will prevent any deficiency. (See table of Recommended Dietary Allowances, page 317.)

VITAMIN B$_6$ DEFICIENCY: It is conceivable that while taking EDTA you will develop a deficiency of vitamin B$_6$, since the drug causes dermatitis with lesions like those associated with a vitamin B$_6$ deficiency. Other symptoms of this deficiency are a sore mouth and tongue, cracks in the lips and corners of the mouth, and patches of itching, scaling skin. A severe vitamin B$_6$ deficiency may cause depression and confusion.

Vitamin B$_6$ deficiencies are often found in the elderly, and marginal deficiencies sometimes occur among smokers. Alcoholics, as well, often experience this deficiency, since alcohol interferes with the body's ability to use B$_6$. It is estimated that one of every two Americans consumes less than 70 percent of the Recommended Dietary Allowance of B$_6$.

Prevention and Treatment: To avoid a B$_6$ deficiency, you should consume a diet featuring food sources of vitamin B$_6$ such as liver (beef, calf, and pork), herring, salmon, walnuts, peanuts, wheat germ, carrots, peas, potatoes, grapes, bananas, and yeast. (See table of Vitamin B$_6$(Pyridoxine)-Rich Foods, page 311.) The vitamin is present in significant amounts in meats, fish, fruits, cereals, and vegetables, and to a lesser extent in milk and other dairy products.

Modern food processing often diminishes dietary sources of the vitamin, since it is decomposed at high temperatures. Consequently, the more processed foods you eat, the more susceptible you will be to a deficiency of this vitamin. The same losses also occur in cooking: meat loses as much as 45 to 80 percent, vegetables 20 to 30 percent.

Keep in mind that you can take too much vitamin B$_6$; people taking over 1 gram have been reported to experience nerve degeneration. However, if you are an oral contraceptive user, you should take a 5 mg supplement of the vitamin per day. It has been observed that 15 to 20 percent of users show direct evidence of vitamin B$_6$ deficiency.

FENFLURAMINE HYDROCHLORIDE

DRUG FAMILY: Appetite suppressant

BRAND NAME: Pondimin

HOW TO TAKE FENFLURAMINE HYDROCHLORIDE: Before meals

FOODS TO AVOID: None

POSSIBLE SIDE EFFECTS: Deficiencies of vitamins A, D, E, and K

ACTION OF FENFLURAMINE HYDROCHLORIDE: Fenfluramine is prescribed as an appetite suppressant for the treatment of obesity.

HIGH-RISK GROUPS: Hypertensives, heart patients

NUTRITIONAL INTERACTIONS

FAT-SOLUBLE VITAMIN DEFICIENCY: The most effective appetite suppressant, fenfluramine does not have the same side effects as other amphetamine-like compounds. It is a sedative rather than a central nervous system stimulant.

However, fenfluramine may impair your absorption of fats, which can in turn lead to greasy diarrhea and to the malabsorption of fat-soluble vitamins. Although unlikely, this could cause mild deficiencies in vitamins A, D, E, and K if the drug is used over a period of several months. Because of its addictive tendencies, fenfluramine should not be prescribed for long periods.

Prevention and Treatment: To avoid a fat-soluble vitamin deficiency, take a vitamin supplement containing the Recommended Dietary Allowance of these vitamins, and balance your diet with foods rich in vitamins A, D, E, and K. (See tables of Vitamin A-, D-, E-, and K-Rich Foods, pages 308, 313, 314, 315.)

WEIGHT-REDUCTION PROGRAMS: Fenfluramine is addictive and should be used only as a short-term aid to weight loss. A reasonable and moderate weight reduction program should aim at a manageable 1 or 2 pound loss per week. An intake reduction of 500 calories per day, for a weekly total of 3,500 calories, will result in the loss of 1 pound per week, regardless of your present weight. Two eggs and a milk shake, 1½ cups of tuna salad, 4 ounces of a roast, 3 frankfurters, 2 cups of ice cream, or 2 pieces of cheesecake all represent approximately 500 calories.

The Weight Watchers exercise and behavior modification program is among those that offer a sensible balance of proper nutrition, exercise, and support in making a dietary change.

OTHER ADVICE: Use of this drug should be avoided when you are taking blood-pressure-lowering drugs, since fenfluramine lowers blood pressure as well, increasing the risk of extremely low blood pressure. The most likely symptom of this is dizziness when you stand up.

FERROUS SUPPLEMENTS

DRUG FAMILY: Mineral supplements

BRAND NAMES: [GENERIC/Brand] FERROUS FUMARATE/Cevi-Fer; Chromagen; Feostat; Ferancee; Ferancee-HP; Ferro-Sequels; Fetrin; Hemocyte; Hemocyte-F; Hemo-Vite; Ircon-FA; Natalins Rx; Natalins; Poly-Vi-Flor 1.0 mg Vitamins w/ Iron & Fluoride; Pramilet FA; Prenate 90; Stuartinic; Trinsicon/Trinsicon M; Zenate; FERROUS GLUCONATE/Albafort; Fergon; Ferralet; Fosfree; Glytinic; I.L.X. B_{12}; Iromin-G; Megadose; Mission Prenatal; Mission Prenatal F.A.; Mission Prenatal H.P.; Mission Pre-Surgical; FERROUS SULFATE/Dayalets plus Iron; Eldec; Feosol; Fermalox; Fero-Folic-500; Fero-Grad-500; Fero-Gradumet; Ferrous Sulfate; Heptuna Plus; Iberet; Iberet-500; Iberet-Folic-500; Irospan; Mevanin-C; Pramet FA

HOW TO TAKE FERROUS COMPOUNDS: At mealtimes with fruit juice

FOODS TO AVOID: Do not take the supplement at a meal containing whole grain foods, eggs, tea, or significant quantities of dairy products.

POSSIBLE SIDE EFFECTS: Gastrointestinal distress

ACTION OF FERROUS COMPOUNDS: These mineral supplements are used to treat iron deficiency anemia.

HIGH-RISK GROUPS: Anyone who takes this drug

NUTRITIONAL INTERACTIONS

IRON ABSORPTION: The absorption of iron supplements is decreased by antacids and by foods rich in phosphates and fiber, while vitamin C and foods rich in vitamin C such as citrus fruit juices enhance absorption.

Prevention and Treatment: You should not take iron supplements with antacids, but rather should take them at mealtimes, preferably with a vitamin C-rich fruit juice or with milk. Foods rich in phosphate (chocolate, cocoa, dried beans and peas, dried fruit, nuts, peanut butter, and whole grains) should not be taken at the same time as the iron supplement. Nor should you take iron supplements with foods rich in fiber, such as oatmeal and other whole grain cereals.

If you take a vitamin C supplement regularly, take it with the ferrous supplement.

GASTROINTESTINAL DISTRESS: Iron supplements are gastrointestinal irritants and can cause stomach discomfort, nausea, diarrhea, and constipation.

Prevention and Treatment: These supplements should always be taken with meals.

FLUOROURACIL

DRUG FAMILY: Anti-cancer

BRAND NAME: Adrucil

HOW TO TAKE FLUOROURACIL: Injection

FOODS TO AVOID: Fatty foods, spicy foods, alcoholic beverages, strong tea, coffee, cola beverages, and chocolate

POSSIBLE SIDE EFFECTS: Nausea, vomiting, impaired taste, mouth sores, poor appetite, and a much-reduced capacity to digest and absorb all foods

ACTION OF FLUOROURACIL: This drug is prescribed as an anti-cancer agent to prevent the cancer cells from dividing.

HIGH-RISK GROUPS: Anyone who takes this drug

NUTRITIONAL INTERACTIONS

DIGESTIVE DIFFICULTIES: Because fluorouracil prevents the synthesis of new cells, areas of the body that continuously need to be repaired are likely to show signs of wear and tear soon after you start taking this drug. The surface of the tongue becomes very sore and smooth due to the atrophy of the surface structures. The lining of the intestine, which is replaced every 3 days in a healthy system, becomes sore and thin, and atrophies as the old cells wear out and are not replaced by new ones. Since these are the cells that produce digestive enzymes, their loss results in diarrhea, and an inability to digest and absorb food.

The two nutrients most affected seem to be protein and glucose, although fluorouracil also directly impairs the activity of thiamin. The inability to absorb protein will further damage the body's ability to replace worn-out tissues, and thus worsen the condition of the intestinal lining.

The lack of glucose absorption will increase body protein losses. You need 100 to 125 grams of glucose per day in order to supply the brain and other tissues with the glucose they require to carry out their normal functions. If this is not supplied, due to a dietary deficiency or an inability to absorb glucose, then the body breaks down muscle and converts it to glucose. This, of course, weakens the body still further.

Prevention and Treatment: Patients in a poor nutritional state should not be given fluorouracil, since it will worsen their degree of undernutrition. A supplement supplying the Recommended Dietary Allowances of both vitamins and minerals will compensate for some of the dietary nutrients malabsorbed but cannot overcome the problem of protein deficiency.

Because of the malabsorption problems with fluorouracil, a large amount of malabsorbed nutrients remain in the intestine, even at the level of the large intestine, where they provide an excellent breeding ground for intestinal bacteria. These bacteria increase the problem of diarrhea even further.

Patients in this situation shoud consume a fairly bland diet. This means avoiding pepper, chili powder, cocoa, cola beverages, coffee (caffeinated and decaffeinated), alcohol, and tea, as well as anything else that they normally find difficult to digest. However, if weight loss is continuous, they should be fed by tube a solution containing a mixture of the essential amino acids and other nutrients. If this is not well tolerated, they should be fed intravenously.

GASTROINTESTINAL DISTRESS: Fluorouracil is likely to cause nausea, vomiting, impaired taste, mouth sores, and anorexia.

Prevention and Treatment: Nausea and vomiting may be controlled by taking several basic steps. First, you should eat smaller meals and limit your intake of high-fat foods. Second, when experiencing nausea, you should slowly sip clear beverages, such as ginger ale. Sucking a Popsicle may also alleviate the condition. You should lie down, loosen your clothes, and get fresh air by lying by an open window.

If you find that you vomit frequently, you should take plenty of liquids to prevent dehydration.

FLURAZEPAM HYDROCHLORIDE

DRUG FAMILY: Sleeping pills

BRAND NAME: Dalmane

HOW TO TAKE FLURAZEPAM HYDROCHLORIDE: At bedtime, with a full glass of water or fruit juice and a snack

FOODS TO AVOID: All alcoholic beverages

POSSIBLE SIDE EFFECTS: Nausea, vomiting, stomachache, and diarrhea

ACTION OF FLURAZEPAM HYDROCHLORIDE: This drug is used in the treatment of all kinds of insomnia.

HIGH-RISK GROUPS: Heavy drinkers

NUTRITIONAL INTERACTIONS

REDUCED REACTION TIME: Flurazepam hydrochloride is likely to cause varying degrees of light-headedness, lassitude, increased reaction time, inability to move in a coordinated fashion, and confusion. All of these effects impair driving skills. The drug also causes slurred speech and a dry mouth. When it is taken immediately before a full night's sleep these effects may not be noticed, but they can persist into the working hours of the next day. The concurrent use of alcohol can make these effects last up to 20 hours.

The drug also has a bitter taste.

Prevention and Treatment: You should not drive, or attempt to run machinery or perform other tasks requiring precise coordination, immediately after taking flurazepam; you should be wary of the effect it has upon you the following day as well.

The drug should not be taken concurrently with alcohol.

Flurazepam should be taken with a large volume of water or fruit juice, which will mask its bitter taste.

GASTROINTESTINAL DISTRESS: The drug also sometimes causes nausea, vomiting, stomachache, and diarrhea.

Prevention and Treatment: It should be taken with a snack to help prevent the possible gastrointestinal discomforts.

FUROSEMIDE

DRUG FAMILY: Diuretic

BRAND NAMES: Lasix; SK-Furosemide

HOW TO TAKE FUROSEMIDE: With milk or meals

FOODS TO AVOID: None

POSSIBLE SIDE EFFECTS: Deficiencies of calcium, magnesium, potassium, and zinc; gastrointestinal disturbances; rarely, gout

ACTION OF FUROSEMIDE: This diuretic increases the excretion of water and of sodium and chloride.

HIGH-RISK GROUPS: The elderly, heart patients, anyone who consumes alcohol, diabetics, vegetarians, oral contraceptive users

NUTRITIONAL INTERACTIONS

CALCIUM DEFICIENCY: Use of furosemide causes an increase in the excretion of calcium, and its long-term use could conceivably lead to a deficiency of calcium. When calcium blood levels are low, the body will take the necessary amounts of calcium from the bones, where it is stored, weakening them and making them more susceptible to fractures.

A condition called osteomalacia can result. This is more likely after middle age, since in older people the body uses dietary calcium less efficiently. Osteomalacia is a weakening of the bones as a consequence of uniform and steady calcium loss. This disease affects millions of older Americans but also many younger people. In fact, one out of every four postmenopausal women suffers from this problem. Prominent symptoms are bone pain in the back, thighs, shoulder region, or ribs; difficulty in walking; and weakness in the muscles of the legs. The condition is reversible once calcium blood levels are raised.

A prolonged period of calcium deficiency could also cause osteoporosis, another condition in which the bones are made weak and brittle. However, osteoporosis, an unexplained and rapid loss of calcium from the bones, is irreversible. Here the first symptoms are backache, a gradual loss of weight, and periodontal disease. In cases of osteoporosis, fractures of the vertebrae, hip, and wrist occur frequently, sometimes spontaneously.

Roughly 7 percent of women fifty years of age and older have osteoporosis, and certain observers believe that the incidence of this disease is on the rise; between 15 and 20 million Americans are said to have osteoporosis today. In some 30 percent of people over sixty-five, the disease is severe enough to result in fractures. By age eighty, virtually all women experience some degree of osteoporosis; early menopause is a strong predictor of the disease. One out of five cases of the disease is found in men, but generally men get it at a later age and less severely than women.

Prevention and Treatment: The Recommended Dietary Allowance for calcium is 800 mg, and all women should consume at least 1,200 mg of calcium per day. The average intake in the United States, however, is only 450 to 550 mg. For the elderly, and women who have already reached menopause or are about to, this should be increased to 1,500 mg by the consumption of foods rich in calcium, particularly milk and dairy products (including yogurt and hard cheeses) and, to a lesser extent, almonds. Three 8-ounce glasses of milk, for example, provide 1,500 mg of calcium. (See table of Calcium-Rich Foods, page 289.)

If calcium foods must be avoided because of an intolerance to lactose, the sugar found in dairy products (a problem for an estimated 30 million Americans), a 1,000 mg daily supplement of calcium should be taken. The best-absorbed supplement is calcium carbonate. (See Calcium Supplements entry page 51.) If magnesium is included in the supplement, the calcium is slightly better absorbed, and any tendency to constipation is reduced. The supplement should be taken in two 500 mg dosages, one of which should be consumed before bedtime because most of the calcium loss from your body occurs while you sleep.

Keep in mind that cigarette smoking leads to loss of body calcium, as does excessive alcohol consumption. On the other hand, vitamin C assists calcium absorption.

Foods that can decrease the absorption of calcium should be temporarily restricted, such as kale, rhubarb, spinach, cocoa, chocolate, beet greens, tea, and coffee. A deficiency might also arise if the ratio of phosphorus to calcium in your diet is very high; processed foods, especially most carbonated beverages, are particularly high in phosphorus. The ideal ratio is essentially 1 to 1, as in dairy products; when the ratio is 15 or 20 to 1, as in meat, very little calcium is absorbed. High-fiber foods may contribute to a calcium deficiency, since fiber binds to calcium and passes it out in the stool. Excess fat and protein in the diet also hinder absorption.

People who take magnesium- or aluminum-based antacids are also more prone to calcium deficiencies, because both magnesium and aluminum in excess impair calcium absorption. Since there is little calcium in strict vegetarian diets (those that avoid dairy products as well as meat), vegetarians are also at greater risk of a calcium deficiency.

Besides a change in dietary habits and the use of calcium supplements, it is recommended that anyone at risk of this deficiency adopt an exercise regimen that causes the bones to support the weight of the body, to strengthen the bones and to counteract the loss of bone density. A regular walking or jogging program, for example, can help prevent the bone degeneration of the spine, hips, and legs. Note, however, that swimming, though good for the heart as an aerobic exercise, is not especially beneficial for bone buildup.

It has been observed that oral contraceptives seem to help calcium absorption, and, that during pregnancy the body absorbs calcium more effectively, making the mother's bones actually stronger despite the calcium needs of the fetus.

MAGNESIUM DEFICIENCY: Furosemide causes increased excretion of magnesium, and it is conceivable that its use will lead to a deficiency if it is taken over prolonged periods of time, especially in elderly patients with congestive heart disease who are anorexic.

Muscle weakness, tremors, depression, emotional instability, and irrational behavior are among the clinical signs of a magnesium deficiency. Alcohol also depletes magnesium.

Prevention and Treatment: A diet containing the four food groups provides the normal amount of magnesium. However, if a magnesium depletion is suspected, your diet should feature foods such as nuts (almonds and cashews are highest), meat, fish, milk, whole grains, and fresh greens, since cooking can wash away some magnesium. (See table of Magnesium-Rich Foods, page 300.) Since alcohol provokes magnesium excretion, its intake should be restricted to no more than two drinks per day while you are on furosemide.

POTASSIUM DEFICIENCY: An increase in the excretion of potassium also occurs with furosemide use, and in the long term it is conceivable that it will lead to a potassium deficiency.

Potassium regulates the amount of water in the cells of the body, and is essential for the proper functioning of the kidneys and the heart muscle, and the secretion of stomach juices. The most alarming symptom of a potassium deficiency is an irregular heartbeat, which can lead to heart failure.

Low blood serum levels of potassium, called hypokalemia, are associated with laxative abuse, because many laxatives promote an increased loss of potassium in the gastrointestinal tract. This risk is especially high in elderly patients who consume diets low in potassium.

People who take the laxatives phenolphthalein, bisacodyl, and senna on a daily basis have been reported to have a much greater chance of experiencing serious hypokalemia. These people, and others with a potassium deficiency, may have such symptoms as weakness, loss of appetite, nausea, vomiting, dryness of the mouth, increased thirst, listlessness, apprehension, and diffuse pain that comes and goes.

Proper potassium levels in your body can also be threatened if this drug is taken concurrently with cortisone-containing drugs.

Prevention and Treatment: Potassium depletion can be avoided by including such potassium-rich foods in your diet as tomato juice, lentils, dried apricots, asparagus, bananas, peanut butter, chicken, almonds, and milk. (See table of Potassium-Rich Foods, page 302.)

Potassium supplements should never be taken unless prescribed by a physician. They can cause anemia by interfering with the absorption of vitamin B_{12}. Just a few grams can also drastically increase the risk of heart failure. If you experience difficulty in swallowing while taking potassium supplements, consult your physician immediately. If supplements are prescribed, be aware that the absorption of the supplements potassium iodide and potassium chloride is decreased by dairy products, and that both are gastric irritants and should be taken with meals.

Too much salt in your diet can also compromise your body's supply of potassium, as can 1 to 3 ounces per day of licorice candy made from natural extract. Usually only imported licorice contains the natural product; check the package.

ZINC DEFICIENCY: Zinc, too, is excreted at a more rapid rate if you are taking furosemide; thus long-term use of this drug could conceivably lead to a deficiency of this mineral.

A shortage of zinc in your system may result in impaired healing of wounds and ulcers, scaly dry skin of the face and limbs, and anorexia associated with the loss of taste.

Prevention and Treatment: Patients using this drug should be sure to get the Recommended Dietary Allowance of zinc. Animal foods are good sources, with the richest being oysters, herring, milk, and egg yolks. Among plant foods, whole grains are richest in zinc, but it is not as well absorbed from them as from meat. Fiber and phytic acid in the cereal grains hinder its absorption. The recommended intake of 15 mg a day for adults is usually easily met by the diet of the average middle-class person, but deficiencies are more likely if animal protein is underemphasized. As a rule of thumb, two small servings of animal protein a day will provide sufficient zinc.

OTHER ADVICE: This drug sometimes causes gastrointestinal disturbances and should be taken with milk or food if such discomfort occurs. It may also precipitate gout in susceptible people.

GENTAMICIN SULFATE

DRUG FAMILY: Antibiotic

BRAND NAME: Garamycin

HOW TO TAKE GENTAMICIN: Injection

FOODS TO AVOID: None

POSSIBLE SIDE EFFECTS: Potassium and magnesium deficiencies

ACTION OF GENTAMICIN: This potent antibiotic is used only in the treatment of life-threatening infections that cannot be effectively treated with other agents.

HIGH-RISK GROUPS: The elderly, anyone who consumes alcohol

NUTRITIONAL INTERACTIONS

POTASSIUM DEFICIENCY: Gentamicin sulfate damages the kidneys, which could conceivably lead to the loss of abnormally high amounts of potassium and magnesium in the urine, and to a deficiency of the two nutrients. Potassium regulates the amount of water in the cells of the body, and is essential for the proper functioning of the kidneys, and the heart muscle, and the secretion of stomach juices. The most alarming symptom of a potassium deficiency is an irregular heartbeat, which can lead to heart failure.

Low blood serum levels of potassium, called hypokalemia, are associated with laxative abuse, because many laxatives promote an increased loss of potassium in the gastrointestinal tract.

People who take laxatives on a daily basis, as many elderly people do, have a much greater chance of developing serious hypokalemia. These people, and others with a potassium deficiency, may have such symptoms as weakness, loss of appetite, nausea, vomiting, dryness of the mouth, increased thirst, listlessness, apprehension, and diffuse pain that comes and goes.

Prevention and Treatment: Potassium depletion can be avoided by including such potassium-rich foods in your diet as tomato juice, lentils, dried apricots, asparagus, bananas, peanut butter, chicken, almonds, and milk. (See table of Potassium-Rich Foods, page 302.)

Diuretics, commonly prescribed for people with heart disease, lower the level of body potassium. Therefore, the risk of a deficiency is significantly increased if diuretics are taken concurrently with this drug.

Potassium supplements may be necessary but should not be taken except under the supervision of a physician. They can cause anemia by interfering with the absorption of vitamin B_{12}. Just a few grams can also drastically increase the risk of heart failure. If you experience difficulty in swallowing while taking potassium supplements, consult your physician immediately. If supplements are prescribed, be aware that the absorption of the supplements potassium iodide and potassium chloride is decreased by dairy products, and that both are gastric irritants and should be taken with meals.

MAGNESIUM DEFICIENCY: Magnesium deficiencies are not common because the average American diet contains appreciable amounts of magnesium. However, given the effects of gentamicin sulfate, it is conceivable that you will develop such a deficiency, especially if you drink alcohol-containing beverages on a regular basis, since these deplete body magnesium.

Clinical signs of magnesium deficiency include muscle weakness, tremors, depression, emotional instability, and irrational behavior.

Prevention and Treatment: A diet containing the four food groups provides the normal amount of magnesium. However, if a magnesium depletion is suspected, your diet should feature foods such as nuts (almonds and cashews are highest), meat, fish, milk, whole grains, and fresh greens, since cooking can wash away some magnesium. (See table of Magnesium-Rich Foods, page 300.)

GLUTETHIMIDE

DRUG FAMILY: Anti-anxiety

BRAND NAME: Doriden

HOW TO TAKE GLUTETHIMIDE: At meals

FOODS TO AVOID: Sweet, sticky foods

POSSIBLE SIDE EFFECTS: Vitamin D deficiency; dry mouth; constipation

ACTION OF GLUTETHIMIDE: This drug decreases anxiety and tension. It can also provide protection against motion sickness, in part by inhibiting salivary secretion and intestinal motility.

HIGH-RISK GROUPS: The elderly

NUTRITIONAL INTERACTIONS

VITAMIN D DEFICIENCY: Glutethimide accelerates the rate at which the liver breaks down vitamin D, permitting it to be excreted before it is fully effective. This can lead to a vitamin D deficiency if glutethimide is used for extended periods.

Vitamin D is needed for the body to absorb calcium and phosphorus, to promote the development of strong teeth and bones. Whenever calcium blood levels are low, the body will liberate the calcium it needs from the bones, where it is stored. The result is osteomalacia, a condition in which the bones are weakened, in severe cases to the degree that they will fracture easily. Prominent symptoms are bone pain in the back, thighs, shoulder region, or ribs; difficulty in walking; and weakness in the muscles of the legs.

The condition is reversible once calcium blood levels are raised.

Long-term losses of calcium may also lead to osteoporosis, another condition where the bones are weakened and made brittle. Osteoporosis, an unexplained and sudden loss of calcium from the bones, is irreversible. The common symptoms are backache, a gradual loss of height, and periodontal disease. Fractures of the vertebrae, hip, and wrist occur, sometimes spontaneously.

Prevention and Treatment: To avoid a vitamin D deficiency while on this drug, you should take 400 to 800 IU of vitamin D per day as a supplement to a diet of foods rich in the vitamin, such as fortified milk, butter, liver, egg yolks, salmon, tuna, and sardines. (See table of Vitamin D-Rich Foods, page 313.)

Vitamin D is initially formed in the skin by exposure to sunlight and activated in the kidneys and liver. The production of vitamin D is dependent upon climatic conditions, air pollution, skin pigmentation (the darker the skin, the lower the production), the area of skin exposed, the duration of exposure to the sun, and the use of sun screens. Adults who are not often exposed to sunlight (e.g. those who are housebound or by custom heavily clothed), require dietary sources of vitamin D to prevent osteomalacia.

In adults, 2,000 IU of the vitamin should be taken if osteomalacia is indicated. If your intake of vitamin D exceeds 4,000 IU per day, vitamin D poisoning can occur. The symptoms are loss of appetite, headache, excessive thirst, irritability, and kidney stones.

If dairy products must be avoided because you have an intolerance to lactose (the sugar present in dairy products), a 1,200 to 1,500 mg daily supplement of calcium should be taken. (See Calcium Supplements entry page 51.)

OTHER PROBLEMS: By decreasing salivary activity, glutethimide can make you more susceptible to dental cavities. As a result, you should avoid sweet, sticky foods, and strict attention shoud be paid to oral hygiene.

This drug should also be taken at meals to avoid stomach and intestinal distress.

Glutethimide can also cause constipation. Constipation is usually safely remedied by an increase in the bulk in the diet. This means consuming larger servings of any of the following: dried fruits, fresh fruits, salad vegetables, cooked vegetables, and whole grain foods (brown rice, whole wheat breads, and cereals). It is not necessary to purchase products that claim "extra fiber" has been added to them.

Persistent constipation may also be relieved by doubling the amount of fluid consumed each day. Wheat bran, if used, should be added to the diet gradually, and fluid should be increased by at least ¾ cup per teaspoon of bran. (See table of Dietary Fiber-Rich Foods, page 293.)

GRISEOFULVIN

DRUG FAMILY: Anti-fungal

BRAND NAMES: Fulvicin P/G; Fulvicin P/G 165 & 330; Fulvicin-U/F; Grifulvin V; Grisactin; Gris-PEG

HOW TO TAKE GRISEOFULVIN: At midday, with a meal that contains fatty foods such as meat sandwiches, hamburgers, milk, ice cream, pizza, nuts, and fried foods

FOODS TO AVOID: None

POSSIBLE SIDE EFFECTS: Poor sense of taste

ACTION OF GRISEOFULVIN: This drug is used against superficial fungal infections of the hair, skin, and nails.

HIGH-RISK GROUPS: Anyone who takes this drug

NUTRITIONAL INTERACTIONS

WEIGHT LOSS: Griseofulvin alters taste sensation and decreases the appreciation of food. You could conceivably find that this tends to reduce the amount of food you eat and that weight loss will result.

Prevention and Treatment: Very flavorful foods should be included in your diet to limit the possible effects of a reduced sense of taste and appetite.

OTHER ADVICE: Griseofulvin is best absorbed at midday, and its absorption is also enhanced by a high fat intake. Thus, you would be well advised to take it at lunch with a meal that contains considerable amounts of fat: meat sandwiches, hamburgers, milk, ice cream, pizza, nuts, or fried foods.

The drug is likely to be poorly absorbed by your body if taken in the morning, and a fatty breakfast will only marginally improve its absorption. In the evening it is not well absorbed, and dietary fat will not facilitate its absorption significantly at the evening meal.

People with gallbladder disease should not take this medication, since it appears to cause gallbladder contraction and severe abdominal pain in such patients.

GUANETHIDINE MONOSULFATE AND GUANETHIDINE SULFATE

DRUG FAMILY: Anti-hypertensive

BRAND NAMES: [GENERIC/Brand] GUANETH-IDINE MONOSULFATE/Esimil; GUANETHI-DINE SULFATE/Ismelin

HOW TO TAKE GUANETHIDINE: With meals or milk

FOODS TO AVOID: Alcoholic beverages

POSSIBLE SIDE EFFECTS: Fainting spells; gastrointestinal distress

ACTION OF GUANETHIDINE: This drug is prescribed in the treatment of high blood pressure. It is one of the most potent of the anti-hypertensive agents.

HIGH-RISK GROUPS: Anyone who consumes alcohol

NUTRITIONAL INTERACTIONS

LOW BLOOD PRESSURE: Fainting spells could conceivably occur while you are taking this drug, particularly if you stand up quickly. The cause is low blood pressure. This reaction seems to be accentuated by alcohol.

Prevention and Treatment: Alcohol, which has a potent vasodilation effect of its own, shoud not be consumed concurrently with guanethidine. A glass (6 ounces) of sherry or 10 ounces of table wine will significantly dilate the blood vessels for 4 hours and tend to lower blood pressure.

OTHER ADVICE: Guanethidine also causes gastrointestinal disturbances and should be taken with meals or milk.

HALOPERIDOL

DRUG FAMILY: Anti-psychotic; anti-hyperactive

BRAND NAME: Haldol

HOW TO TAKE HALOPERIDOL: As directed by your physician

FOODS TO AVOID: All alcoholic beverages

POSSIBLE SIDE EFFECTS: Impaired mental and physical ability, and loss of appetite

ACTION OF HALOPERIDOL: This tranquilizer is used to sedate psychotic patients and also in the short-term treatment of severely hyperactive children who show conduct disorders.

HIGH-RISK GROUPS: Heavy drinkers

NUTRITIONAL INTERACTIONS

ALCOHOL INTERACTION: Alcohol taken concurrently with haloperidol increases the sedative effect of the drug and is also likely to lead to hypotension. Loss of appetite is also a common side effect of the drug.

Prevention and Treatment: You should not consume alcohol while taking haloperidol. You should also carefully monitor your weight to avoid unwanted weight loss.

OTHER ADVICE: This drug is likely to impair the mental and/or physical ability required for the performance of hazardous tasks such as driving a car and operating machinery. While you are on haloperidol you should take care to avoid such situations.

HEPARIN

DRUG FAMILY: Anti-coagulant

BRAND NAMES: Heparin Sodium; Hep-Lock; Hep-Lock PF; Calciparine

HOW TO TAKE HEPARIN: Injection

FOODS TO AVOID: Alcoholic beverages

POSSIBLE SIDE EFFECTS: Vitamin K deficiency

ACTION OF HEPARIN: Commonly referred to as a blood thinner, heparin decreases the rate at which blood clots; it is taken by arteriosclerosis patients whose blood tends to clot more readily than normal—a condition that can lead to the blockage of blood vessels. If this happens in the brain or heart, a stroke or heart attack will occur.

HIGH-RISK GROUPS: The elderly, pregnant women, heavy drinkers.

NUTRITIONAL INTERACTIONS

VITAMIN K DEFICIENCY: An improper balance of this drug and vitamin K in the body can cause interrelated problems. Heparin can prevent vitamin K from producing blood-clotting substances in the liver, but a diet that features excessive amounts of vitamin K-rich foods can actually reduce the effectiveness of the drug.

People with an abnormally low dietary intake of vitamin K should be careful regarding long-term use of heparin, because they run the risk of easy hemorrhaging. Bleeding may take place in the gastrointestinal tract (causing black or blood-stained stools), in the urinary tract (causing blood in the urine), and in the uterus (causing blood loss at times other than the normal menstrual periods). Excessive blood loss may occur from an injury or surgery. Another sign of a deficiency of this vitamin is more frequent and more visible bruising than normal.

Half the vitamin K in humans comes from dietary sources: predominantly green leafy vegetables, and to a lesser extent fruit, cereals, dairy products, and meat. The rest of the vitamin K in our bodies is synthesized by the bacteria in the intestines. The daily need for the vitamin is in the range of 70 to 140 mcg.

Newborn babies have negligible amounts of vitamin K in their bodies, since they do not have a bacterial population in the large intestine to help make vitamin K and do not develop the capacity to do so for the first week of life. Consequently, most newborns are given vitamin K shots at birth. Heparin is the drug of choice for pregnant women, since it does not pass into the fetus and hence does not effect its vitamin K status.

Women who have had several pregnancies or whose menstrual periods are heavy should also be careful. Many elderly people are also at risk of a vitamin K deficiency because they have a problem of poor fat absorption, and vitamin K, a fat-soluble vitamin, must be accompanied by sufficient dietary fat to be properly absorbed.

Remember, however, that although heparin can prevent vitamin K from producing blood-clotting substances in the liver, a diet that features excessive amounts of vitamin K-rich foods can actually threaten the effectiveness of the drug.

Prevention and Treatment: A vitamin K deficiency can be countered by a vitamin K supplement of 100 mcg per day and a diet that includes foods rich in the vitamin, such as kale, spinach, cabbage, cauliflower, leafy green vegetables, liver (especially pork liver), and fish. (See table of Vitamin K-Rich Foods, page 315.) Pregnant women on this drug should take 5 mg of vitamin K per day for 3 days prior to anticipated delivery—but only under the guidance of a physician—to reduce blood losses at delivery.

Vitamin E supplements should not be taken when at risk of a vitamin K shortage, because vitamin E impairs the absorption of this vitamin.

OTHER ADVICE: Do not drink alcohol concurrently with this medication. Alcohol and heparin are broken down in the liver by the same mechanism. If there is a high level of alcohol present, it is likely that less of the drug will be broken down. Hence, higher levels of this anti-coagulant will build up in the body, which can be extremely dangerous since it can lead to hemorrhaging.

HYDRALAZINE

DRUG FAMILY: Anti-hypertensive

BRAND NAMES: [GENERIC/Brand] HYDRALAZINE/ H-H-R; Hydralazine-Thiazide; Hydralazine w/Hydrochlorothiazide; HYDRALAZINE HYDROCHLORIDE/Apresazide; Apresoline Hydrochloride; Apresoline-Esidrix; Hydralazine Hydrochloride; Hydrochlorothiazide, Hydralazine Hydrochloride, Reserpine; Ser-Ap-Es; Serpasil-Apresoline; Unipres

HOW TO TAKE HYDRALAZINE: With meals or milk

FOODS TO AVOID: Foods rich in tyramine or dopamine should not be eaten in large quantities. These include aged cheeses, raisins, avocados, liver, bananas, eggplant, sour cream, salami, meat tenderizers, yeast, soy sauce, chocolate, and alcoholic beverages; licorice candy made from natural extract should also be avoided.

POSSIBLE SIDE EFFECTS: Vitamin B_6 deficiency; loss of appetite, nausea

ACTION OF HYDRALAZINE: This drug relaxes the muscles in the walls of the blood vessels and reduces blood pressure. It is prescribed for long-term treatment of high blood pressure.

HIGH-RISK GROUPS: Heavy drinkers, users of oral contraceptives, smokers, the elderly

NUTRITIONAL INTERACTIONS

VITAMIN B_6 DEFICIENCY: Hydralazine causes an increase in the excretion of vitamin B_6, so users are likely to experience a deficiency. Common symptoms of this deficiency are a sore mouth and tongue, cracks in the lips and corners of the mouth, and patches of itching, scaling skin. A severe vitamin B_6 deficiency may cause depression and confusion.

Vitamin B_6 deficiencies are common among the elderly. Alcoholics, as well, often experience this deficiency, since alcohol interferes with the body's ability to use B_6. It is estimated that one of every two Americans consumes less than 70 percent of the Recommended Dietary Allowance of B_6. Smokers tend to have lower body levels of this vitamin than nonsmokers. Oral contraceptive users sometimes show signs of vitamin B$_6$ deficiency.

Prevention and Treatment: To avoid a B$_6$ deficiency, you should consume a diet featuring such food sources of vitamin B$_6$ as liver (beef, calf, and pork), herring, salmon, walnuts, peanuts, wheat germ, carrots, peas, potatoes, grapes, bananas, and yeast. (See table of Vitamin B$_6$(Pyridoxine)-Rich Foods, page 311.) The vitamin is present in significant amounts in meats, fish, fruits, cereals, and vegetables, and to a lesser extent in milk and other dairy products.

Since vitamin B$_6$ is decomposed at high temperatures, modern food processing often diminishes dietary sources of the vitamin. Consequently, the more processed foods you eat, the more susceptible you will be to a deficiency of this vitamin. The same losses also occur in cooking: meat loses as much as 45 to 80 percent, vegetables 20 to 30 percent.

If you show signs of a B$_6$ deficiency, you should take 25 to 100 mg of vitamin B$_6$ per day at a time of day other than when the drug is taken. However, keep in mind that you can take too much vitamin B$_6$; people taking over 1 gram per day have been reported to experience nerve degeneration.

TYRAMINE-RICH FOODS: Foods that are high in tyramines elevate blood pressure when consumed in quantity and make this drug less effective.

Prevention and Treatment: Tyramine-containing foods must be restricted while you are being treated with hydralazine. Tyramine is common in many foods, but it is found in the greatest amount in high-protein foods that have undergone some decomposition, like aged cheese. Tyramine is also found in chicken and beef livers, bananas, eggplant, sour cream, alcoholic beverages, salami, meat tenderizers, chocolate, yeast, and soy sauce. (See table of Tyramine-Rich Foods, page 307.) Raisins and avocados should also be avoided, because they contain dopamine, which has the same effect as tyramine.

Licorice candy made with natural extract contains glycyrrhizic acid, which also can elevate blood pressure by causing sodium and water retention. As little as 3 ounces is enough to induce such a reaction, so it is best to avoid eating licorice when taking this drug. Only imported licorice is usually made with natural extract, and it is unusual in the case of domestic products. However, check the package.

OTHER ADVICE: Hydralazine is likely to cause a loss of appetite and nausea. The drug should always be taken with meals or milk to minimize the discomfort. Doing so will also improve the drug's absorption.

Careful attention should be paid to body weight and appetite while taking this drug, to avoid unwanted weight loss.

HYDROCODONE

DRUG FAMILY: Cough medicine

BRAND NAMES: [GENERIC/Brand] HYDROCODONE BITARTRATE/ Amacodone; Bancap HC; Citra Forte; Codiclear DH; Codimal DH; Co-Gesic; Damacet-P; Damason-P; Detussin; Di-Gesic; Donatussin DC; Duradyne DHC; Entuss; Hycodan; Hycodaphen; Hycomine; Hyco-Pap; Hycotuss; Hydrocodone; P-V-Tussin; Ru-Tuss; S-T Forte; Tussend; Vicodin; HYDROCODONE RESIN COMPLEX/Tussionex

HOW TO TAKE HYDROCODONE: At mealtimes

FOODS TO AVOID: None

POSSIBLE SIDE EFFECTS: Nausea and constipation

ACTION OF HYDROCODONE: This medication is used to treat coughing. A dose of this agent is effective for 12 hours.

HIGH-RISK GROUPS: The elderly

NUTRITIONAL INTERACTIONS

GASTROINTESTINAL DISTRESS: You could conceivably experience nausea or mild constipation while taking hydrocodone. Since the elderly are more prone to constipation, this side effect is more likely to occur among older consumers of this drug.

Prevention and Treatment: In order to avoid nausea, the drug should be taken at mealtimes.

Constipation is usually safely remedied by an increase in the bulk in the diet. This means consuming larger servings of any of the following: dried or fresh fruits (especially unpeeled apples or pears), salad vegetables, radishes, oatmeal, and whole grain foods (brown rice, whole wheat breads, and cereals). It is not necessary to purchase products that claim "extra fiber" has been added to them.

Persistent constipation may also be relieved by doubling the amount of fluid consumed each day. Bran, if used, should be added to the diet gradually, and fluid should be increased by at least ¾ cup per teaspoon of bran. (See table of Dietary Fiber-Rich Foods, page 293.)

IBUPROFEN

DRUG FAMILY: Analgesic

BRAND NAMES: Motrin; Rufen

HOW TO TAKE IBUPROFEN: With meals or milk

FOODS TO AVOID: None

POSSIBLE SIDE EFFECTS: Nausea, stomachache, heartburn, sensation of fullness

ACTION OF IBUPROFEN: This analgesic is used in the treatment of rheumatoid arthritis and osteoarthritis. It can also be used for mild to moderate pain caused by other ailments, and is especially effective in treating the pain of dysmenorrhea (the pain in the back and lower abdomen associated with menstruation).

HIGH-RISK GROUPS: Anyone who takes this drug

NUTRITIONAL INTERACTIONS

GASTROINTESTINAL DISTRESS: Side effects of this drug may include nausea, stomach pain, heartburn, abdominal discomfort, and sensations of fullness. Such symptoms occur in up to 15 percent of the people who take the drug. However, at comparable doses these effects are less acute than with aspirin or indomethacin.

Prevention and Treatment: Ibuprofen should always be taken with milk or food to reduce the gastrointestinal effects.

INDOMETHACIN

DRUG FAMILY: Anti-inflammatory

BRAND NAMES: Indocin Capsules; Indocin SR Capsules

HOW TO TAKE INDOMETHACIN: With meals or milk

FOODS TO AVOID: None

POSSIBLE SIDE EFFECTS: Iron deficiency

ACTION OF INDOMETHACIN: This anti-inflammatory drug is prescribed for patients with arthritis and related diseases.

HIGH-RISK GROUPS: The elderly, premenopausal women, vegetarians

NUTRITIONAL INTERACTIONS

IRON DEFICIENCY: Indomethacin causes gastric irritation and microscopic bleeding. Consequently, iron in the blood is lost, and it is conceivable that, while you are on this drug, you will experience an iron deficiency. Iron is important to the oxygen-carrying cells of the blood and muscles, which use two thirds of the iron your body needs. Thus, an iron shortage reduces the blood's oxygen-carrying capacity, and the result is an anemia signaled by such symptoms as tiredness, general feelings of malaise, irritability, decreased attention span, pale complexion, rapid heart rhythm, headaches, loss of concentration, and breathlessness on exertion. A mild iron deficiency will also impair the functioning of your immune system.

For iron to be absorbed from any vegetable source, it must first be converted to another form by the action of the hydrochloric acid produced in the stomach. Many elderly people secrete less hydrochloric acid than normal, so they absorb iron poorly even under normal circumstances. The diets of many Americans lack adequate quantities of this mineral for their normal needs. For example, 10 percent of American women suffer from an iron deficiency, and up to 30 percent have inadequate iron stores. Other people who are at significant risk of an iron deficiency are women who have had several pregnancies and those whose menstrual periods are heavy. The shortage of iron in many diets is due not only to the selection of foods that are poor sources of the mineral, but also to the switch from cast-iron cookware to aluminum, stainless steel, and nonstick surfaces. The acids in food used to leach iron from iron pots and pans, and the nutrient then became available as dietary iron.

Prevention and Treatment: To counteract an iron deficiency, iron-rich foods should be included in your diet: liver, whole grain products, oysters, dried apricots, prunes, peaches, leafy green vegetables, and lean red meat. (See table of Iron-Rich Foods, page 299.)

Other foods and drugs have a considerable impact on the way your body absorbs (or does not absorb) iron. There are two kinds of iron in food sources: heme iron in meat and ionic iron in vegetables. Up to 30 percent of the iron from meat, fish, and poultry is absorbed, but less than 10 percent is absorbed from eggs, whole grains, nuts, and dried beans. Only 10 percent of ionic iron is absorbed from vegetable sources, with as little as 2 percent being absorbed from spinach. Antacids will interfere with iron absorption from vegetables, as will commercial black and pekoe tea, taken in substantial quantities, because of its tannin content. Coffee also seems to decrease iron absorption but not to the same degree as tea. Vitamin C supplements or citrus juices increase the absorption of iron from vegetable sources by two to three times if taken simultaneously.

If your diet is high in fiber-containing foods, you will have impaired iron absorption because the fiber will bind to the iron and pass it out in the stool. This same action contributes to the poor absorption of iron from vegetable sources. Foods high in phosphorus (e.g. meat) interfere with iron absorption, which explains why only 30 percent of the iron in meat is captured. (However, meat and fish facilitate iron absorption from vegetables.) For that matter, any use of large quantities of mineral supplements, such as zinc, will impair iron absorption. Because iron can be leached from vegetables if they are cooked in large amounts of water, it is preferable to steam them.

Iron supplements should not be taken without a physician's recommendation, because an accumulation of too much iron can lead in extreme cases to such serious problems as anemia, malfunctioning of the pancreas and the heart, cirrhosis of the liver, a brown cast to the skin, and depression.

OTHER ADVICE: Indomethacin should always be taken with milk, meals, or an antacid to reduce gastric irritation.

INSULIN

DRUG FAMILY: Anti-diabetic

BRAND NAMES: Humulin N; Humulin R; Novolin N; Novolin R; Novolin L; Insulatard NPH; Mixtard; NPH Iletin I; NPH Insulin; NPH Purified Pork Isophane Insulin Suspension; Regular Purified Pork Insulin; Iletin I, Lente; Iletin I, Semilente; Iletin I, Ultralente; Lente Insulin; Lente Purified Pork Insulin Zinc Suspension; Protamine, Zinc & Iletin; Semilente Insulin; Semilente Purified Pork Prompt Insulin Zinc Suspension; Ultralente Insulin; Ultralente Purified Beef Extended Insulin Zinc Suspension

HOW TO TAKE INSULIN: As directed by your physician

FOODS TO AVOID: Foods rich in animal fat and cholesterol

POSSIBLE SIDE EFFECTS: Hypoglycemia

ACTION OF INSULIN: Used to control diabetes, insulin restores the body's ability to use sugar normally by replacing the insulin that the pancreas normally produces. Insulin is also prescribed to lower blood potassium levels.

HIGH-RISK GROUPS: Anyone who takes this drug

NUTRITIONAL INTERACTIONS

HYPOGLYCEMIA AND HYPERGLYCEMIA: Diabetes occurs when the pancreas fails to produce the proper amount of insulin to clear the blood of glucose. If you are diabetic, you must match the amount of food you consume to the number of units of insulin administered.

If too little insulin is taken for a given amount of food, you will experience hyperglycemia or too much sugar in the blood. If there is insufficient insulin to allow the cells in the body to absorb glucose, the cells are starved of the energy they need. In this instance, coma can result.

If too little food is taken for a given amount of insulin, hypoglycemia—the opposite problem—will occur. Hypoglycemia is a condition in which there is too little sugar (glucose) in the blood. If your blood sugar levels drop to below 30 mg/100 ml of blood (a normal level is 100 mg/100 ml of blood), you may become mentally confused, due to a lack of glucose reaching the brain. Other early symptoms are headaches, hunger, and a general sensation resembling mild drunkenness. Below 10 mg/100 ml, you can go into a diabetic coma and, if the situation is not corrected within a few minutes, permanent brain damage may occur.

Prevention and Treatment: If you are diabetic, you must monitor your food intake to avoid an excess of carbohydrates in the form of simple sugars, such as cookies, canides, sodas, honey, and table sugar. These foods are absorbed very rapidly and will increase your blood sugar to very high levels. If you are diabetic, such high blood sugar levels are dangerous, because the insulin administered may not be sufficient to bring the levels back into the normal range. A preferred diet is low in fats but with plenty of complex carbohydrates, such as starches, cereals, and vegetables. (See table of Simple and Complex Carbohydrate Foods, page 305.)

Diabetics carry sugar cubes with them to take in the event they experience hypoglycemia.

Recent studies have demonstrated that a high-fiber diet may cause a slower and more sustained release of glucose from the gastrointestinal tract into the bloodstream, preventing the wide swings in blood sugar levels. It also increases the intestine's ability to absorb glucose. If you are diabetic, it is recommended that you remain physically active and exercise daily, because by doing so your cells are made more susceptible to insulin. Finally, a change in eating schedule from the standard three meals per day to five or six smaller meals will also help keep blood sugar levels within normal range.

ALCOHOL INTERACTION: Insulin requirements may be increased if you consume alcohol, which is a sugar and requires insulin for absorption like other sugars. However, alcohol can also lead to hypoglycemia in some people taking insulin.

Prevention and Treatment: As a diabetic, you should never forget when calculating your insulin requirements that alcohol is a sugar that contains 7 calories per gram.

ISONIAZID

DRUG FAMILY: Anti-tubercular

BRAND NAMES: INH; Rifamate

HOW TO TAKE ISONIAZID: On an empty stomach either 1 hour before or 2 to 3 hours after eating

FOODS TO AVOID: Alcoholic beverages; large quantities of foods containing tyramine, or dopamine, such as aged cheeses, raisins, avocados, liver, bananas, eggplant, sour cream, salami, meat tenderizers, yeast, and soy sauce

POSSIBLE SIDE EFFECTS: Deficiencies of calcium, vitamins B_6 and B_{12}, folic acid, niacin, magnesium

ACTION OF ISONIAZID: This drug kills the bacteria that cause tuberculosis.

HIGH-RISK GROUPS: Heavy drinkers, users of oral contraceptives, the elderly, vegetarians, children, anyone who consumes alcohol, hypertensives, smokers, teenagers

NUTRITIONAL INTERACTIONS

CALCIUM DEFICIENCY: Isoniazid decreases the absorption of calcium, and its long-term use could conceivably lead to a calcium deficiency. Whenever calcium blood levels are low, the body will liberate the necessary amounts of calcium from the bones, where it is stored, thereby weakening them and making them more susceptible to fractures. A condition called osteomalacia can result. This is more likely after middle age, since in older people the body uses dietary calcium less efficiently.

Osteomalacia is a weakening of the bones as a consequence of uniform and steady calcium loss. This disease affects millions of older Americans but also many younger people. In fact, one out of every four postmenopausal women suffers from this problem. Prominent symptoms are bone pain in the back, thighs, shoulder region, or ribs; difficulty in walking; and weakness in the muscles of the legs. The condition is reversible once calcium blood levels are raised.

Osteoporosis is another condition in which bones are made weak and brittle, and which may develop as a result of a calcium deficiency. But osteoporosis, an unexplained and rapid loss of calcium from the bones, is irreversible. Here the first symptoms are backache, a gradual loss of height, and periodontal disease. In cases of osteoporosis, fractures of the vertebrae, hip, and wrist occur frequently, sometimes spontaneously.

Approximately 7 percent of women fifty years of age and older have osteoporosis, and certain observers believe that the incidence of this disease is on the rise; between 15 and 20 million Americans are said to have osteoporosis today. In some 30 percent of people over sixty-five, the disease is severe enough to result in fractures. By age eighty, virtually all women experience some degree of osteoporosis; early menopause is a strong predictor of the disease. One out of five cases of the disease is found in men, but generally men get it at a later age and less severely than women.

If this drug is given to children, a condition known as rickets can occur. Again, the effect is on the bones, which become bent or malformed. Children under four years of age may develop pigeon breast, bowlegs, a protruding abdomen due to a weakness of stomach muscles, and poorly formed teeth that tend to decay.

Prevention and Treatment: The Recommended Dietary Allowance for calcium is 800 mg, and all women should consume at least 1,200 mg of calcium per day. The average intake in the United States, however, is only 450 to 550 mg. For the elderly, and women who have already reached menopause or are about to, this should be increased to 1,500 mg by the consumption of foods rich in calcium, particularly milk and dairy products (including yogurt and hard cheeses) and, to a lesser extent, almonds. Three 8-ounce glasses of milk, for example, provide 1,500 mg of calcium. (See table of Calcium-Rich Foods, page 289.)

If calcium foods must be avoided because of an intolerance to lactose, the sugar present in dairy products (a problem for an estimated 30 million Americans), a 1,000 mg daily supplement of calcium should be taken. The best-absorbed supplement is calcium carbonate. (See Calcium Supplements entry page 51.) If magnesium is included in the supplement, the calcium is slightly better absorbed, and any tendency to constipation is reduced. The supplement should be taken in two 500 mg doses, one of which should be consumed before bedtime, because most of the calcium loss from your body occurs while you sleep.

Keep in mind that vitamin C assists calcium absorption, while cigarette smoking tends to deplete body calcium, as does excessive alcohol consumption. Isoniazid users should temporarily avoid foods that can decrease the absorption of calcium, such as kale, rhubarb, spinach, cocoa, chocolate, beet greens, tea, and coffee. A deficiency might also arise if the ratio of phosphorus to calcium in your diet is very high; processed foods, especially carbonated beverages, are particularly high in phosophorus. The ideal ratio is essentially 1 to 1, as in dairy products; when the ratio is 15 or 20 to 1, as in meat, very little calcium is absorbed. High-fiber foods may contribute to a calcium deficiency, since fiber binds to calcium and passes it out in the stool. Excess

fat and protein in the diet also hinder absorption.

Since there is little calcium in strict vegetarian diets (those that avoid dairy products as well as meats), vegetarians are at greater risk of a calcium deficiency. People who take magnesium- or aluminum-based antacids are also more prone to calcium deficiencies, because both magnesium and aluminum in excess impair calcium absorption.

Besides a change in dietary habits and the use of calcium supplements, it is recommended that anyone at risk of this deficiency adopt an exercise regimen that causes the bones to support the weight of the body, to strengthen the bones, and to counteract the loss of bone density. A regular walking or jogging program, for example, can help prevent the bone degeneration of the spine, hips, and legs. Note, however, that swimming, though good for the heart as an aerobic exercise, is not especially beneficial for bone buildup.

It has been observed that oral contraceptives seem to help calcium absorption, and that during pregnancy the body absorbs calcium more effectively, making the mother's bones actually stronger despite the calcium needs of the fetus.

All patients taking isoniazid should take a vitamin D supplement of 400 to 800 IU daily to enhance calcium absorption.

VITAMIN B6 AND NIACIN DEFICIENCIES: Isoniazid both inactivates vitamin B_6 and causes an increased excretion of the vitamin, and is likely to create a deficiency. At least 20 percent of all people who take the drug report a deficiency of B_6.

Common symptoms of this deficiency are

a sore mouth and tongue, cracks in the lips and corners of the mouth, and patches of itching, scaling skin. A severe vitamin B_6 deficiency may cause depression and confusion.

Vitamin B_6 deficiencies are common among the elderly. Alcoholics, as well, often experience this deficiency, since alcohol interferes with the body's ability to use B_6. In addition, smokers seem to have an increased need for the vitamin. It is established that one of every two Americans consumes less than 70 percent of the Recommended Dietary Allowance of B_6.

As vitamin B_6 and niacin work in conjunction with one another, the B_6 deficiency also leads to a niacin deficiency in large numbers of isoniazid users. The vitamin B_6 deficiency impairs your body's ability to produce niacin from tryptophan, which is a constitutent of proteins. The most often experienced symptoms of a niacin deficiency are a scaly dermatitis on areas of the skin exposed to sunlight, a confused mental state, and diarrhea.

Prevention and Treatment: To avoid a B_6 deficiency, you should consume a diet featuring food sources of vitamin B_6, such as liver (beef, calf, and pork), herring, salmon, walnuts, peanuts, wheat germ, carrots, peas, potatoes, grapes, bananas, and yeast. (See table of Vitamin B_6(Pyridovine)-Rich Foods, page 311.) The vitamin is present in significant amounts in meats, fish, fruits, cereals, and vegetables, and to a lesser extent in milk and other dairy products.

Since vitamin B_6 is decomposed at high temperatures, modern food processing often diminishes dietary sources of the vitamin. Consequently, the more processed foods you eat, the more susceptible you will be to a deficiency of this vitamin. The same losses also occur in cooking: meat loses as much as 45 to 80 percent, vegetables 20 to 30 percent.

It has been observed that 15 to 20 percent of oral contraceptive users show direct evidence of vitamin B_6 deficiency.

A daily supplement of 5 mg of vitamin B_6 should be taken to maintain vitamin B_6 levels in your body. No more than 100 mg of B_6 should be taken in any one day, however, since it counteracts the action of the drug above this level.

To maintain niacin levels in your body, your diet should include such niacin-rich foods as asparagus, peas, and peanut butter. (Refer to the table of Vitamin B_3(Niacin)-Rich Foods, page 310.) A supplement of 15 to 25 mg of niacin should be taken by anybody using isoniazid.

VITAMIN B_{12} DEFICIENCY: Isoniazid decreases the absorption of vitamin B_{12} and could conceivably cause a deficiency. Vitamin B_{12} is needed for the normal development of red blood cells and for the healthy functioning of all cells, in particular those of the bone marrow, nervous system, and intestines.

The most common result of a B_{12} deficiency is pernicious anemia, which is characterized by listlessness, fatigue (especially following such physical exertion as climbing a flight of stairs), a numbness and tingling in the fingers and toes, palpitations, angina, light-headedness, and a pale complexion. A vitamin B_{12} deficiency can also lead to an irreversible breakdown of the brain membranes, causing loss of coordination, confusion, memory loss, paranoia, apathy, tremors, and hallucinations. In extreme cases, degeneration of the spinal cord can also result.

Since vitamin B_{12} can be obtained only from animal food sources, strict vegetarians are at particular risk here. Oral contraceptive users, too, have a greater chance of experiencing this deficiency, since they often have a poor vitamin B_{12} status to begin with, as do smokers. Heavy consumers of alcohol, as well, frequently lack B_{12}, because alcohol impairs the absorption of the vitamin. Many elderly people also have a reduced ability to absorb the vitamin. In any case, anyone who is likely to have a vitamin B_{12} absorption problem should be alert for signs of pernicious anemia while taking isoniazid.

Prevention and Treatment: A balanced diet containing plenty of vitamin B_{12} sources is advised. Only animal products, including dairy foods and fish and shellfish, contain natural vitamin B_{12}. However, some vegetarian products are supplemented with the vitamin; many soy products, for example, are enriched with vitamin B_{12} to safeguard vegetarians. (See table of Vitamin B_{12}-Rich Foods, page 312.)

Vitamin B_{12} is stored in the liver, so one meal that includes a B_{12}-rich source such as calf's liver will normally fulfill your body's need for this vitamin for 2 to 3 weeks. (One 3-ounce serving of calf's liver contains 100 mcg of vitamin B_{12}.) If none of these products figures prominently in your diet, you should take a 6 mcg supplement each day while on isoniazid.

People who use major amounts of vitamin C should be aware that vitamin C supplements of more than 500 mg per day can damage B_{12} and contribute to a B_{12} deficiency. However, anyone who eats red meat two times a week has a three- to five-year supply of B_{12} in his liver.

The use of baking soda in cooking will destroy vitamin B_{12} and should be avoided whenever possible. B_{12} also degrades at high temperatures, as when meat is placed on a hot griddle. The pasteurization of milk and the sterilization in boiling water of a bottle of milk also cause the loss of some B_{12}.

FOLIC ACID DEFICIENCY: Isoniazid decreases your body's ability to use folacin efficiently and could lead to a deficiency. Often the first sign of a folic acid or folacin deficiency is inflamed and bleeding gums. The symptoms that follow are a sore, smooth tongue; diarrhea; forgetfulness; apathy; irritability; anemia; and a reduced resistance to infection. Despite the fact that folacin is found in a variety of foods, folacin deficiency is still the most common vitamin deficiency in the United States.

In adults, deficiencies are limited almost exclusively to the elderly and women, 30 percent of whom have intakes below the recommended daily allowance, and 5 to 7 percent of whom also have severe anemia. There are several factors that account for this bias, but one of the most obvious reasons is that oral contraceptive use decreases the absorption of folic acid. Constant dieting also limits folacin intake, and alcohol interferes with the body's absorption and use of folic acid, as well. Folacin is not stored by the body in any appreciable amounts, so an adequate supply must be consumed on a daily basis.

Folacin is required for the production of new cells, and a deficiency during pregnancy can lead to birth defects. Folic acid is also crucial to the normal metabolism of proteins.

Prevention and Treatment: To counteract a deficiency in folic acid, your diet should contain liver, yeast, and leafy vegetables such as spinach, kale, parsley, cauliflower, brussels sprouts, and broccoli. The fruits that are highest in folic acid are oranges and cantaloupes. To a lesser degree, folacin is found in almonds and lima beans, corn, parsnips, green peas, pumpkins, sweet potatoes, bran, peanuts, rye, and whole grain wheat. (See table of Folacin-Rich Foods, page 297.) Approximately one half of the folic acid you consume is absorbed by your body.

Normal cooking temperatures (110 to 120 degrees for 10 minutes) reduce the amount of useful folacin in your food by as much as 65 percent. Your daily diet, therefore, should include some raw vegetables and fruits. Cooking utensils made out of copper speed up folacin's destruction.

The recommended daily consumption of folacin is 400 mcg. Oral contraceptive users should consume 800 mcg daily.

MAGNESIUM DEFICIENCY: Magnesium deficiencies are not common because the average American diet contains appreciable amounts of magnesium. However, the level of magnesium absorption is decreased as a result of the presence of isoniazid in your system, and, though unlikely, such deficiencies do occur, particularly in the elderly patient with a congestive heart condition. (A congestive heart condition results from the heart's inability to pump adequate amounts of blood, which causes a backup or congestion.) Compounding the problem is

the fact that these patients are often taking other drugs that further deplete the body of magnesium.

Heavy drinkers, as well, are more likely to experience this deficiency, since alcohol depletes magnesium. Clinical signs of magnesium deficiency include muscle weakness, tremors, depression, emotional instability, and irrational behavior.

Prevention and Treatment: A diet containing the four food groups provides the normal amount of magnesium. However, while taking isoniazid, your daily diet should include such foods as nuts (almonds and cashews are highest), meat, fish, milk, whole grains, and fresh greens, since cooking can wash away some magnesium. Since alcohol provokes magnesium excretion, its intake should be restricted to two drinks per day while you are on this drug.

HIGH BLOOD PRESSURE: Isoniazid can cause an increase in blood pressure if it is taken with tyramine-containing foods. Normally, ingested tyramine is inactivated in the liver by an enzyme called monoamine oxidase, but when this enzyme is partially blocked by isoniazid, the tyramine can remain in the blood in large quantities and raise blood pressure.

Prevention and Treatment: Your intake of tyramine-containing foods must be restricted while you are being treated with isoniazid. Tyramine is common in many foods, but it is found in the greatest amounts in aged cheeses, chicken and beef livers, bananas, eggplant, yogurt, sour cream, alcoholic beverages, salami, meat tenderizers, yeast, and soy sauce. (See table on Tyramine-Rich Foods, page 307.) Raisins and avocados should also be avoided, because they contain dopamine, which has the same effect as tyramine.

OTHER ADVICE: Alcohol speeds up the rate at which isoniazid is broken down and makes it less effective. If you consume alcohol regularly, you should inform your doctor; he may increase your dosage of the drug.

Ideally, isoniazid is most rapidly absorbed by an empty stomach, so it should be taken either 1 hour before or 2 to 3 hours after eating. When it is taken with foods, its effectiveness is reduced by up to 40 percent.

Isoniazid should not be taken at the same time of day as antacids, since they are likely to delay its absorption.

ISOPROPAMIDE IODIDE

DRUG FAMILY: Anti-spasmodic

BRAND NAMES: Combid; Darbid; Ornade; Prochlor-Iso; Pro-Iso

HOW TO TAKE ISOPROPAMIDE IODIDE: In the morning before breakfast and at bedtime

FOODS TO AVOID: None

POSSIBLE SIDE EFFECTS: Constipation

ACTION OF ISOPROPAMIDE IODIDE: This drug reduces gastric secretion of acids and digestive enzymes, inhibits contractions of the intestine, prevents intestinal spasms (acute pains due to a violent contraction of the muscles in the intestine), relieves anxiety and tension, and controls nausea and vomiting.

Isopropamide iodide is used in the therapy of peptic ulcers, irritable colon, spastic colon, colitis, and functional gastrointestinal disorders.

HIGH-RISK GROUPS: The elderly

NUTRITIONAL INTERACTIONS

CONSTIPATION: Isopropamide iodide could conceivably cause you to become constipated.

Prevention and Treatment: Constipation is usually safely remedied by an increase in the bulk in the diet. This means consuming larger servings of any of the following: dried or fresh fruits (especially unpeeled apples or pears), salad vegetables (especially unpeeled carrots), radishes, oatmeal, and whole grain foods (brown rice, whole wheat breads, and cereals). It is not necessary to purchase products that claim "extra fiber" has been added to them.

Persistent constipation may also be relieved by doubling the amount of fluid consumed each day. Bran, if used, should be added to the diet gradually, and fluid should be increased by at least ¾ cup per teaspoon of bran. (See table of Dietary Fiber-Rich Foods, page 293.)

ISOSORBIDE DINITRATE

DRUG FAMILY: Vasodilator

BRAND NAMES: Dilatrate-SR; Iso-Bid; Isochron; Isordil; Isordil Oral Titradose, 5mg, 10 mg, 20 mg, and 30 mg; Isordil Sublingual, 2.5 mg, 5 mg, and 10 mg; Isosorbide Dinitrate T.D.; Isotrate Timecelles; Sorate-5; Sorate-10; Sorbide; Sorbitrate

HOW TO TAKE ISOSORBIDE DINITRATE: With meals

FOODS TO AVOID: Alcoholic beverages

POSSIBLE SIDE EFFECTS: Dizziness; gastrointestinal disturbances

ACTION OF ISOSORBIDE DINITRATE: This drug decreases the frequency and severity of angina pectoris attacks by dilating the coronary arteries. It is used for the treatment of acute angina attacks and as a preventive measure in situations likely to provoke such attacks.

HIGH-RISK GROUPS: Anyone who consumes alcohol

NUTRITIONAL INTERACTIONS

LOW BLOOD PRESSURE: Passing episodes of dizziness and weakness due to low blood pressure could conceivably develop while you are taking isosorbide dinitrate, particularly if you are standing still for any length of time. In some cases, the dizziness may progress to a loss of consciousness. This reaction seems to be accentuated by alcohol.
Prevention and Treatment: Alcohol should not be consumed concurrently with isosorbide dinitrate.

OTHER ADVICE: This drug causes gastrointestinal disturbances in some users. To prevent this, isosorbide dinitrate should be taken with meals whenever possible.

ISOTRETINOIN

DRUG FAMILY: Acne treatment

BRAND NAMES: Accutane

HOW TO TAKE ISOTRETINOIN: In 2 equal portions with breakfast and the evening meal

FOODS TO AVOID: Foods rich in saturated fat and cholesterol; more than 2 drinks of any alcoholic beverage per day

POSSIBLE SIDE EFFECTS: Hardening of the arteries; Vitamin A toxicity

ACTION OF ISOTRETINOIN: This drug is used in the treatment of severe cystic acne.

HIGH-RISK GROUPS: Heart patients, diabetics, anyone who consumes alcohol regularly, people with a family history of heart disease, people who are overweight

NUTRITIONAL INTERACTIONS

HEART DISEASE: Isotretinoin is likely to elevate plasma triglycerides and blood cholesterol levels, and to reduce HDL, or high density lipoproteins, which clean the arteries of cholesterol deposits. The reduction in HDL increases the risk of heart disease.
Prevention and Treatment: Animal fat should be limited in the diet. No more than 2 drinks of alcohol per day should be consumed, since it tends to raise triglyceride and cholesterol levels.

VITAMIN A TOXICITY: Isotretinoin is closely related to vitamin A, and patients on the drug are likely to exhibit signs of vitamin A toxicity: joint pain; dysmenorrhea; easily induced bleeding; loss of appetite; irritability; fatigue; restlessness; headache; nausea; muscle weakness; stomach pain; diarrhea; weight loss; dry; itching; peeling skin; rashes, dry; scaling lips; loss of hair; brittle nails.
Prevention and Treatment: Under no circumstances should any form of vitamin A supplement be taken concurrently with the drug.

ISOXAZOLYL PENICILLINS

DRUG FAMILY: Antibiotic

BRAND NAMES: [GENERIC/Brand] CLOXACIL-LIN/Tegopen; DICLOXACILLIN/Dynapen; Pathocil; OXACILLIN/Prostaphlin

HOW TO TAKE ISOXAZOLYL PENICILLINS: On an empty stomach 1 hour before or 2 to 3 hours after eating, with water and never with acidic beverages such as fruit juices, sodas, or wine

FOODS TO AVOID: Fruit juices, sodas, and wine should not be drunk within 1 hour of taking the drug

POSSIBLE SIDE EFFECTS: Gastrointestinal disturbances

ACTION OF ISOXAZOLYL PENICILLINS: These antibiotics are used against bacterial infections of *Staphylococcus aureus* that are resistant to regular penicillin.

HIGH-RISK GROUPS: Anyone who takes this drug

NUTRITIONAL INTERACTIONS

GENERAL ADVICE: This drug is best absorbed on an empty stomach and should be taken 1 hour before or 2 to 3 hours after eating. However, it does sometimes cause gastrointestinal disturbances.

KANAMYCIN

DRUG FAMILY: Antibiotic

BRAND NAME: Kantrex

HOW TO TAKE KANAMYCIN: With meals

FOODS TO AVOID: Fatty and very sweet foods

POSSIBLE SIDE EFFECTS: Deficiencies in vitamins A, K, and B$_{12}$; diarrhea, nausea, and vomiting

ACTION OF KANAMYCIN: This drug is prescribed to suppress the growth of intestinal bacteria prior to surgery. It is also used to treat severe infections caused by gram negative bacilli in children and as an adjunct to the treatment of hepatic coma, tuberculosis, and urinary-tract infections.

HIGH-RISK GROUPS: Vegetarians, the elderly, heavy drinkers, users of oral contraceptives, children, teenagers

NUTRITIONAL INTERACTIONS

VITAMIN A DEFICIENCY: When you are taking kanamycin, it may impair the absorption of fat and lead to the malabsorption of vitamins A and K.

Vitamins A and K are two of the fat-soluble vitamins that are stored in the fat in your body. Deficiencies can occur when kanamycin is used for several weeks by patients whose vitamin stores and dietary intake are marginal—a condition found in a large number of people in the United States, especially in relation to vitamin A.

Prevention and Treatment: Fat-soluble vitamins do not have to be consumed every day, because they are stored in the body, but it is advised not to take major doses of vitamin A (over 10,000 IU per day). An overdose can be toxic and can lead to diarrhea, nausea, hair loss, extreme fatigue, and menstrual irregularities. A small dose of vitamin A such as the 5,000 IU's found in a multivitamin should counteract a vitamin A deficiency.

Vitamin A can be found in foods such as fish oils, liver, whole milk, whole milk products, egg yolks, fortified margarine, green vegetables (spinach), and yellow fruit (cantaloupe). (See table for Vitamin A-Rich Foods, page 308.) Unlike most vitamins, vitamin A is not easily destroyed by cooking or exposure to high temperatures, but long exposure to sunlight will damage it. Therefore, you should keep milk stored in opaque containers and cover vegetables.

A substance called citral is found in orange peel and marmalade. Citral, in large quantities, can decrease the effectiveness of vitamin A, so consumption of foods containing orange peel should be limited while at risk of contracting a vitamin A shortage.

VITAMIN K DEFICIENCY: People with abnormally low dietary intake of vitamin K should be aware that they could conceivably develop a deficiency of the vitamin while on kanamycin; they are at risk of bleeding with unusual ease if they do. Normally vitamin K helps produce blood-clotting substances in the liver. Without sufficient levels of vitamin K in the diet, however, bleeding may take place in the gastrointestinal tract (causing black or blood-stained stools), in the urinary tract (causing blood in the urine), and in the uterus (causing blood loss at times other than the normal menstrual periods). Excessive blood loss may occur from an injury or surgery. Another sign of a deficiency of this vitamin is more frequent and visible bruising than normal.

Many of the elderly are at risk of a vitamin K deficiency because they have a problem of poor fat absorption, and vitamin K, a fat-soluble vitamin, must be accompanied by sufficient dietary fat to be properly absorbed.

Prevention and Treatment: A vitamin K deficiency can be countered by a vitamin K supplement of 100 mcg per day, and a diet that includes foods rich in the vitamin, such as kale, spinach, cabbage, cauliflower, leafy green vegetables, liver (especially pork liver), and fish.

Vitamin E supplements should not be taken at this time, because vitamin E impairs the absorption of vitamin K.

VITAMIN B$_{12}$ DEFICIENCY: Kanamycin also inhibits the absorption of Vitamin B$_{12}$, though it is highly unlikely that it will do so to the degree that you will develop a deficiency of the vitamin. Vitamin B$_{12}$ is needed for the normal development of red blood cells, and for the healthy functioning of all cells, in particular those of the bone marrow, nervous system, and intestines.

Prevention and Treatment: If plenty of animal foods, (or vegetarian-type foods supplemented with vitamin B$_{12}$) are included in the diet, this will not occur. (See table of Vitamin B$_{12}$-Rich Foods, page 312.)

GASTROINTESTINAL DISTRESS: It is conceivable that while taking kanamycin you will experience one or more of the several kinds of gastrointestinal problems reported by other users. Kanamycin can reduce your body's ability to absorb fats and carbohydrates, which can result in diarrhea. The drug also can produce nausea and vomiting in some people.

Prevention and Treatment: Kanamycin should be taken with meals to minimize these discomforts.

LEVODOPA

DRUG FAMILY: Anti-Parkinsonian

BRAND NAMES: Larodopa; Sinemet

HOW TO TAKE LEVODOPA: With food or milk

FOODS TO AVOID: No more than 1 to 2 servings of protein-rich foods per day; licorice candy made from natural extract

POSSIBLE SIDE EFFECTS: Deficiencies of vitamins B_6 and B_{12}, folacin, and potassium; nausea, vomiting, and anorexia

ACTION OF LEVODOPA: This drug is used to relieve the symptoms of Parkinson's disease. There are over half a million sufferers of this disease in America today.

HIGH-RISK GROUPS: The elderly

NUTRITIONAL INTERACTIONS

PROTEIN INTERACTION: The pharmacological action of levodopa is modified by dietary protein; a high-protein diet diminishes the effects of the drug, and a lack of protein is likely to increase it.

Levodopa is thought to be absorbed and transported to the brain by the same mechanism that transports amino acids, the building blocks of protein. In a sense, the drug and the amino acid tryptophan compete for absorption into the body and the brain. As a result of this "competition" between levodopa and the amino acids, some patients taking the drug have developed mental depression and, in extreme cases, even dementia. This occurs because tryptophan is used by the brain to make serotonin, the chemical messenger that is responsible for elevating mood. When there is a lot of levodopa in the blood, there will be less tryptophan entering the brain. This means less serotonin is produced, and depression can set in.

Prevention and Treatment: A low-protein diet is suggested for people taking levodopa. The optimum level of protein consumption seems to be .5 gram of protein per kilogram of body weight, with a total intake that should not exceed 35 to 40 grams per day. This means limiting your protein intake to no more than 1 to 2 servings per day. (See the table of Protein-Rich Foods, page 304.) If depression is experienced as a result of taking this drug, do not take tryptophan supplements but seek the advice of your doctor.

VITAMIN B_6 AND NIACIN INTERACTION: Vitamin B_6 nullifies the beneficial effects of levodopa in the control of Parkinson's disease. The vitamin causes the drug to be broken down in the tissues of the body as the blood containing the drug passes through them, and as a result, less levodopa reaches the brain where it is supposed to do its work.

Vitamin B_6 also binds to the drug in the tissues and reduces the amount available to enter the brain. In the same way that vitamin B_6 binds to levodopa and prevents its action, levodopa binds to vitamin B_6 and prevents it from carrying out its normal functions. Many patients who take levodopa develop the classic sign of vitamin B_6 deficiency, scaly dermatitis of the face and scalp.

As vitamin B_6 and niacin work in conjunction with one another, a B_6 deficiency can also lead to a niacin deficiency. The most common symptoms are a scaly dermatitis on areas of the skin exposed to sunlight, a confused mental state, and diarrhea.

Prevention and Treatment: No vitamin supplement containing any vitamin B_6 should be taken without a doctor's advice.

Good sources of vitamin B_6 should be included in the diet. Such sources are liver (beef, calf, and pork), herring, salmon, walnuts, peanuts, wheat germ, carrots, peas, potatoes, grapes, bananas, and yeast. The vitamin is present in significant amounts in meats, fish, fruits, cereals, and vegetables, and to a lesser extent in milk and other dairy products.

You should maintain a vitamin B_6 intake of about 1.5 to 2 mg per day. A drug called carbidopa can also be prescribed, for it prevents the breakdown of levodopa in the peripheral tissues and so prevents the loss of the drug's effects produced by dietary vitamin B_6.

Keep in mind that, since vitamin B_6 is decomposed at high temperatures, modern food processing often diminishes dietary sources of the vitamin.

Niacin-containing foods must also be present in your diet while you are taking levodopa. (Refer to the table of Vitamin B_3 (Niacin)-Rich Foods, page 310.) Several good sources are asparagus, peas, and peanut butter.

VITAMIN B_{12} AND FOLACIN INTERACTIONS: Both vitamin B_{12} and folacin are indirectly involved in the breakdown of levodopa. As a result, Parkinson's disease patients have increased needs for these vitamins and are likely to develop deficiencies if their diet contains very little of these nutrients.

Prevention and Treatment: As long as your diet contains the Recommended Dietary Allowance of both of these vitamins, however, no special dietary supplementation should be necessary. Good folacin sources are green, leafy vegetables; beets; and members of the cabbage family such as cauliflower, broccoli, and brussels sprouts.

As for vitamin B_{12}, if you eat any animal products at all, you should get sufficient B_{12} for your needs. Vegetarians who eat no animal products must include some soy foods enriched with B_{12}, or some other B_{12}-supplemented food, in their diets.

GASTROINTESTINAL DISTRESS: Levodopa causes some unpleasant gastrointestinal disturbances in most people who take it. Nausea, vomiting, and anorexia are common problems.

Prevention and Treatment: These side effects can be alleviated by taking the drug with food or milk. However, the side effects normally lessen over time.

POTASSIUM DEFICIENCY: Levodopa causes an increase in the excretion of potassium in the urine, which can in some instances lead to a potassium deficiency. The likelihood of this deficiency occurring is greater if you are taking other drugs that increase potassium excretion, like the thiazide diuretics.

Potassium regulates the amount of water in the cells of the body and is essential for the proper functioning of the kidneys and the heart muscle, and the secretion of stomach juices. The most alarming symptom of a potassium deficiency is an irregular heartbeat, which can lead to heart failure.

Low blood serum levels of potassium, called hypokalemia, are associated with laxative abuse, because many laxatives promote an increased loss of potassium from the gastrointestinal tract. This risk is especially high in elderly patients who consume diets low in potassium.

People who take laxatives phenolphthalein, bisacodyl, and senna on a daily basis have been reported to have a much greater chance of experiencing serious hypokalemia. These people, and others with a potassium deficiency, may have such symptoms as weakness, loss of appetite, nausea, vomiting, dryness of the mouth, increased thirst, listlessness, apprehension, and diffuse pain that comes and goes.

Proper potassium levels in your body can also be threatened if this drug is taken concurrently with cortisone-containing drugs.

Prevention and Treatment: Potassium depletion can be avoided by including such potassium-rich foods in your diet as tomato juice, lentils, dried apricots, asparagus, bananas, peanut butter, chicken, almonds, and milk. (See table of Potassium-Rich Foods, page 302.)

Potassium supplements should never be taken unless prescribed by a physician. They can cause anemia by interfering with the absorption of vitamin B_{12}. Just a few grams can also drastically increase the risk of heart failure. If you experience difficulty in swallowing while taking potassium supplements, consult your physician immediately. If supplements are prescribed, be aware that the absorption of the supplements potassium iodide and potassium chloride is decreased by dairy products, and that both are gastric irritants and should be taken with meals.

Too much salt in your diet can also compromise your body's supply of potassium, as can 1 to 3 ounces per day of licorice candy made from natural extract. Imported licorice contains the natural extract, but the domestic brands usually use synthetic flavorings, which are not harmful. Check the package.

LINCOMYCIN

DRUG FAMILY: Antibiotic

BRAND NAME: Lincocin

HOW TO TAKE LINCOMYCIN: On an empty stomach at least 1 hour before or 2 hours after a meal, with nothing but water

FOODS TO AVOID: None

POSSIBLE SIDE EFFECTS: Gastrointestinal distress; vitamin B_6 deficiency

ACTION OF LINCOMYCIN: This anti-bacterial agent is prescribed for serious infections where less toxic anti-bacterial agents are not effective. It is normally reserved for patients who are allergic to penicillin.

HIGH-RISK GROUPS: Anyone who takes this drug

NUTRITIONAL INTERACTIONS

GASTROINTESTINAL DISTRESS: Use of lincomycin is usually associated with nausea, vomiting, and diarrhea. The drug also impairs the sense of taste and can lead to a loss of appetite.

Prevention and Treatment: If persistent diarrhea occurs, you should discontinue use of lincomycin and consult your physician regarding a substitute.

You should carefully monitor your body weight to prevent significant weight loss.

VITAMIN B$_6$ DEFICIENCY: Since lincomycin is an antagonist of vitamin B$_6$, users of this drug are likely to experience a B$_6$ deficiency. Common symptoms of this deficiency are a sore mouth and tongue, cracks in the lips and corners of the mouth, and patches of itching, scaling skin. A severe vitamin B$_6$ deficiency may cause depression and confusion.

Vitamin B$_6$ deficiencies are common among the elderly, and also among alcoholics, since alcohol interferes with the body's ability to use B$_6$. It is estimated that one of every two Americans consumes less than 70 percent of the Recommended Dietary Allowance of B$_6$.

Prevention and Treatment: To avoid a B$_6$ deficiency, you should consume a diet featuring such food sources of vitamin B$_6$ as liver (beef, calf, and pork), herring, salmon, walnuts, peanuts, wheat germ, carrots, peas, potatoes, grapes, bananas, and yeast. (See table of Vitamin B$_6$(Pyridoxine)-Rich Foods, page 311.) The vitamin is present in significant amounts in meats, fish, fruits, cereals, and vegetables, and to a lesser extent in milk and other dairy products.

Since vitamin B$_6$ is decomposed at high temperatures, modern food processing often diminishes dietary sources of the vitamin. Consequently, the more processed foods you eat, the more susceptible you will be to a deficiency of this vitamin. The same losses also occur in cooking: meat loses as much as 45 to 80 percent, vegetables 20 to 30 percent.

It has been observed that 15 to 20 percent of oral contraceptive users show direct evidence of vitamin B$_6$ deficiency. If you are among these people, you should take a 5 mg supplement of vitamin B$_6$ per day.

All users of lincomycin should take a B complex with C vitamin supplement containing the Recommended Dietary Allowance of each vitamin.

OTHER INTERACTIONS: Despite lincomycin's adverse gastrointestinal effects, this drug should be given with nothing but water. Food should not be consumed for 1 to 2 hours before and after taking the drug, since any food present in the digestive system reduces the absorption of the drug.

LITHIUM

DRUG FAMILY: Anti-psychotic, anti-depressant

BRAND NAMES: [GENERIC/Brand] LITHIUM CARBONATE/Eskalith; Eskalith CR; Lithane; Lithobid; LITHIUM CITRATE/Cibalith-S.

HOW TO TAKE LITHIUM: As directed by your physician

FOODS TO AVOID: None

POSSIBLE SIDE EFFECTS: Gastrointestinal distress

ACTION OF LITHIUM: This drug is used in treating manic-depressive illness and mania. It normalizes the swings in norepinephrine levels in the brain, responsible for the periods of depression and excitement shown by manic patients.

HIGH-RISK GROUPS: People taking diuretics, low-salt dieters

NUTRITIONAL INTERACTIONS

SODIUM BALANCE: Low blood sodium levels could conceivably enhance the action of lithium by decreasing its excretion, producing a toxic buildup of the drug. In many people, the toxic effect, generally mild, will occur 2 to 4 hours after taking the drug, when it is at its maximum concentration in the bloodstream. However, people on severely restricted sodium diets, such as those taking diuretics (spironolactone and the thiazides in particular), may suffer from much more serious reactions.

A mild toxic reaction is characterized by nausea, abdominal pain, diarrhea, vomiting, sedation, and a slight tremor. More acute toxicity results in an extreme thirst and frequent urination, and sometimes in an enlarged thyroid gland. Severe toxicity leads to vomiting, profuse diarrhea, loss of control of the voluntary movements of everyday life, irregular heartbeats, abnormally low blood-pressure, a gross tremor, mental confusion, difficulty in articulating words, seizures, and even coma, which can eventually cause death.

Prevention and Treatment: Patients on lithium should not be on sodium-restricted diets, or on other drugs that cause body depletion of sodium, such as diuretics.

MAGNESIUM ANTACIDS

DRUG FAMILY: Antacids

BRAND NAMES: Aludrox; Aluminum & Magnesium Hydroxides with Simethicone; Camalox; Gelusil; Gelusil-M; Gelusil-II; Kudrox; Maalox; Magnesia & Alumina; Milk of Magnesia; Mygel; Mylanta; Mylanta-II; Phillips' Milk of Magnesia; Simeco

HOW TO TAKE MAGNESIUM ANTACIDS: Between meals and at bedtime

FOODS TO AVOID: Acid-containing foods such as fruit juices, sodas and wine; foods containing caffeine such as cola, coffee, tea, and chocolate

POSSIBLE SIDE EFFECTS: Deficiencies of calcium, phosphorus, vitamin B_1, folacin, and iron; diarrhea; kidney stones

ACTION OF MAGNESIUM ANTACIDS: These drugs are used to reduce the acidity of the stomach.

HIGH-RISK GROUPS: The elderly, kidney patients, heavy drinkers, young women, pregnant or lactating women, vegetarians, teenagers, smokers, users of oral contraceptives

NUTRITIONAL INTERACTIONS

PHOSPHATE AND CALCIUM DEFICIENCIES: Excess consumption of antacids containing magnesium hydroxide could conceivably cause you to experience phosphate and, to a lesser degree, calcium depletion from your body. This occurs because magnesium combines with phosphate in the diet, forming magnesium phosphate, which passes out of the body in the stool. On rare occasions, hypophosphatemia, or dangerously low blood phosphate levels, can also develop. It is difficult to diagnose because it is indicated by a slow development of weakness, a common symptom of many metabolic disorders in the elderly.

To replace the lost phosphate, the body

withdraws the mineral from the bones to maintain optimal blood phosphate levels. As phosphate cannot be drawn from the bones without also removing calcium, the calcium loss, if protracted, can lead to osteomalacia and possibly osteoporosis.

Osteomalacia is a weakening of the bones that results from a uniform and steady calcium loss. Prominent symptoms are bone pain in the back, thighs, shoulder region, or ribs; difficulty in walking; and weakness in the muscles of the legs. The condition is reversible once calcium blood levels are raised.

Osteoporosis is an unexplained and rapid loss of calcium from the bones. Characteristic symptoms are a loss of height, periodontal disease, and backache. Fractures too are common, usually of the hip, wrist, or vertebrae.

Prevention and Treatment: In order to guard against low phosphate levels, plenty of phosphate-rich foods should be included in the diet. (See table of Phosphorus-Rich Foods, page 302.) Such foods include liver, nuts, beans, peas, whole grains, and cereals.

OTHER ADVICE: Magnesium products tend to cause diarrhea in some patients. It is conceivable this is so in your case, and if it is, you should switch to an antacid that combines aluminum and magnesium compounds, and has little or no effect on bowel movements.

Magnesium antacids should be used with extreme caution in kidney disease patients. They may have difficulty in excreting the excess magnesium and suffer from magnesium toxicity, characterized by nausea, vomiting, flushing, problems in breathing, and eventually heart failure. Antacids that contain magnesium trisilicate can cause kidney stones.

Malnutrition can result from excessive self-medication with antacids, as a result of malabsorption of nutrients, especially vitamin B_1, folacin, and iron. It should be emphasized that nutrient depletion from antacid use is gradual, and evidence of malnutrition does not make its appearance until nutrient stores are exhausted. If you are a regular user of magnesium antacids, you should take a one-a-day vitamin to guard against deficiencies.

People taking antacids therapeutically should avoid large amounts of acid-containing foods such as fruit juices and foods containing caffeine, which irritate the stomach wall.

MAGNESIUM-BASED SALINE CATHARTICS

DRUG FAMILY: Laxatives

BRAND NAMES: Milk of Magnesia; Magnesium Citrate; Magnesium Sulfate; any brand of Epsom salts.

HOW TO TAKE MAGNESIUM-BASED SALINE CATHARTICS: Preferably at bedtime but never within 2 hours of taking a meal

FOODS TO AVOID: None

POSSIBLE SIDE EFFECTS: Magnesium toxicity

ACTION OF MAGNESIUM-BASED SALINE CATHARTICS: These act as laxatives by increasing the action of the muscles lining the intestines, and so reduce the time required for food to pass through the intestinal tract. Saline cathartics, including those that are magnesium-based, act partly by drawing water into the colon and so increasing the bulk of the stools. They also act by releasing cholecystokinin from the small intestine. This is a hormone that is responsible for causing bile to be secreted into the intestine. Bile contains sodium, which further increases the amount of water drawn into the colon, adding additional bulk to the stool.

HIGH-RISK GROUPS: Kidney patients

NUTRITIONAL INTERACTIONS

MAGNESIUM TOXICITY: One third of all the prescriptions for laxatives are for milk of magnesia. Just 30 ml of milk of magnesia provides 1,000 mg of magnesium, which is three to four times the average dietary intake. Only 20 percent to 30 percent of a 1,000 mg laxative dose is absorbed but, added to the 300 mg of magnesium commonly found in the diet, these magnesium laxatives, if frequently used, could conceivably result in excessive absorption and toxic levels of magnesium in your system. The early symptoms are drowsiness, lethargy, profuse sweating, slurring of speech, and unsteadiness. Magnesium salts are most likely to induce toxicity if you are unable to excrete magnesium at a normal rate, which is often true in patients with kidney disease.

Prevention and Treatment: If you have a serious kidney impairment, do not use magnesium-based saline cathartics because the higher levels of magnesium in your blood can cause heart failure.

NUTRITIONAL DEFICIENCIES: All the saline cathartics produce small increases in the ex-cretion of sodium, potassium, protein, and fat, no matter when they are taken, although the effect is usually only modest. The effect could be intensified if taken with meals or shortly thereafter.

Prevention and Treatment: No magnesium-based saline cathartics should be taken with meals or within 2 hours of a meal. Epsom salts have a bitter taste and can be taken in lemon juice, which helps mask the taste.

MAPROTILINE HYDROCHLORIDE

DRUG FAMILY: Anti-depressant

BRAND NAME: Ludiomil

HOW TO TAKE MAPROTILINE HYDROCHLORIDE: As directed by your physician

FOODS TO AVOID: All alcoholic beverages

POSSIBLE SIDE EFFECTS: Dry mouth, nausea, and constipation

ACTION OF MAPROTILINE HYDROCHLORIDE: This drug is prescribed for the treatment of depressive and manic-depressive illnesses. It is also effective in relieving anxiety associated with depression.

HIGH-RISK GROUPS: The elderly; heavy drinkers

NUTRITIONAL INTERACTIONS

SALIVA SUPPRESSION: In 22 percent of all users of maprotiline, dry mouth has been experienced as a result of the drug's inhibiting the secretion of saliva. This impairs the ability to swallow food. In addition, in 2 percent of users nausea occurs.

Prevention and Treatment: You should

drink lots of fluids while taking this drug, to reduce the discomfort of the dry mouth. Other methods of dealing with dry mouth are the use of gum, hard candy, or mints, and the consumption of substantial amounts of dietary fiber. The fiber stimulates the salivary glands. Maprotiline should be taken with meals to reduce the risk of nausea.

A shortage of saliva also makes the mouth more susceptible to the growth of bacteria responsible for tooth decay and gum disease. You should take special care to brush and floss your teeth often.

CONSTIPATION: In 6 percent of those using maprotiline, constipation has been observed. The drug slows down the rate at which the muscles in the intestines contract, and so reduces the rate at which food passes down the gastrointestinal tract.

Prevention and Treatment: Constipation is usually safely remedied by an increase in the bulk in the diet. This means consuming larger servings of any of the following: dried or fresh fruits (especially unpeeled apples or pears), salad vegetables, radishes, oatmeal, and whole grain foods (brown rice, whole wheat breads, and cereals). It is not necessary to purchase products that claim "extra fiber" has been added to them.

Persistent constipation may also be relieved by doubling the amount of fluid consumed each day. Bran, if used, should be added to the diet gradually, and fluid should be increased by at least ¾ cup per teaspoon of bran. (See table of Dietary Fiber-Rich Foods, page 293.)

ALCOHOL INTERACTION: Alcohol increases the depressant effects of maprotiline, which can seriously impair the already-compromised mental and physical abilities, making driving and other such tasks extremely hazardous.

Prevention and Treatment: Alcohol should not be consumed by people taking this drug.

MECHLORETHAMINE HYDROCHLORIDE

DRUG FAMILY: Anti-cancer

BRAND NAME: Mustargen

HOW TO TAKE MECHLORETHAMINE HYDROCHLORIDE: Injection

FOODS TO AVOID: Sweet foods such as cookies, candies, and cake

POSSIBLE SIDE EFFECTS: Glucose malabsorption, nausea, vomiting, impaired taste, mouth sores, and loss of appetite

ACTION OF MECHLORETHAMINE HYDROCHLORIDE: This alkylating agent acts by preventing tumor cells from proliferating.

HIGH-RISK GROUPS: Anyone who takes this drug

NUTRITIONAL INTERACTIONS

GLUCOSE MALABSORPTION: These drugs decrease your glucose absorption, which can result in diarrhea. They can also decrease your absorption of all nutrients and have a weakening effect.

Prevention and Treatment: If you experience diarrhea when using mechlorethamine hydrochloride, you should reduce the amount of simple sugars in your diet and increase the starches you eat. If you are being tube-fed, the dietician should likewise decrease the level of simple sugars being given to you via the tube feedings.

GASTROINTESTINAL DISTRESS: Mechlorethamine hydrochloride is likely to cause nausea, vomiting, impaired taste, mouth sores, and anorexia.

Prevention and Treatment: Nausea and vomiting may be controlled by taking several basic steps. First, you should eat smaller meals and limit your intake of high-fat foods. Second, when you experience nausea, you should slowly sip clear beverages, such as ginger ale. Sucking a Popsicle may also alleviate the condition. You should lie down, loosen your clothes, and get fresh air as well.

You should take plenty of liquids to prevent dehydration if you find that you vomit frequently.

MECLIZINE HYDROCHLORIDE

DRUG FAMILY: Anti-histamine, anti-nausea

BRAND NAMES: Antivert; Bonine; Meclizine Hydrochloride MLT; Ru-Vert-M

HOW TO TAKE MECLIZINE HYDROCHLORIDE: At mealtimes

FOODS TO AVOID: All alcoholic beverages

POSSIBLE SIDE EFFECTS: Dry mouth, difficulty in swallowing

ACTION OF MECLIZINE HYDROCHLORIDE: This drug is effective against nausea, vomiting, and the dizziness associated with motion sickness. It is also used to treat the vertigo that frequently accompanies ear infections.

HIGH-RISK GROUPS: Anyone who consumes alcohol

NUTRITIONAL INTERACTIONS

ALCOHOL INTERACTION: Alcohol enhances the somnolent effects of meclizine, and impairs mental and motor functions. It is dangerous to drive after having taken this drug concurrently with even a small amount of alcohol.

Prevention and Treatment: Patients should not drink alcoholic beverages while taking this drug.

OTHER ADVICE: Meclizine should be taken at mealtimes. Plenty of liquids should be consumed when taking the drug, since it also has been reported to cause dry mouth and some difficulty in swallowing.

MEFENAMIC ACID

DRUG FAMILY: Analgesic and anti-inflammatory

BRAND NAME: Ponstel

HOW TO TAKE MEFENAMIC ACID: With meals or milk

FOODS TO AVOID: None

POSSIBLE SIDE EFFECTS: Diarrhea

ACTION OF MEFENAMIC ACID: This analgesic agent is used to treat pain arising from rheumatic conditions; soft-tissue injuries; other painful, musculoskeletal conditions; and dysmenorrhea (painful menstrual periods).

HIGH-RISK GROUPS: People with a history of abdominal distress

NUTRITIONAL INTERACTIONS

GASTROINTESTINAL DISTRESS: Mefenamic acid causes irritation of the gastrointestinal tract, which can result in some discomfort. Severe diarrhea sometimes occurs and can result in some impairment in the absorption of fat-soluble vitamins.

Prevention and Treatment: Mefenamic acid should always be taken with meals or milk. If severe diarrhea results, you should advise your physician, and he will probably switch you to an alternative drug in order to prevent the risk of any vitamin-deficient state.

MEPROBAMATE

DRUG FAMILY: Anti-anxiety

BRAND NAMES: Deprol; Equagesic; Equanil; Mepro Compound; Meprospan; Milpath; Miltown; Miltown 600; PMB 200; PMB 400; Pathibamate; SK-Bamate

HOW TO TAKE MEPROBAMATE: With milk or meals

FOODS TO AVOID: All alcoholic beverages

POSSIBLE SIDE EFFECTS: Nausea, vomiting, and diarrhea

ACTION OF MEPROBAMATE: This drug is prescribed as an anti-anxiety drug and as a treatment for insomnia.

HIGH-RISK GROUPS: The elderly; heavy drinkers

NUTRITIONAL INTERACTIONS

VARIATIONS IN POTENCY: Alcohol increases the depressant effects of meprobamate, leading to poor motor coordination, slow reactions, and memory impairment. Elderly people seem to break down the drug much more slowly than younger people. This can lead to a toxic buildup of the drug, exacerbating the above effects. Blood pressure may also drop below normal, causing light-headedness.

Prevention and Treatment: Alcohol should only be used in moderation while taking meprobamate. Inform your doctor if you consume alcohol on a regular basis.

GASTROINTESTINAL DISTRESS: In some people, this drug causes gastrointestinal discomforts such as nausea, vomiting, and diarrhea.

Prevention and Treatment: This drug should always be taken with milk or food to avoid any adverse digestive disturbances.

MERCAPTOPURINE

DRUG FAMILY: Anti-leukemia

BRAND NAME: Purinethol

HOW TO TAKE MERCAPTOPURINE: With meals or milk

FOODS TO AVOID: Those rich in purines such as anchovies, kidneys, liver, meat extracts, sardines, sweetbreads, beans, and lentils

POSSIBLE SIDE EFFECTS: Niacin deficiency; gout; nausea, loss of appetite

ACTION OF MERCAPTOPURINE: This drug, which prevents cells from dividing and increasing in number, is used in the treatment of leukemia and is especially effective in the treatment of children.

HIGH-RISK GROUPS: Anyone who takes this drug

NUTRITIONAL INTERACTIONS

NIACIN DEFICIENCY: It is conceivable that you will develop a niacin deficiency while taking mercaptopurine, since some cases have been reported.

The characteristic symptoms of a deficiency of niacin (vitamin B_3) are a smooth, sore, and swollen tongue; diarrhea; mental confusion; and irritability. You should remember, however, that many of these symptoms commonly occur in cases of vitamin B_6 and folacin deficiency.

Prevention and Treatment: Good sources of niacin (as well as vitamin B_6 and folic acid) should be included in the diet. (See table of Vitamin B_3(Niacin)-Rich Foods, page 310.)

Niacin is needed by the body for the conversion of food into energy, to satisfy the needs of all the tissues and to enable them to make proteins and fats. Niacin is found in foods in two forms: nicotinic acid and nicotinamide (also known as niacinamide).

Recommended niacin intakes are stated in "equivalents." This is because niacin is unique among the B vitamins in that it can also be made from protein. Tryptophan, one of the amino acids (the constituent building blocks of protein), can be converted to niacin in the body. Six grams of protein in the diet contain 60 mg of tryptophan, which may be converted to 1 mg of niacin. Thus, a food that supplies 1 mg niacin and 60 mg tryptophan contains the equivalent of 2 mg of niacin. However, not all the tryptophan in the diet is made into niacin, since the tryptophan is also needed to build body proteins.

Milk, eggs, meat, poultry, and fish contribute about half the niacin equivalents consumed by most people, and about a fourth come from enriched breads and cereals. Vegetarians are well advised to emphasize nuts and legumes in their diets, since these are good sources of niacin and protein.

OTHER ADVICE: Mercaptopurine tends to cause a buildup of uric acid, which could conceivably lead to the development of gout. Alkaline urine helps the kidneys to excrete the uric acid from the body, so foods causing the production of alkaline urine should be present in the diet. Such foods are milk, buttermilk, cream, almonds, chestnuts, coconuts, all vegetables except corn and lentils, and all fruits except cranberries, prunes, and plums.

Approximately one in four adults taking this drug experiences nausea and loss of appetite. Mercaptopurine should be taken with meals or milk to reduce this side affect. Adults should also monitor their weight carefully to safeguard against weight loss.

Persistent nausea may also be controlled by taking several basic steps. First, you should eat smaller meals and limit your intake of high-fat foods. Second, when you experience nausea, you should slowly sip clear beverages, such as ginger ale. Sucking a Popsicle may also alleviate the condition. Relief can also be obtained by loosening your clothes and lying down by an open window so that you get plenty of fresh air.

MERCURIAL DIURETICS

DRUG FAMILY: Anti-glaucoma, anti-epileptic, diuretic

BRAND NAMES: [GENERIC/Brand] ACETAZO-LAMID/Diamox; DICHLORPHENAMIDE/Daranide; METHAZOLAMIDE/Neptazane.

HOW TO TAKE MERCURIAL DIURETICS: With meals or milk

FOODS TO AVOID: None

POSSIBLE SIDE EFFECTS: Deficiencies of potassium, vitamin B_1, calcium, and magnesium; gastrointestinal disturbances

ACTION OF MERCURIAL DIURETICS: These drugs reduce fluid retention and increase urine excretion, and are effective and most commonly used in the treatment of glaucoma. They also are used to treat seizures and occasionally as diuretics.

HIGH-RISK GROUPS: Anyone who takes this drug

NUTRITIONAL INTERACTIONS

POTASSIUM DEFICIENCY: Long-term use of this drug is likely to result in a potassium depletion in your body, due to increased potassium excretion. Potassium regulates the amount of water in the cells of the body and is essential for the proper functioning of the kidneys and the heart muscle, and the secretion of stomach juices. The most alarming symptom of a potassium deficiency is an irregular heartbeat, which can lead to a heart attack.

Hypokalemia, as low blood serum levels of potassium are called, is associated with laxative abuse because many laxatives promote an increased loss of potassium from the gastrointestinal tract. People who take laxatives on a daily basis have been reported to have a much greater chance of experiencing serious hypokalemia. These people, and others with a potassium deficiency, may have such symptoms as weakness, loss of appetite, nausea, vomiting, dryness of the mouth, increased thirst, listlessness, apprehension, and diffuse pain that comes and goes.

Proper potassium levels in your body can also be threatened if this drug is taken concurrently with cortisone-containing drugs.

Prevention and Treatment: Potassium depletion can be avoided by including such potassium-rich foods in your diet as tomato juice, lentils, dried apricots, asparagus, bananas, peanut butter, chicken, almonds, and milk. (See table of Potassium-Rich Foods, page 302.)

Do not take potassium supplements unless they have been prescribed by a physician. They can cause anemia by interfering with the absorption of vitamin B_{12}. Just a few grams can also cause heart failure. If you experience difficulty in swallowing while taking potassium supplements, consult your physician immediately. If supplements are prescribed, be aware that the absorption of the supplements potassium iodide and potassium chloride is decreased by dairy products, and that both are gastric irritants and should be taken with meals.

If there is too much salt in your diet, your body's supply of potassium can also be compromised. Licorice candy containing natural extract can have the same effect. Imported licorice falls under this category, but domestic brands rarely use the natural extract. Check the package.

VITAMIN B_1 DEFICIENCY: Mercurial diuretics could conceivably lead to a deficiency of vitamin B_1 (thiamin), due to increased excretion of the vitamin.

Vitamin B_1 is essential to the body's ability to metabolize carbohydrates, for muscle coordination, and to keep the nerves healthy. A deficiency in this vitamin may cause heart palpitations, along with mental confusion, moodiness, and tiredness. Other symptoms of a B_1 deficiency are difficuty in walking, weight loss, and water retention, especially at the ankles. Consumers of alcohol tend to be deficient in this vitamin since alcohol interferes with the body's ability to absorb thiamin. Heavy drinkers are at higher risk of a thiamin deficiency. Antacids taken at mealtime destroy dietary thiamin and can also contribute to a deficiency.

Frequently, older Americans are found to be marginally deficient in this vitamin. A severe deficiency in those in this age group can be the cause of symptoms resembling senility, which are reversible when the supply of B_1 is replenished. This vitamin is also said to stimulate appetite.

Prevention and Treatment: To avoid a thiamin deficiency, significant food sources of the vitamin should be included in your diet, such as whole grain cereals, oatmeal, nuts, peas, lima beans, oysters, liver, pork (especially ham), beef, lamb, poultry, and eggs. (See table of Vitamin B_1(Thiamin)-Rich Foods, page 309.)

The use of baking soda in cooking will result in the destruction of both vitamins B_1 and B_{12}, so it should be avoided when possible. High temperatures too are very destructive to B_1. Blackberries, brussels sprouts, beets, red cabbage, and spinach contain the enzyme thiaminase, which inactivates the vitamin. Large quantities of these foods should not be consumed raw. The consumption of chocolate should be avoided, as it will have the same effect.

CALCIUM DEFICIENCY: Prolonged use of this drug could conceivably lead to a deficiency of calcium in your body, because it results in increased calcium excretion. Whenever calcium blood levels are low, the body liberates necessary amounts of calcium from the bones, where it is stored, thereby weakening them and making them more susceptible to fractures. A condition called osteomalacia can result. This is more likely after middle age, since in older people the body uses dietary calcium less efficiently.

Osteomalacia is a weakening of the bones as a consequence of a uniform and steady calcium loss. This disease affects millions of older Americans, but also many younger people. In fact, one out of every four postmenopausal women suffers from this problem. Prominent symptoms are bone pain in the back, thighs, shoulder region, or ribs; difficulty in walking; and weakness in the muscles of the legs. The condition is reversible once calcium blood levels are raised.

Long periods of calcium deficiency also seem to cause osteoporosis, another condition in which the bones are made weak and brittle. However, osteoporosis, an unexplained and rapid loss of calcium from the bones, is irreversible. Here the first symptoms are backache, a gradual loss of height, and periodontal disease. In cases of osteoporosis, fractures of the vertebrae, hip, and wrist occur frequently, sometimes spontaneously.

Roughly 7 percent of women fifty years of age and older have osteoporosis, and certain observers believe that the incidence of this disease is on the rise; between 15 and 20 million Americans are said to have osteoporosis today. In some 30 percent of people over sixty-five, the disease is severe enough to result in fractures. By age eighty, virtually all women experience some degree of osteoporosis; early menopause is a strong predictor of the disease. One out of five cases of the disease is found in men, but generally men get it at a later age and less severely than women.

Prevention and Treatment: The Recommended Dietary Allowance for calcium is 800 mg and all women should consume at least 1,200 mg of calcium per day. The average intake in the United States, however, is only 450 to 550 mg. For the elderly, and women who have already reached menopause or are about to, this should be increased to 1,500 mg by the consumption of foods rich in calcium, particularly milk and dairy products (including yogurt and hard cheeses) and, to a lesser extent, almonds. Three 8-ounce glasses of milk, for example, provide 1,500 mg of calcium. (See table of Calcium-Rich Foods, page 289.)

If you cannot consume calcium foods because of an intolerance to lactose, the sugar found in dairy products (a problem for an estimated 30 million Americans), a 1,000 mg daily supplement of calcium should be taken. The best absorbed supplement is calcium carbonate. (See Calcium Supplements entry, page 51.) If magnesium is included in the supplement, the calcium is slightly better absorbed, and any tendency to constipation is reduced. The supplement should be taken in two 500 mg dosages, one of which should be consumed before bedtime,

because most of the calcium loss from your bones occurs while you sleep.

Keep in mind that vitamin C assists calcium absorption, while cigarette smoking leads to depletion of body calcium, as does excessive alcohol consumption. The patient using mercurial diuretics should temporarily avoid foods that can decrease the absorption of calcium, such as kale, rhubarb, spinach, cocoa, chocolate, beet greens, tea, and coffee. A deficiency might also arise if the ratio of phosphorus to calcium in your diet is very high; processed foods, especially most carbonated beverages, are particularly high in phosphorus. The ideal ratio is essentially 1 to 1, as in dairy products; when the ratio is 15 or 20 to 1, as in meat, very little calcium is absorbed. High-fiber foods may contribute to a calcium deficiency, since fiber binds to calcium and passes it out in the stool. Excess fat and protein in the diet also hinder absorption.

Since there is little calcium in strict vegetarian diets (those that avoid dairy products as well as meat), vegetarians are at greater risk of a calcium deficiency. People who take magnesium- or aluminum-based antacids are also more prone to calcium deficiencies because both magnesium and aluminum in excess impair calcium absorption.

Besides a change in dietary habits and the use of calcium supplements, it is recommended that anyone at risk of this deficiency adopt an exercise regimen that causes the bones to support the weight of the body, to strengthen the bones and to counteract the loss of bone density. A regular walking or jogging program, for example, can help prevent the bone degeneration of the spine, hips, and legs. Note, however, that swimming, though good for the heart as an aerobic exercise, is not especially beneficial for bone buildup.

MAGNESIUM DEFICIENCY: Once again, these drugs cause the body to excrete a lot of magnesium in the urine, and a deficiency of magnesium could conceivably occur, though magnesium deficiencies are not common since the average American diet contains appreciable amounts of the mineral. However, the high level of magnesium excretion resulting from the interaction with mercurial diuretics makes such a deficiency far more likely.

The clinical signs of magnesium deficiency include muscle weakness, tremors, depression, emotional instability, and irrational behavior. Alcohol also increases magnesium excretion and puts the regular drinker at increased risk for these symptoms.

Prevention and Treatment: A diet containing the four food groups provides the normal amount of magnesium. However, if a magnesium depletion is suspected, your diet should feature foods such as nuts (almonds and cashews are highest), meat, fish, milk, whole grains, and fresh greens, since cooking can wash away some magnesium. (See table of Magnesium-Rich Foods, page 300.) Alcohol intake should be restricted to no more than 2 drinks per day when one is taking this drug.

GASTROINTESTINAL DISTRESS: Mercurial diuretics also damage the lining of the stomach and can lead to gastrointestinal disturbances.

Prevention and Treatment: This drug should be taken with meals or milk.

METAPROTERENOL SULFATE

DRUG FAMILY: Anti-asthmatic

BRAND NAME: Alupent

HOW TO TAKE METAPROTERENOL SULFATE: With fruit juice after meals

FOODS TO AVOID: None

POSSIBLE SIDE EFFECTS: Gastrointestinal distress

ACTION OF METAPROTERENOL SULFATE: This drug is used as a bronchodilator in the treatment of bronchitis, emphysema, and asthma.

HIGH-RISK GROUPS: Anyone who takes this drug

NURTIONAL INTERACTIONS

GASTROINTESTINAL DISTRESS: This drug could conceivably cause you to experience nausea, nervousness, and tremor. The drug also has a very unpleasant taste, which can affect your appetite.

Prevention and Treatment: Metaproterenol sulfate should be taken with fruit juices, just after a meal, to avoid gastrointestinal disturbances and to prevent the bad taste of the drug from affecting your appetite.

METHADONE HYDROCHLORIDE

DRUG FAMILY: Analgesic

BRAND NAME: Dolophine Hydrochloride

HOW TO TAKE METHADONE HYDROCHLORIDE: As directed by your physician

FOODS TO AVOID: All alcoholic beverages; large quantities of alkaline foods should be avoided, like milk, buttermilk, cream, almonds, chestnuts, coconut, all vegetables except corn and lentils, and all fruit except cranberries, prunes, and plums.

POSSIBLE SIDE EFFECTS: Constipation; nausea, vomiting, light-headedness, dizziness, drowsiness, and sweating

ACTION OF METHADONE HYDROCHLORIDE: This drug is used to treat severe pain. It is also given to prevent the withdrawal symptoms that occur from opioid abstinence (morphine, heroin, and codeine after long-term usage).

HIGH-RISK GROUPS: Anyone who consumes alcohol, the elderly

NUTRITIONAL INTERACTIONS

ALCOHOL INTERACTION: The effects of methadone are likely to be enhanced by the concurrent consumption of alcohol. In fact, alcohol consumption could depress the brain to such an extent that a coma could result.

Prevention and Treatment: Alcohol should not be taken in any amount by people taking this drug.

CONSTIPATION: Methadone could conceivably cause constipation.

Prevention and Treatment: Constipation is usually safely remedied by an increase in the bulk in the diet. This means consuming larger servings of any of the following: dried or fresh fruits, salad vegetables, radishes, oatmeal, and whole grain foods (brown rice, whole wheat breads, and cereals). It is not necessary to purchase products that claim "extra fiber" has been added to them.

Persistent constipation may also be relieved by doubling the amount of fluid consumed each day. Bran, if used, should be added to the diet gradually, and fluid should be increased by at least ¾ cup per teaspoon of bran. (See table of Dietary Fiber-Rich foods, page 293.)

ALKALINE URINE: Methadone reduces the acid secretion in the stomach. Since methadone is alkaline, it is excreted at a normal rate only if your urine is acidic. However, if the quantity of alkaline foods in your diet is high, particularly given the decrease in acid secretion in the stomach, your urine may lose its acidity, and the excretion of this drug will be slowed. The effects of the drug will be prolonged, and a toxic buildup can result. The symptoms of such a buildup or overdose are light-headedness, dizziness, drowsiness, nausea, vomiting, and sweating.

Prevention and Treatment: Fruits, vegetables, and dairy products tend to be alkaline, and high-protein foods tend to be acidic. Foods causing the production of alkaline urine include milk, buttermilk, cream, almonds, chestnuts, coconuts, all vegetables except corn and lentils, and all fruits except cranberries, prunes, and plums.

Antacids that neutralize the acid in the stomach will also neutralize the acid in the urine, causing it to turn alkaline. Therefore, you should avoid taking antacids while you are on methadone.

METHENAMINE

DRUG FAMILY: Antibiotic

BRAND NAMES: [GENERIC/Brand] METHENAMINE/Trac Tabs 2X; Urised; Uroblue; Uro-

Phosphate; METHENAMINE HIPPURATE/Hiprex; Urex; METHENAMINE MANDELATE/Mandelamine; Thiacide; Uroqid-Acid

HOW TO TAKE METHENAMINE: With fruit juice or soda pop

FOODS TO AVOID: Large quantities of alkaline foods such as almonds, buttermilk, chestnuts, coconuts, cream, fruits except cranberries, prunes, and plums, milk, and vegetables except corn and lentils

POSSIBLE SIDE EFFECTS: Gastrointestinal distress

ACITON OF METHENAMINE: This drug is used to treat chronic, recurring urinary tract infections. When in the presence of acid urine, it breaks down to formaldehyde, which kills the bacteria.

HIGH-RISK GROUPS: Anyone who takes this drug

NUTRITIONAL INTERACTIONS

ACID URINE: While using this drug, you should take care to maintain your urine in an acidic state. If the quantity of acidic foods in your diet is high, your urine will also be acidic, and this drug will be able to kill the unwanted bacteria in the urinary tract.

Prevention and Treatment: Foods that tend to be acidic, such as high-protein foods, should be well represented in the diet, and fruits, vegetables, and dairy products, which tend to be alkaline, should be limited. Foods causing the production of acid urine include meat, fish, poultry, eggs, cheese, peanut butter, corn, lentils, bacon, nuts, cranberries, plums, prunes, bread, crackers, macaroni, spaghetti, cakes and cookies. (See table of Acidic Foods, page 288.)

Supplementation with vitamin C can also result in acidic urine. Antacids will make the urine alkaline, and their use will inactivate this drug.

METHOTREXATE

DRUG FAMILY: Anti-cancer

BRAND NAMES: Folex; Mexate

HOW TO TAKE METHOTREXATE: As directed by your physician

FOODS TO AVOID: All alcoholic beverages

POSSIBLE SIDE EFFECTS: Deficiencies of folic acid, vitamin B_{12}, and calcium; nausea, vomiting, lack of appetite, diarrhea; liver damage

ACTION OF METHOTREXATE: This drug is used in the treatment of leukemia, cancer, and psoriasis, and other malignant and benign diseases that are resistant to other forms of treatment. It prevents the cancerous cells from multiplying by impairing the activity of folic acid, which is required by all cells if they are to reproduce.

HIGH-RISK GROUPS: Anyone who takes this drug

NUTRITIONAL INTERACTIONS

FOLIC ACID DEFICIENCY: The direct antagonism between methotrexate and folic acid in the diet leads to the excretion of folic acid in the urine and to a folic acid deficiency if the drug is used over extended periods of time without rest periods.

The typical sign of a toxicity due to a deficiency of folacin is anemia characterized by pallor, lethargy, irritability, and breathlessness on exertion.

This drug also causes a loss of appetite, nausea, stomach pain, ulceration of the mouth and intestine, and, eventually, diarrhea. When the diarrhea sets in, the use of the drug should be discontinued immediately.

Prevention and Treatment: Because of the anorexia, gastrointestinal upset, and gastrointestinal lesions caused by the drug, there is a danger both of a failure to eat enough food and of an inability to absorb the nutrients from the food that is consumed.

With a cancer patient who needs to be on the drug for long periods of time, periodic injections or the oral administration of the active form of folic acid called folinic acid will prevent the occurrence of these symptoms. With the noncritical patient, such as one who is suffering from psoriasis, a daily .8 mg supplement of folic acid for a week before treatment should prevent the symptoms.

While you are on the drug, it is pointless to take folic acid supplements. The body cannot use the vitamin, and it will simply be excreted.

VITAMIN B$_{12}$ DEFICIENCY: There have been reports of vitamin B$_{12}$ malabsorption in those taking methotrexate. Over a short course of methotrexate treatment, B$_{12}$ deficiency should not be a problem, since everybody except strict vegetarians has a three- to five-year supply of vitamin B$_{12}$ stored in his liver. However, strict vegetarians could conceivably get into a deficiency state since their stores tend to be much lower.

A B$_{12}$ deficiency is also associated with anemia, characterized by lethargy, pallor, irritability, and breathlessness on exertion.

Prevention and Treatment: Vitamin B$_{12}$ is unique among nutrients in that it is found almost exclusively in animal flesh and animal products. Anyone who eats meat is guaranteed an adequate intake, and lacto-ovovegetarians (who include milk, cheese, and eggs in their diets) are also protected from this deficiency. Strict vegetarians, however, must use vitamin B$_{12}$-fortified soy milk or other such products, or take B$_{12}$ supplements, to ensure their supply of the vitamin.

CALCIUM DEFICIENCY: Methotrexate damages the lining of the intestine and causes general malabsorption of all nutrients. If taken over a prolonged period, the drug is likely to lead to a calcium deficiency.

If your calcium blood levels are low, your body will liberate the necessary amounts of calcium from the bones, where it is stored, thereby weakening them and making them more susceptible to fractures. A condition called osteomalacia can result. This is more likely after middle age, since in older people the body uses dietary calcium less efficiently.

Osteomalacia is a weakening of the bones as a consequence of uniform and steady calcium loss. This disease affects millions of older Americans, but also many younger people. In fact, one out of every four postmenopausal women suffers from this problem. Prominent symptoms are bone pain in the back, thighs, shoulder region, or ribs; difficulty in walking; and weakness in the muscles of the legs. The condition is reversible once calcium blood levels are raised.

Osteoporosis may result if a calcium deficiency persists over a long period of time. Osteoporosis is another condition in which the bones are made weak and brittle. However, osteoporosis, an unexplained and rapid loss of calcium from the bones, is irreversible. Here the first symptoms are backache, a gradual loss of height, and periodontal disease. In cases of osteoporosis, fractures of the vertebrae, hip, and wrist occur frequently, sometimes spontaneously.

Approximately 7 percent of women fifty years of age and older have osteoporosis, and certain observers believe that the incidence of this disease is on the rise; between 15 and 20 million Americans are said to have osteoporosis today. In some 30 percent of people over sixty-five, the disease is severe enough to result in fractures. By age eighty, virtually all women experience some degree of osteoporosis; early menopause is a strong predictor of the disease. One out of five cases of the disease is found in men, but generally men get it at a later age and less severely than women.

Prevention and Treatment: The Recommended Dietary Allowance for calcium is 800 mg, and all women should consume at least 1,200 mg of calcium per day. The average intake in the United States, however, is only 450 to 550 mg. For the elderly, and women who have already reached menopause or are about to, this should be increased to 1,500 mg by the consumption of foods rich in calcium, particularly milk and dairy products (including yogurt and hard cheeses) and, to a lesser extent, almonds. Three 8-ounce glasses of milk, for example, provide 1,500 mg of calcium. (See table of Calcium-Rich Foods, page 289.)

If calcium foods must be avoided because of an intolerance to lactose, the sugar found in dairy products (a problem for an estimated 30 million Americans), a 1,000 mg daily supplement of calcium should be taken. The best-absorbed supplement is calcium carbonate. (See Calcium Supplements entry page 51.) If magnesium is included in the supplement, the calcium is slightly better absorbed and any tendency to constipation is reduced. The supplement should be taken in two 500 mg doses, one of which should be consumed before bedtime, because most of the calcium loss from your body occurs while you sleep.

Vitamin C assists calcium absorption, while cigarette smoking increases body losses of calcium, as does excessive alcohol consumption. Users of methotrexate should temporarily avoid foods that can decrease the absorption of calcium, such as kale, rhubarb, spinach, cocoa and chocolate, beet greens, tea, and coffee. A deficiency might also arise if the ratio of phosphorus to calcium in your diet is very high; processed foods, especially carbonated beverages, are particularly high in phosphorus. The ideal ratio is essentially 1 to 1, as in dairy products; when the ratio is 15 or 20 to 1, as in meat, very little calcium is absorbed. High-fiber foods may contribute to a calcium deficiency, since fiber binds to calcium and passes it out in the stool. Excess fat and protein in the diet also hinder absorption.

Since there is little calcium in strict vegetarian diets (those that avoid dairy products as well as meat), vegetarians are at greater risk of a calcium deficiency. People who take magnesium- or aluminum-based antacids are also more prone to calcium deficiencies because both magnesium and aluminum in excess impair calcium absorption.

Besides a change in dietary habits and the use of calcium supplements, it is recommended that anyone at risk of this deficiency adopt an exercise regimen that causes the bones to support the weight of the body, to strengthen the bones and to counteract the loss of bone density. A regular walking or jogging program, for example, can help prevent the bone degeneration of the spine, hips, and legs. Note, however, that swimming, though good for the heart as an aerobic exercise, is not especially beneficial for bone buildup.

It has been observed that during pregnancy the body absorbs calcium more effectively, making the mother's bones stronger despite the calcium needs of the fetus. Oral contraceptives also seem to help calcium absorption.

GASTROINTESTINAL DISTRESS: Methotrexate causes nausea, vomiting, impaired taste, mouth sores, and anorexia.

Prevention and Treatment: Nausea and vomiting may be controlled by taking several basic steps. First, you should eat smaller meals and limit your intake of high-fat foods. Second, when you experience nausea, you should slowly sip clear beverages, such as ginger ale. Sucking a Popsicle may also alleviate the condition. You should lie down, loosen your clothes, and get fresh air as well.

If you find that you vomit frequently, you should take plenty of liquids to prevent dehydration.

OTHER ADVICE: Aspirin and other salicylate-containing drugs decrease the excretion of

methotrexate and make it more potent and hence more toxic.

Both alcohol and methotrexate damage the liver and eventually cause cirrhosis. Regular consumers of alcohol are more disposed to methotrexate liver damage than teetotalers.

METHYLPHENIDATE HYDROCHLORIDE

DRUG FAMILY: Stimulant

BRAND NAME: Ritalin

HOW TO TAKE METHYLPHENIDATE HYDROCHLORIDE: Preferably 30 to 45 minutes before meals (usually breakfast and lunch)

FOODS TO AVOID: None

POSSIBLE SIDE EFFECTS: Loss of appetite leading to stunted growth

ACTION OF METHYLPHENIDATE HYDROCHLORIDE: A central nervous system stimulant, methylphenidate is used in the treatment of hyperactive children.

HIGH-RISK GROUPS: Children

NUTRITIONAL INTERACTIONS

ANOREXIA AND GROWTH RETARDATION: This drug causes anorexia (loss of appetite) and can lead to the stunting of growth.

Prevention and Treatment: Children on long-term methylphenidate therapy should be carefully monitored for height and weight. The use of the drug should be discontinued to induce catch-up growth during vacation periods, when the hyperactivity, lack of concentration, and short attention span do not interfere with the educational process.

METOCLOPRAMIDE HYDRO-CHLORIDE

DRUG FAMILY: Gastrointestinal

BRAND NAME: Reglan

HOW TO TAKE METOCLOPRAMIDE HYDROCHLO-RIDE: Injection by the physician, or taken orally 30 minutes before each meal and at bedtime

FOODS TO AVOID: Alcoholic beverages

POSSIBLE SIDE EFFECTS: None

ACTION OF METOCLOPRAMIDE HYDROCHLO-RIDE: This drug enhances the motility of the upper gastrointestinal tract and accelerates the rate at which the stomach empties. It is used to treat stasis of the gut, which sometimes occurs in diabetics; to facilitate the transit of a barium meal used for X-ray purposes; and to prevent nausea associated with cancer chemotherapy cures involving the drug cisplatin.

HIGH-RISK GROUPS: Anyone who consumes alcohol

NUTRITIONAL INTERACTIONS

ALCOHOL INTERACTION: This drug is likely to have a sedative effect when it is taken with alcohol.

Prevention and Treatment: Metoclopramide should not be taken concurrently with alcohol.

METOPROLOL TARTRATE

DRUG FAMILY: Anti-hypertensive

BRAND NAME: Lopressor

HOW TO TAKE METOPROLOL TARTRATE: At mealtimes

FOODS TO AVOID: Sugary foods such as cookies, candies, sodas, honey, and table sugar should not be eaten to excess.

POSSIBLE SIDE EFFECTS: Hyperglycemia

ACTION OF METOPROLOL TARTRATE: This anti-hypertensive agent causes the dilation of blood vessels.

HIGH-RISK GROUPS: Diabetics

NUTRITIONAL INTERACTIONS

HYPERGLYCEMIA: Metoprolol inhibits the release of insulin in your system, and as a result blood glucose levels can rise above normal levels. This could be a problem for the diabetic.

Diabetes occurs when the pancreas fails to produce enough insulin to clear the blood of excess glucose, or sugar. The metabolism of fat and protein is also disordered. Blood vessels are damaged, and, as a result, the kidneys, eyes, and heart can sustain long-term damage, as can the nervous system in some cases.

Symptoms of high blood glucose levels are headaches, excessive hunger and thirst, and a need to urinate frequently.

In diabetics who have not stabilized on a given amount of insulin, the varied glucose levels caused by metoprolol can lead the physician to administer higher dosages of insulin. This, in turn, can cause blood glucose levels to fall below normal, leading to hypoglycemia.

Prevention and Treatment: While on this drug, diabetics should be carefully monitored.

If you are diabetic—and 2 million Americans are, over 80 percent of them over the age of forty-five—you must carefully monitor your food intake under any circumstances to avoid an excess of carbohydrates. The worst of the dietary culprits are the simple sugars in cookies, candies, sodas, honey, and table sugar. These foods are absorbed very rapidly and will increase your blood sugar to very high levels. If you are diabetic, such high blood sugar levels are dangerous, because the insulin administered may not be sufficient to bring the levels back into the normal range. A preferred diet is low in fats, but with plenty of complex carbohydrates, such as starches, cereals, and vegetables. (See table of Simple and Complex Carbohydrate Foods, page 305.) This is particularly true when taking metoprolol.

Recent studies have demonstrated that a high-fiber diet may cause a slower and more sustained release of glucose from the gastrointestinal tract into the bloodstream, preventing the wide swings in blood sugar levels. After a prolonged period on a high-fiber diet, the intestines also absorb sugar more readily. For the diabetic, it is recommended that you remain physically active and exercise daily, because the cells are thereby made more susceptible to the insulin. A change in eating schedule from the standard three meals per day to five or six smaller meals may also help keep blood sugar levels within normal range.

OTHER ADVICE: Metoprolol is best absorbed with food, so it should always be taken at mealtime.

METRONIDAZOLE

DRUG FAMILY: Anti-microbial

BRAND NAMES: Flagyl; Protostat; Sātric

HOW TO TAKE METRONIDAZOLE: With meals or milk

FOODS TO AVOID: Foods and beverages containing alcohol

POSSIBLE SIDE EFFECTS: Gastrointestinal disturbances, especially nausea and loss of appetite

ACTION OF METRONIDAZOLE: This drug is the preparation of choice for the treatment of certain venereal infections caused by the organism *T. vaginalis.* This drug is also used in the treatment of a wide variety of gastrointestinal infections caused by intestinal parasites such as giardia and amoeba.

HIGH-RISK GROUPS: Anyone who takes this drug

NUTRITIONAL INTERACTIONS

GASTROINTESTINAL DISTRESS: This drug is likely to cause gastrointestinal disturbances.

Prevention and Treatment: Although food delays its absorption, it does not reduce the effectiveness of the drug and so metronidazole is best taken with food.

ALCOHOL INTERACTION: Metronidazole prevents the complete breakdown of alcohol. This can lead to a rapid buildup of acetaldehyde, a by-product of alcohol as it is metabolized, in the blood. If alcohol is consumed after this drug is taken, it will cause symptoms such as headaches, flushing, nausea, vomiting, low blood pressure, blurred vision, and possibly vertigo.

The reaction begins within 5 to 10 minutes of one's consuming the alcohol. In sensitive people, this reaction may result from consuming just 1 or 2 sips of an alcoholic beverage, or if they consume foods flavored with wine or liquor.

Prevention and Treatment: No food or beverage containing alcohol should be consumed while you are taking this drug.

MINERAL OIL

DRUG FAMILY: Laxative

BRAND NAMES: Agoral; Liqui-Doss; Milk of Magnesia-Mineral Oil Emulsion; Milkinol; Whirl-Sol

HOW TO TAKE MINERAL OIL: With fruit juice or some other strong-tasting liquid, between meals and not within 2 hours of taking a meal; bedtime is the ideal time to take mineral oil.

FOODS TO AVOID: None

POSSIBLE SIDE EFFECTS: Deficiencies of vitamins D, K, and A, potassium, and calcium

ACTION OF MINERAL OIL: Mineral oil softens and lubricates the stool. It reduces the reabsorption of water from the stools that normally takes place in the large intestine and, in this way, increases the volume of the stool, which facilitates its movement through the intestine. It also softens the stool directly, since the oil is not absorbed and becomes a constituent of the stool itself. Mineral oil is a mixture of liquid hydrocarbons obtained from petroleum.

HIGH-RISK GROUPS: The elderly

NUTRITIONAL INTERACTIONS

VITAMIN D DEFICIENCIES: Mineral oil is indigestible and largely nonabsorbable from the intestine, but it decreases the absorption of vitamins D, A, and K and can lead to deficiencies in people who use it regularly. (The occasional user should not experience these problems.) These fat-soluble vitamins are dissolved in the mineral oil, carried straight through the intestine, and excreted in the feces without being absorbed by the body. If taken at meals in a normal dosage of 30 to 60 ml, mineral oil will dissolve an even greater amount of the dietary supply of all three of these vitamins.

Vitamin D is needed by the body to enable it to absorb calcium and phosphorus, and so to promote the development of strong teeth and bones. Whenever calcium blood levels are low, the body will liberate the necessary amounts of calcium from the bones, where it is stored. As a result, the bones will be weakened and made more susceptible to fractures. A condition called osteomalacia can result. This is more likely after middle age, since in older people the body uses dietary calcium less efficiently.

Osteomalacia is a weakening of the bones as a consequence of uniform and steady calcium loss. This disease affects millions of older Americans but also many younger people. In fact, one out of every four postmenopausal women suffers from this problem. Prominent symptoms are bone pain in the back, thighs, shoulder region, or ribs; difficulty in walking; and weakness in the muscles of the legs. The condition is reversible once calcium blood levels are raised.

Osteoporosis is another condition that may develop as a result of a calcium deficiency. Osteoporosis also leads to the bones being weakened and made brittle, but osteoporosis, an unexplained and rapid loss of calcium from the bones, is irreversible. The first symptoms are backache, a gradual loss of height, and periodontal disease. Fractures of the vertebrae, hip, and wrist occur, sometimes spontaneously.

Approximately 7 percent of women fifty years of age and older have osteoporosis, and certain observers believe that the incidence of this disease is on the rise; between 15 and 20 million Americans are said to have osteoporosis today. In some 30 percent of people over sixty-five, the disease is severe enough to result in fractures. By age eighty, virtually all women experience some degree of osteoporosis; early menopause is a strong predictor of the disease. One out of five cases of the disease is found in men, but generally men get it at a later age and less severely than women.

In children, a vitamin D deficiency can result in a condition known as rickets, in which the bones become bent or malformed. Children under four years of age may also develop pigeon breast, bowlegs, a protruding abdomen due to a weakness of stomach muscles, and poorly formed teeth that tend to decay.

Prevention and Treatment: To avoid a vitamin D deficiency while you are on mineral oil, you should take 400 to 800 IU of vitamin D per day as a supplement to a diet of foods rich in vitamin D, such as fortified milk, butter, liver, egg yolks, salmon, tuna, and sardines. (See table of Vitamin D-Rich Foods, page 313.)

Vitamin D is initially formed in the skin as a result of exposure to sunlight and is activated in the liver and kidneys. The production of vitamin D is dependent upon climatic conditions, air pollution, skin pigmentation (the darker the skin, the lower the production), the area of skin exposed, the duration of exposure to the sun, and the use of sun screens. Adults who are not often exposed to sunlight (e.g. those who are housebound or by custom heavily clothed), require dietary sources of vitamin D to prevent osteomalacia.

Vitamin D is also indispensable to infants, children, and to pregnant or lactating women, whose requirements are high due to bone growth or skeletal mineral replacement. Supplementation for pregnant women is crucial, since vitamin D deficiencies can cause fetal abnormalities. However, no more than 800 IU of the vitamin should be taken by pregnant women, because excessive consumption can cause kidney damage. In nonpregnant adults, 2,000 IU of the vitamin should be taken if osteomalacia is indicated. If your intake of vitamin D exceeds 4,000 IU per day, toxicity of vitamin D poisoning can occur. The symptoms are loss of appetite, headache, excessive thirst, irritability, and kidney stones.

In all of these cases, foods rich in calcium should be included in the diet, especially dairy products. (See table of Calcium-Rich Foods, page 289.)

VITAMIN K DEFICIENCY: People with an abnormally low dietary intake of vitamin K are at risk of bleeding with unusual ease if they use mineral oil for a long period of time or in substantial dosages.

Normally, vitamin K helps produce blood-clotting substances in the liver. Without sufficient levels of vitamin K in the diet, however, bleeding may take place in the gastrointestinal tract (causing black or blood-stained stools), in the urinary tract (causing blood in the urine), and in the uterus (causing blood loss at times other than the normal menstrual periods), and excessive blood loss may also occur after an injury or surgery. Another sign of a deficiency of this vitamin is more frequent and more visible bruising than normal.

Half the vitamin K intake in humans comes from dietary sources, predominantly green leafy vegetables and to a lesser extent fruit, cereals, dairy products, and meat. The rest of the vitamin K in our bodies is synthesized by the bacteria in the intestines. The daily need for the vitamin is in the range of 70 to 140 mcg.

Pregnant women are at high risk because a vitamin K deficiency can lead to hemorrhaging in the fetus. A fetus is more susceptible than an adult, since it does not have a bacterial population in its large intestine to make vitamin K and does not develop the capacity to do so for the first week of life. Women who have had several pregnancies or whose menstrual periods are heavy should also be careful. Many of the elderly are at risk of a vitamin K deficiency because they have a problem of poor fat absorption, and vitamin K, a fat-soluble vitamin, must be accompanied by sufficient dietary fat to be properly absorbed. Finally, anyone suffering from a kidney disease or cancer, or who is on a prolonged antibiotic therapy, may be at risk.

Prevention and Treatment: A vitamin K deficiency can be countered by a vitamin K supplement of 100 mcg per day and a diet that includes foods rich in the vitamin, such as kale, spinach, cabbage, cauliflower, leafy green vegetables, liver (especially pork liver), and fish. (See table of Vitamin K-Rich Foods, page 315.)

Vitamin E supplements should not be taken when at risk of a vitamin K shortage, because vitamin E impairs the absorption of K.

VITAMIN A DEFICIENCY: A deficiency in vitamin A takes a long time to develop and is not usually seen in people taking mineral oil. Carotene is the red pigment in plants, obvious in carrots, yellow maize, and red palm oil. It is converted into vitamin A in the body. One milligram of carotene in the diet is equivalent to one sixth of a milligram of vitamin A in the body. Night blindness is one early sign of a vitamin A deficiency.

Vitamin A increases your resistance to infection. In fact, it is thought that this vitamin also lowers susceptibility to certain forms of cancer. It keeps the eyes healthy and is required for your body to maintain the nails, hair, bones, and glands.

Symptoms of a vitamin A deficiency are an impaired ability to see in dim light and an increased susceptibility to skin disorders and a variety of other diseases.

Prevention and Treatment: If your daily dose of a mineral oil preparation equals or exceeds 30 ml, a vitamin A supplement is required. A small dosage of vitamin A such as the 5,000 IU's found in a multivitamin should counteract this deficiency. Vitamin A is one of the fat-soluble vitamins and hence does not have to be consumed everyday, because it is stored in the body. It is advised not to take major doses (over 10,000 IU per day). An overdose can be toxic and can lead to diarrhea, nausea, hair loss, extreme fatigue, and menstrual irregularities.

Vitamin A can be found in foods such as fish oils, liver, whole milk, whole milk products, egg yolks, fortified margarine, green vegetables (especially spinach), and yellow fruit (cantaloupes). (See table of Vitamin A-Rich Foods, page 308.) Unlike most vitamins, vitamin A will not be easily destroyed by cooking or exposure to high temperatures, but long exposure to sunlight and freeze drying will damage it. Therefore, you should keep milk stored in opaque containers and cover vegetables. Frying calf or chicken livers will also destroy the vitamin, and cooking green, yellow, or red vegetables for a long period of time will reduce the vitamin's potency.

Orange peel and marmalade contain a substance called citral, which in large quantities can decrease the effectiveness of vitamin A; the consumption of orange peel should be moderated while at risk of a vitamin A shortage.

POTASSIUM AND CALCIUM DEPLETION: Mineral oil should never be taken habitually, or with meals, because chronic misuse could conceivably lead to a loss of body potassium and calcium. As discussed above, calcium depletion can lead to osteomalacia.

Potassium regulates the amount of water in the cells of the body and is essential for the proper functioning of the kidneys and the heart muscle, and the secretion of digestive juices.

The most alarming symptom of a potassium deficiency is an irregular heartbeat, which can lead to heart failure. Other symptoms include weakness, loss of appetite, nausea, vomiting, listlessness, apprehension, and diffuse pain that comes and goes.

Proper potassium levels in your body can also be threatened if this drug is taken concurrently with cortisone-containing drugs or diuretics.

Prevention and Treatment: Potassium depletion can be avoided by including such potassium-rich foods in your diet as tomato juice, lentils, dried apricots, peanut butter, chicken, almonds, and milk. (See table of Potassium-Rich Foods, page 302.)

Potassium supplements should never be taken unless prescribed by a physician. They can cause anemia by interfering with the absorption of vitamin B_{12}. In addition, just a few grams can drastically increase the risk of heart failure. If you experience difficulty in swallowing while taking potassium supplements, consult your physician immediately.

Too much salt in your diet can also compromise your body's supply of potassium, as can 1 to 3 ounces per day of natural licorice. As a rule only imported licorice contains the natural extract, since domestic brands use synthetic flavorings.

Prevention and Treatment: The Recommended Dietary Allowance for calcium is 800 mg, and all women should consume at least 1,200 mg of calcium per day. The average intake in the United States, however, is only 450 to 550 mg. For the elderly, and women who have already reached menopause or are about to, this should be increased to 1,500 mg by the consumption of foods rich in calcium, particularly milk and dairy products (including yogurt and hard cheeses) and, to a lesser extent, almonds. Three 8-ounce glasses of milk, for example, provide 1,500 mg of calcium. (See table of Calcium-Rich Foods, page 289.)

If calcium foods must be avoided because of an intolerance to lactose, the sugar present in dairy products (a problem for an estimated 30 million Americans), a 1,000 mg daily supplement of calcium should be taken. The best-absorbed supplement is calcium carbonate. (See Calcium Supplements entry, page 51.) If magnesium is included in the supplement, the calcium is slightly better absorbed, and any tendency to constipation is reduced. The supplement should be taken in two 500 mg dosages, one of which should be consumed before bedtime because most of the calcium loss from your body occurs while you sleep.

Keep in mind that vitamin C assists calcium absorption, while cigarette smoking tends to deplete body calcium, as does excessive alcohol consumption. Users of mineral oil should temporarily avoid foods that can decrease the absorption of calcium, such as kale, rhubarb, spinach, cocoa, chocolate, beet greens, tea, and coffee. A deficiency might also arise if the ratio of phosphorus to calcium in your diet is very high; processed foods, especially carbonated beverages, are particularly high in phosphorus. The ideal ratio is essentially 1 to 1, as in dairy products; when the ratio is 15 or 20 to 1, as in meat, very little calcium is absorbed. High-fiber foods may contribute to a calcium deficiency, since fiber binds to calcium and passes it out in the stool. Excess fat and protein in the diet also hinder absorption.

Since there is little calcium in strict vegetarian diets (those that avoid dairy products as well as meat), vegetarians are at greater risk of a calcium deficiency. People who take magnesium- or aluminum-based antacids are also more prone to calcium deficiencies because both magnesium and aluminum in excess impair calcium absorption.

Besides a change in dietary habits and the use of calcium supplements, it is recommended that anyone at risk of this deficiency adopt an exercise regimen that causes the bones to support the weight of the body, to strengthen the bones and counteract the loss of bone density. A regular walking or jogging program, for example, can help prevent the bone degeneration of the spine, hips, and legs. Note, however, that swimming, though good for the heart as an aerobic exercise, is not especially beneficial for bone buildup.

OTHER ADVICE: Mineral oil should be used infrequently and never within 2 hours of meals. The ideal time to take mineral oil is at bedtime.

If taken with fruit juice, the tasteless consistency can be masked and the medication be made more palatable.

MONOAMINE-OXIDASE INHIBITORS

DRUG FAMILY: Anti-depressant

BRAND NAME: [GENERIC/Brand] ISOCARBOX-AZID/Marplan; PHENELZINE SULFATE/Nardil; TRANYLCYPROMINE SULFATE/Parnate

HOW TO TAKE MONOAMINE-OXIDASE INHIBITORS: With meals or milk

FOODS TO AVOID: Tyramine- and dopamine-containing foods such as aged cheeses, raisins, avocados, chicken and beef livers, bananas, eggplant, sour cream, alcoholic beverages (especially sherry, beer, and Chianti wine), salami, meat tenderizers, pickled herring, broad beans, natural chocolate, canned figs, yeast, and soy sauce; all alcoholic beverages

POSSIBLE SIDE EFFECTS: Gastrointestinal distress

ACTION OF MONOAMINE-OXIDASE INHIBITORS: MAO inhibitors are mood-elevating agents used in the treatment of severe depression. They prevent the breakdown of the chemical messengers (neurotransmitters) in the brain responsible for elevating mood (serotonin and norepinephrine).

HIGH-RISK GROUPS: Anyone who takes this drug

NUTRITIONAL INTERACTIONS

TYRAMINE-RICH FOODS: Toxic reactions to cheese and other tyramine-containing foods are likely to occur in patients using this drug. Attacks are characterized by transient high blood pressure, headaches, palpitations, nausea, and vomiting.

The severity of the attacks has been related to the level of tyramine in particular foods. The ingested tyramine is usually converted in the liver to an inactive form through the action of monoamine oxidase (MAO). However, drugs in the MAO inhibitor class leave tyramine in its active form. As a result, the tyramine remains in the blood and can increase blood pressure to dangerous levels. Reactions usually occur within a half hour of the ingestion of the offending food or drink.

Other foods that contain dopa or dopamine have similar effects. Both tyramine and dopamine enter the general circulation and release norepinephrine from nerve endings in the body. This potentiates the elevated norepinephrine effect of the monoamine-oxidase inhibitors. Other anti-depressant drugs, such as amphetamines, also act as MAO inhibitors and when combined with tyramine- and dopamine-containing foods can precipitate severe or even lethal side effects.

Similar effects have also been observed with caffeine in animals. The effect of alcohol is intensified, since MAO inhibitors slow the rate at which the body detoxifies it.

Prevention and Treatment: Foods containing tyramine and related substances must be restricted while you are being treated with MAO inhibitors. Tyramine is common in many foods, but it is found in the greatest amounts in high-protein foods that have undergone some decomposition, like aged cheese, especially Swiss, cheddar, processed American, Brie, Camembert, Gruyère, and blue cheeses. Tyramine is also found in raisins, avocados, chicken and beef livers, bananas, eggplant, sauerkraut, yogurt, sour cream, alcoholic beverages (especially sherry, beer, and such wines as Chianti), salami, meat tenderizers, coffee, pickled herring, broad beans, cola, natural chocolate, canned figs, pineapples, yeast, and soy sauce. (See table of Tyramine-Rich Foods, page 307.) Raisins and avocados should also be avoided, because they contain dopamine, which has the same effect as tyramine.

Alcohol should not be consumed by people taking MAO inhibitors.

OTHER ADVICE: Since these drugs sometimes cause gastrointestinal distress, they should be taken with food or milk.

MORPHINE SULFATE

DRUG FAMILY: Analgesic

BRAND NAMES: RMS Suppositories; Roxanol

HOW TO TAKE MORPHINE SULFATE: As directed by your physician

FOODS TO AVOID: All alcoholic beverages; large quantities of alkaline foods such as milk, buttermilk, cream, almonds, chestnuts, coconuts, all vegetables except corn and lentils, and all fruits except cranberries, prunes, and plums

POSSIBLE SIDE EFFECTS: Constipation

ACTION OF MORPHINE SULFATE: This drug is used to relieve pain, coughing, and also diarrhea.

HIGH-RISK GROUPS: Anyone who consumes alcohol, the elderly

NUTRITIONAL INTERACTIONS

ALCOHOL INTERACTION: The effects of morphine sulfate are likely to be enhanced by the concurrent consumption of alcohol. This can lead to cessation of breathing and cardiac arrest.

Prevention and Treatment: Alcohol should not be taken in any amount by people on this drug.

CONSTIPATION: Morphine sulfate could conceivably cause you to become constipated.

Prevention and Treatment: Constipation is usually safely remedied by an increase in the bulk in the diet. This means consuming larger servings of any of the following: dried or fresh fruits, salad vegetables, radishes, oatmeal, and whole grain foods (brown rice, whole wheat breads, and cereals). It is not necessary to purchase products that claim "extra fiber" has been added to them.

Persistent constipation may also be relieved by doubling the amount of fluid consumed each day. Bran, if used, should be added to the diet gradually, and fluid should be increased by at least ¾ cup per teaspoon of bran. (See table of Dietary Fiber-Rich Foods, page 293.)

ALKALINE URINE: Morphine sulfate reduces the acid secretion in the stomach. Since morphine sulfate is alkaline, it is excreted at a normal rate only if your urine is acidic. However, if the quantity of alkaline foods in your diet is high, particularly given the decrease in acid secretion in the stomach, your urine may lose its acidity, and the excretion of this drug will be slowed. The effects of the drug will be prolonged, and a toxic buildup could conceivably occur, resulting in light-headedness, dizziness, drowsiness, nausea, vomiting, and sweating.

Prevention and Treatment: Fruits, vegetables, and dairy products tend to be alkaline, and high-protein foods tend to be acidic. Foods causing the production of alkaline urine include milk, buttermilk, cream, almonds, chestnuts, coconuts, all vegetables except corn and lentils, and all fruits except cranberries, prunes, and plums.

Antacids that neutralize the acid in the stomach will also neutralize the acid in the urine, causing it to turn alkaline. Therefore, you should avoid taking antacids while you are on this drug.

NADOLOL

DRUG FAMILY: Vasodilator

BRAND NAMES: Corgard; Corzide

HOW TO TAKE NADOLOL: With meals

FOODS TO AVOID: None

POSSIBLE SIDE EFFECTS: Gastrointestinal distress; weight gain

ACTION OF NADOLOL: This drug dilates the blood vessels and is used in the long-term treatment of patients with angina pectoris and in the management of high blood pressure.

HIGH-RISK GROUPS: Diabetics

NUTRITIONAL INTERACTIONS

GASTROINTESTINAL DISTRESS: Approximately five in every thousand of those who use this medication experience gastrointestinal disturbances. A similar percentage also tend to gain weight.

Prevention and Treatment: Nadolol should be taken with meals to minimize the threat of gastrointestinal discomfort and increase absorption. Body weight should be carefully monitored.

OTHER ADVICE: Nadolol tends to mask the rapid heartbeat associated with dangerously low blood glucose levels, which sometimes occurs in diabetics as a result of taking too much insulin or other drug used to control blood glucose levels. If this happens, a person can fall suddenly into a coma, without having enough warning to seek help.

Prevention and Treatment: Anyone susceptible to periods of hypoglycemia should be very watchful for signs of the disorder, including anxiety, irritability, sweating, hunger, and trembling. If any of these symptoms are experienced, you should eat a sugar cube, a spoonful of sugar, or some other very sweet food, and seek help immediately from a physician.

NALIDIXIC ACID

DRUG FAMILY: Antibiotic

BRAND NAME: NegGram

HOW TO TAKE NALIDIXIC ACID: Always with food or milk

FOODS TO AVOID: None

POSSIBLE SIDE EFFECTS: Iron deficiency; gastric irritation

ACTION OF NALIDIXIC ACID: This antibiotic drug is usually prescribed for the treatment of bacterial urinary tract infections.

HIGH-RISK GROUPS: Premenopausal women, the elderly, children, vegetarians

NUTRITIONAL INTERACTIONS

IRON DEFICIENCY ANEMIA: Nalidixic acid is a gastric irritant that often causes gastric bleeding. This can lead to a loss of iron from the body.

Since this drug is only taken for short periods of time, it is unlikely that you will develop iron deficiency anemia unless your body has low iron stores to begin with. However, if you experience such symptoms as lethargy, apathy, tiredness, and a pale complexion, your problem may well be iron deficiency anemia.

Iron is especially important to the oxygen-carrying cells of the blood and muscles, which consume two thirds of your body's iron requirement. As a result, an iron deficiency can cause an anemia by reducing the oxygen-carrying capacity of the blood; its symptoms are tiredness, general feelings of malaise, irritability, decreased attention span, pale complexion, and breathlessness on exertion.

In order for iron to be absorbed from any vegetable source, it must be converted to another form by the action of the hydrochloric acid produced in the stomach. Since many elderly people secrete less hydrochloric acid than normal, they absorb iron poorly even under normal circumstances. The diets of many Americans, young and old, lack adequate quantities of this mineral for their normal needs, let alone the increased need that results from blood loss. For example, 10 percent of American women suffer from an iron deficiency, and up to 30 percent have inadequate iron stores.

The shortage of iron in many diets is due not only to the selection of foods that are poor sources of iron, but also to the switch from cast-iron cookware to aluminum, stainless steel, and nonstick surfaces. Iron used to be leached from the surface of iron pots and pans by the acids in foods and was made available as dietary iron.

Other people who are at significant risk for iron deficiency are women who have had several pregnancies and those whose menstrual periods are heavy. There is also a good deal of evidence that teenagers eat too little iron-rich foods, because of the popularity of fast foods, and many suffer from anemia.

Prevention and Treatment: To counteract iron deficiency, iron-rich foods should be included in your diet: beans, enriched bran flakes, tuna, chicken, oysters, dried apricots, prunes, strawberries, leafy green vegetables, and lean red meat and liver. (See table of Iron-Rich Foods, page 299.)

Other foods and drugs have a considerable impact on the way your body absorbs iron. There are two kinds of iron in food sources: heme iron in meat and ionic iron in vegetables. Only 30 percent of heme iron from meat sources is absorbed, and only 10 percent of ionic iron from vegetable sources. Antacids will interfere with iron absorption in vegetables, as will commercial black and pekoe tea, taken in substantial quantities. Vitamin C supplements or citrus juices will favorably affect absorption if taken at the same time. If your diet is rich in high-fiber foods, the fiber will impair iron absorption, because it binds with the iron and passes it out in the stool. It is this same action with fiber that contributes to the poor iron absorption from vegetable sources. Foods high in phosphorus (e.g. meat) interfere with iron absorption, which explains why only 30 percent of the iron in meat is captured. For that matter, any use of large quantities of mineral supplements, such as zinc, will impair iron absorption.

Iron supplements should not be taken without a physician's recommendation, because an accumulation of too much iron can damage the pancreas and the heart, and can also cause cirrhosis of the liver.

OTHER ADVICE: Nalidixic acid should always be taken with food or milk to limit the gastric irritation.

NAPROXEN AND SODIUM NAPROXEN

DRUG FAMILY: Anti-inflammatory

BRAND NAMES: Naprosyn; Anaprox

HOW TO TAKE NAPROXEN: With meals or milk

FOODS TO AVOID: None

POSSIBLE SIDE EFFECTS: Constipation, heartburn, stomach pain, nausea, diarrhea, and indigestion

ACTION OF NAPROXEN: This anti-inflammatory and painkilling drug is prescribed to reduce joint swellings, pain, and the duration of morning stiffness in patients with arthritis.

HIGH-RISK GROUPS: Anyone who takes this drug

NUTRITIONAL INTERACTIONS

GASTROINTESTINAL DISTRESS: One in seven people taking naproxen is reported to suffer from gastrointestinal disturbances. The most common symptoms are constipation, heartburn, stomach pain, and nausea, although diarrhea and indigestion also occur.

Prevention and Treatment: Naproxen should always be taken with meals to reduce the chances of heartburn, stomach pains, and nausea.

Constipation is usually safely remedied by an increase in the bulk in the diet. This means consuming larger servings of any of the following: dried or fresh fruits (especially unpeeled apples or pears), salad vegetables, radishes, oatmeal, and whole grain foods (brown rice, whole wheat breads, and cereals). It is not necessary to purchase products that claim "extra fiber" has been added to them.

Persistent constipation may also be relieved by doubling the amount of fluid consumed each day. Bran, if used, should be added to the diet gradually, and fluid should be increased by at least ¾ cup per teaspoon of bran. (See table of Dietary Fiber-Rich Foods, page 293.)

POTENCY: Naproxen is most rapidly absorbed when it is taken with milk or food. Sodium bicarbonate increases the rate of absorption, and aluminum hydroxide decreases the rate.

Prevention and Treatment: You should take naproxen with meals, which will increase its absorption as well as help limit the gastrointestinal discomforts.

NEOMYCIN

DRUG FAMILY: Antibiotic

BRAND NAMES: Coly-Mycin; Neomycin Sulfate

HOW TO TAKE NEOMYCIN: As directed by your physician

FOODS TO AVOID: Milk and other dairy products, and sweet foods such as cookies, candies, and cake should not be eaten in large quantities.

POSSIBLE SIDE EFFECTS: Inability to digest food properly; diarrhea; deficiencies of vitamin B$_6$, folacin, and iron

ACTION OF NEOMYCIN: This broad-based antibiotic is mainly used to suppress the growth of intestinal bacteria.

HIGH-RISK GROUPS: Heavy drinkers, users of oral contraceptives, vegetarians, premenopausal women, smokers

Nutritional Interactions

DEFICIENCIES RESULTING FROM LONG-TERM USE: Although neomycin impairs the absorption of most nutrients, it does not usually cause deficiencies in short-term treatment. However, it is conceivable that multiple deficiencies could occur as a result of a two-week or longer use of neomycin.

Neomycin damages the lining of the intestine and in so doing inhibits the action of the disaccharidase enzymes that are found in the lining. These are responsible for breaking down carbohydrates such as sucrose and lactose (milk sugar) to facilitate their absorption. The drug decreases your ability to digest lactose by as much as 75 percent, and as a result, consumption of milk and sugary foods can lead to diarrhea and should be restricted in the diet.

VITAMIN B$_6$ DEFICIENCY: Neomycin inactivates vitamin B$_6$, and could conceivably lead to a deficiency. Common symptoms of this deficiency are a sore mouth and tongue, cracks in the lips and corners of the mouth, and patches of itching, scaling skin. A severe vitamin B$_6$ deficiency may cause depression and confusion.

Vitamin B$_6$ deficiencies are common among the elderly. Alcoholics, as well, often experience this deficiency, since alcohol interferes with the body's ability to use B$_6$. Smokers also have an increased need for the vitamin. It is estimated that one of every two Americans consumes less than 70 percent of the Recommended Dietary Allowance of B$_6$.

Prevention and Treatment: To avoid a B$_6$ deficiency, you should consume a diet featuring foods sources of vitamin B$_6$ such as liver (beef, calf, and pork), herring, salmon, walnuts, peanuts, wheat germ, carrots, peas, potatoes, grapes, bananas, and yeast. (See table of Vitamin B$_6$(Pyridoxine)-Rich Foods, page 311.) The vitamin is present in significant amounts in meats, fish, fruits, cereals, and vegetables, and to a lesser extent in milk and other dairy products.

Since vitamin B$_6$ is decomposed at high temperatures, modern food processing often diminishes dietary sources of the vitamin. Consequently, the more processed foods you eat, the more susceptible you will be to a deficiency of this vitamin. Similar losses also occur in cooking: meat loses as much as 45 to 80 percent, vegetables 20 to 30 percent.

It has been observed that 15 to 20 percent of oral contraceptive users show direct evidence of vitamin B$_6$ deficiency. If you are among these people, you should take a 5 mg supplement of vitamin B$_6$ per day. Smokers should take a daily supplement of 5 mg. However, keep in mind that you can take too much vitamin B$_6$; people taking over 1 gram per day have been reported to experience nerve degeneration.

FOLIC ACID DEFICIENCY: Neomycin decreases folate absorption. In long-term use, this could conceivably lead to a deficiency. Often the first sign of a folic acid or folacin deficiency is inflamed and bleeding gums. The symptoms that follow are a sore, smooth tongue; diarrhea; forgetfulness; apathy; irritability; anemia; and a reduced resistance to infection. Despite the fact that folacin is found in a variety of foods, folacin deficiency is still the most common vitamin deficiency in the United States.

Folacin deficiencies are limited in adults almost exclusively to the elderly and women, 30 percent of whom have intakes below the recommended daily allowance, and 5 to 7 percent of whom also have severe anemia. There are several factors that account for this bias, but one of the most obvious reasons is that oral contraceptive use decreases the absorption of folic acid. Constant dieting also limits folacin intake. Alcohol interferes with the absorption and utilization of the vitamin by the body. Folacin is not stored by the body in any appreciable amounts, so an adequate supply must be consumed on a daily basis.

Folic acid is crucial to the normal metabolism of proteins. It is also required for cell growth, so a deficiency during pregnancy can lead to birth defects.

Prevention and Treatment: To counteract a deficiency in folic acid, your diet should contain liver, yeast, and leafy vegetables such as spinach, kale, parsley, cauliflower, brussels sprouts, and broccoli. The fruits that are highest in folic acid are oranges and cantaloupes. To a lesser degree, folacin is found in almonds and lima beans, corn, parsnips, green peas, pumpkins, sweet potatoes, bran, peanuts, rye, and whole grain wheat. (See table of Folacin-Rich Foods, page 297.) Approximately one half of the folic acid you consume is absorbed by your body.

Normal cooking temperatures (110 to 120 degrees for 10 minutes) destroy 65 percent of the vitamin in food. Your daily diet, therefore, should include some raw vegetables and fruits. Cooking utensils made out of copper speed up folacin's destruction.

The recommended daily consumption of folacin is 400 mcg. Oral contraceptive users should consume 800 mcg daily.

IRON DEFICIENCY: Neomycin use can create the risk of an iron deficiency by decreasing iron absorption. Iron is especially important to the oxygen-carrying cells of the blood and muscles, which account for two thirds of the iron your body requires. An iron shortage reduces the blood's oxygen-carrying capacity. The result is an anemia signaled by such symptoms as tiredness, general feelings of malaise, irritability, decreased attention span, pale complexion, rapid heart rhythm, headaches, loss of concentration, and breathlessness on exertion. A mild iron deficiency will also impair the functioning of your immune system.

In order for iron to be absorbed from any vegetable source, it must be converted to another form by the action of the hydrochloric acid produced in the stomach. Some elderly people secrete less hydrochloric acid than normal, so they absorb iron poorly even under normal circumstances. The diets of many Americans lack adequate quantities of the mineral for their normal needs. For example, 10 percent of American women suffer from an iron deficiency, and up to 30 percent have inadequate iron stores. Other people who are at significant risk of an iron deficiency are women who have had several pregnancies and those whose menstrual periods are heavy.

The shortage of iron in many diets is due not only to the selection of foods that are poor sources of iron, but also to the switch away from cast-iron cookware to aluminum, stainless steel, and recently nonstick surfaces. Iron used to be leached from iron pots and pans, and became available as dietary iron.

Prevention and Treatment: To counteract an iron deficiency, iron-rich foods should be included in your diet: liver, whole grain products, oysters, dried apricots, prunes, peaches, leafy green vegetables, and lean red meat. (See table of Iron-Rich Foods, page 299.)

Other foods and drugs have a considerable impact on the way your body absorbs (or does not absorb) iron. There are two kinds of iron in food sources: heme iron in meat and ionic iron in vegetables. Up to 30 percent of the iron from meat, fish, and poultry is absorbed, but less than 10 percent is absorbed from eggs, whole grains, nuts, and dried beans. Only 10 percent of ionic iron is absorbed from vegetable sources, with as little as 2 percent being absorbed from spinach. Antacids will interfere with iron absorption in vegetables, as will commercial black and pekoe tea, taken in substantial quantities, because of its tannin content.

Coffee also seems to decrease iron absorption, but not to the same degree as tea. Vitamin C supplements or citrus juices increase the absorption of iron from vegetable sources by two to three times if taken simultaneously.

If your diet is rich in high-fiber foods, you will have impaired iron absorption, because the fiber will bind to the iron and pass it out in the stool. The same action contributes to the poor absorption of iron from vegetable sources. Foods high in phosphorus (e.g. meat) interfere with iron absorption, which explains why only 30 percent of the iron in meat is captured. (However, meat and fish facilitate iron absorption from vegetables.) For that matter, any use of large quantities of mineral supplements, such as zinc, will impair iron absorption. Because iron can be leached from vegetables if they are cooked in large amounts of water, it is preferable to steam them.

Iron supplements should not be taken without a physician's recommendation because an accumulation of too much iron can lead in extreme cases to such serious problems as anemia, malfunctioning of the pancreas and the heart, cirrhosis of the liver, a brown cast to the skin, and depression.

OTHER ADVICE: Milk and dairy products should not be consumed in large amounts by people taking neomycin. Sweet foods should also be limited in the diet, because they will provoke diarrhea.

NITROFURANTOIN MACROCRYSTALS

DRUG FAMILY: Antibiotic

BRAND NAME: Macrodantin

HOW TO TAKE NITROFURANTOIN MACROCRYSTALS: With food or milk

FOODS TO AVOID: None

POSSIBLE SIDE EFFECTS: Nausea, vomiting, and diarrhea

ACTION OF NITROFURANTOIN MACROCRYSTALS: This drug is prescribed for treating urinary tract infections.

HIGH-RISK GROUPS: People with a history of abdominal distress

NUTRITIONAL INTERACTIONS

GASTROINTESTINAL DISTRESS: It is likely that while taking nitrofurantoin macrocrystals you will experience nausea, vomiting, or diarrhea as a side effect of the drug.

Prevention and Treatment: Nitrofurantoin macrocrystals should always be taken with milk or meals. This will not only reduce the risk of gastrointestinal disturbances, but will aid in the absorption of this drug.

NITROGLYCERIN

DRUG FAMILY: Vasodilator

BRAND NAMES: Nitro-Bid; Nitro-Bid IV; Nitrodisc; Nitro-Dur; Nitroglycerin S.R.; Nitroglyn; Nitrol; Nitrolin; Nitrong; Nitrospan; Nitrostat; Nitrostat IV; Transderm-Nitro; Tridil

HOW TO TAKE NITROGLYCERIN: As directed by your physican

FOODS TO AVOID: Most people needing to take this drug would benefit from restricting their sodium intake by cutting down on pickled foods and salty foods such as luncheon meats, snack chips, and processed cheeses; also, all types of alcoholic beverages should be limited.

POSSIBLE SIDE EFFECTS: Light-headedness, increased heart rate, throbbing in the head, flushed face

ACTION OF NITROGLYCERIN: This drug dilates the arteries and veins, including the large coronary arteries supplying the heart. This reduces the work load on the heart muscle and alleviates the pain associated with angina pectoris.

HIGH-RISK GROUPS: Anyone who takes this drug

NUTRITIONAL INTERACTIONS

HYPERTENSION: Hypertension, or high blood pressure, is the major cause of angina. Hypertension affects 60 million Americans— roughly 75 percent of all Americans have hypertension at age sixty-five. It increases the work load of the heart and the risk of a heart attack by two or three times and the risk of a stroke by seven times.

Sodium causes water retention in some people, particularly in combination with a low potassium intake. Water retention increases the volume of fluid in the arteries and elevates the blood pressure. Hence patients with hypertension should restrict their sodium intake.

Prevention and Treatment: Anybody on nitroglycerin should restrict his sodium intake to less than 2 grams, or 1 teaspoon, of salt per day. This means not adding salt at the table and using no more than ½ teaspoon in cooking. In addition, pickled foods (such as sauerkraut) and extremely salty foods (such as luncheon meats, snack chips, and processed cheeses) should be eliminated. (See table of Sodium-Rich Foods, page 306.)

Other sources of sodium such as monosodium glutamate should also be avoided. Water that has been passed through a softener also contains significant amounts of sodium.

To sharpen your awareness of the sodium content of food products, read the list of ingredients that appears on the label of all packaged foods. Sodium can be present in a food as either common salt or sodium chloride, or as any other sodium-containing compound, monosodium glutamate being a common one. If sodium appears as one of the first ingredients on the label, the food will contain a significant amount of the mineral. If, on the other hand, it appears very near the end of the list (as in bread), then it need not be a concern.

To avoid the problems of water retention through the use of this drug, your diet should contain natural diuretics, foods rich in potassium, such as citrus fruits, bananas, almonds, dates, dairy products, apricots, and bamboo shoots. (See table of Potassium-Rich Foods, page 302.) Recent evidence points to a protective value for calcium against the harmful effects of sodium, so eat plenty of calcium-containing foods such as dairy products.

ALCOHOL INTERACTION: Alcohol increases the blood-pressure-lowering effect of the drug and is likely to reduce the blood pressure below normal, causing light-headedness, dizziness, and feelings of faintness upon standing or sitting up.

Prevention and Treatment: Alcohol should not be consumed by patients taking nitroglycerin. Alcohol has a potent vasodilation effect of its own. A glass of sherry (6 ounces) or 10 ounces of table wine will significantly dilate the blood vessels for 4 hours and tends to lower blood pressure. Alcohol taken with other drugs accounts for a considerable amount of abuse after age fifty. Alcohol consumption among the elderly is on the increase; some 54 percent of those over fifty use alcohol. According to several studies, between 1 and 2 percent of those over age sixty-five have a drinking problem. You must be honest with your physician about your drinking habits.

OTHER ADVICE: Many people taking this drug suffer from light-headedness when they stand up, increased heart rate, a throbbing in the head, and flushing in the face, which are unavoidable effects of the drug.

NITROUS OXIDE

DRUG FAMILY: Anesthetic gas

FOODS TO AVOID: All foods for at least a 2-hour period prior to its use

POSSIBLE SIDE EFFECTS: Vitamin B_{12} deficiency; nausea and vomiting

ACTION OF NITROUS OXIDE: This anesthetic is used in dental procedures and in other situations where a general anesthesia is required.

HIGH-RISK GROUPS: Children

NUTRITIONAL INTERACTIONS

VITAMIN B_{12} DEFICIENCY: Nitrous oxide breaks down vitamin B_{12} when mixed with an equal volume of oxygen as it is in practice. This has been known to produce B_{12} deficiency in children having extensive dental work.

Vitamin B_{12} is needed for the normal development of red blood cells and for the healthy functioning of all cells, in particular those of the bone marrow, nervous system, and intestines.

The most common result of a B_{12} deficiency is pernicious anemia, which is characterized by listlessness, fatigue (especially following such physical exertion as climbing a flight of stairs), numbness and tingling in the fingers and toes, palpitations, light-headedness, and a pale complexion. A vitamin B_{12} deficiency can also lead to an irreversible breakdown in the brain membranes (called myelin), causing loss of coordination, confusion, memory loss, paranoia, apathy, tremors, and hallucinations. In extreme cases, degeneration of the spinal cord can also result.

Since vitamin B_{12} can be obtained only from animal food sources, strict vegetarians are at particular risk here.

Prevention and Treatment: A balanced diet containing plenty of vitamin B_{12} sources is advised. Only animal products, including dairy foods and fish and shellfish, contain natural vitamin B_{12}. However, some vegetable products are supplemented with vitamin B_{12}; many soy products, for example, are enriched with B_{12} to safeguard vegetarians. (See table of Vitamin B_{12}-Rich Foods, page 312.)

Vitamin B_{12} is stored in the liver, so one meal that includes a B_{12}-rich source such as calf's liver will normally fulfill your body's need for this vitamin for 2 or 3 weeks. (One 3-ounce serving of calf's liver contains 100 mcg of vitamin B_{12}.) If none of these products figures prominently in your diet, you should take a 6 mcg supplement each day while on nitrous oxide.

People who use major amounts of vitamin C should be aware that vitamin C supplements of more than 500 mg per day can damage B_{12} and contribute to a B_{12} deficiency. Copper and thiamin also seem to decrease its availability. However, anyone who eats red meat two times a week has a three- to five-year supply of B_{12} in his liver.

The presence of baking soda in cooking will destroy vitamin B_{12} and should be avoided whenever possible. B_{12} also degrades at high temperatures, as when meat is placed on a hot griddle. The pasteurization of milk and the sterilization in boiling water of a bottle of milk also cause the loss of some B_{12}.

OTHER INTERACTIONS: Vomiting and nausea occur in 15 percent of all people after the use of nitrous oxide.

Prevention and Treatment: This can be limited by not eating for at least a 2-hour period prior to the use of the drug.

OLIVE OIL

DRUG FAMILY: Laxative

HOW TO TAKE OLIVE OIL: Not within 2 hours of consuming a meal and optimally at bedtime

FOODS TO AVOID: None

POSSIBLE SIDE EFFECTS: Iron deficiency

ACTION OF OLIVE OIL: Olive oil is used as a stool softener by people with constipation. The oil promotes the secretion of cholecystokinin, a hormone, from the intestine, which causes bile to be secreted. Because the bile has a high salt content, the salt draws water into the intestine and so increases the bulk of the stool and relieves constipation.

HIGH-RISK GROUPS: The elderly, young women, children (especially teenagers), vegetarians

NUTRITIONAL INTERACTIONS

BALANCED FAT INTAKE: This digestible oil will increase your caloric intake, as will any fat oil. One gram of olive oil contains 9 calories. Olive oil, the pressings of the ripe fruit of the olive tree, is used in cooking, as salad oil, and for canning sardines, among other things.

Olive oil is mainly monounsaturated fat, which does not raise your blood cholesterol levels, and as a result does not heighten your risk of heart disease. It is also the one vegetable oil that contains only small amounts of polyunsaturated fat, which tends to lower blood cholesterol levels but which, in excess, can increase your risk of cancer. The optimal diet has a 1 to 1 to 1 ratio of monounsaturated to saturated to polyunsaturated fats. (See table of Commonly Used Fats and Oils, page 295.) Obviously, since olive oil constitutes a source of calories and very little else, it could add a significant number of calories to your diet.

IRON DEFICIENCY: The use of olive oil decreases iron absorption and over a prolonged period could conceivably lead to an iron deficiency. Iron is especially important to the oxygen-carrying cells of the blood and muscles, which consume two thirds of the iron your body requires. An iron shortage reduces the blood's oxygen-carrying capacity. The result is an anemia signaled by such symptoms as tiredness, general feelings of malaise, irritability, decreased attention span, pale complexion, rapid heart rhythm, headaches, loss of concentration, and breathlessness on exertion. A mild iron deficiency will also impair the functioning of your immune system and will cause your nails to be brittle and ridged.

To be absorbed from any vegetable source, the iron must be converted to another form by the action of the hydrochloric acid produced in the stomach. Some elderly people secrete less hydrochloric acid than normal, so they absorb iron poorly even under normal circumstances. The diets of many Americans lack adequate quantities of the mineral for their normal needs. For example, 10 percent of American women suffer from an iron deficiency, and up to 30 percent have inadequate iron stores. Other people who are at significant risk of an iron deficiency are women who have had several pregnancies and those whose menstrual periods are heavy.

The shortage of iron in many diets is due not only to the selection of foods that are poor sources of iron, but also to the switch away from cast-iron cookware to aluminum, stainless steel, and nonstick surfaces. The acid in foods used to leach iron from the surface of the pots and pans, and provided a significant source of dietary iron.

Prevention and Treatment: To counteract an iron deficiency, iron-rich foods should be included in your diet: liver, whole grain products, oysters, dried apricots, prunes, peaches, leafy green vegetables, and lean red meat. (See table of Iron-Rich Foods, page 299.)

Many foods and drugs have a considerable impact on the way your body absorbs (or does not absorb) iron. There are two kinds of iron in foods sources: heme iron in meat and ionic iron in vegetables. Up to 30 percent of the iron from meat, fish, and poultry is absorbed, but less than 10 percent is absorbed from eggs, whole grains, nuts, and dried beans. Only 10 percent of ionic iron is absorbed from vegetable sources, with as little as 2 percent being absorbed from spinach. Antacids will interfere with iron absorption in vegetables, as will commercial black and pekoe tea, taken in substantial quantities, because of its tannin content. Coffee also seems to decrease iron absorption, but not to the same degree as tea. Vitamin C supplements or citrus fruit juices increase the absorption of iron from vegetable sources by two to three times if taken simultaneously.

You will have impaired iron absorption if your diet is rich in high-fiber foods, since the fiber will bind with the iron and pass it out in the stool. This is the same action that partially accounts for the poor absorption of iron from vegetable sources. Foods high in phosphorus (e.g. meat) interfere with iron absorption, which explains why only 30 percent of the iron in meat is captured. (However, meat and fish facilitate iron absorption from vegetables.) For that matter, any use of large quantities of mineral supplements, such as zinc, will impair iron absorption. Because iron can be leached from vegetables if they are cooked in large amounts of water, it is preferable to steam them.

Iron supplements should not be taken without a physician's recommendation because an accumulation of too much iron can lead in extreme cases to such serious problems as anemia, malfunctioning of the pancreas and the heart, cirrhosis of the liver, a brown cast to the skin, and depression.

OTHER ADVICE: Olive oil should never be consumed within 2 hours of a meal, since it decreases gastric secretion of digestive juices. The optimal time to take it would be bedtime.

Since olive oil slows the rate at which the stomach secretes acid, it should not be used as a laxative by elderly people, who often have a reduced gastric-acid secretion.

OXYCODONE

DRUG FAMILY: Analgesic

BRAND NAMES: [GENERIC/Brand] OXYCODONE HYDROCHLORIDE/Oxycodone Hydrochloride and Acetaminophen; Percocet; Percodan & Percodan-Demi; SK-Oxycodone with Acetaminophen; SK-Oxycodone with Aspirin; Tylox; OXYCODONE TEREPHTHALATE/Oxycodone Terephthalate & Aspirin; Oxycodone Hydrochloride, Oxycodone Terephthalate and Aspirin

HOW TO TAKE OXYCODONE: With meals or milk

FOODS TO AVOID: All alcoholic beverages

POSSIBLE SIDE EFFECTS: Nausea, diarrhea, vomiting, and stomachache

ACTION OF OXYCODONE: This drug is prescribed for the relief of moderate to moderately severe pain.

HIGH-RISK GROUPS: People with a history of abdominal distress

NUTRITIONAL INTERACTIONS

GENERAL ADVICE: The chronic and extensive use of these drugs could conceivably result in the development of unwanted side effects, including such gastrointestinal disorders as nausea, diarrhea, vomiting, and stomachache. The chances of these problems occurring can be limited by taking oxycodone with meals or milk.

The consumption of alcoholic beverages increases the depression of the central nervous system and can make such actions as driving dangerous. As a result, you should never drink while you are taking these drugs.

OXYPHENBUTAZONE

DRUG FAMILY: Anti-inflammatory

BRAND NAMES: Oxalid; Tandearil

HOW TO TAKE OXYPHENBUTAZONE: After meals

FOODS TO AVOID: Foods rich in sodium such as anchovies, dill pickles, sardines, green olives, canned soups and vegetables, TV dinners, soy sauce, processed cheeses, salty snack foods, and cold cuts

POSSIBLE SIDE EFFECTS: Stomach upset; edema

ACTION OF OXYPHENBUTAZONE: This drug is used in the treatment of an acute attack of gout and for the relief of severe symptoms of rheumatoid arthritis that are not relieved by other medications.

HIGH-RISK GROUPS: Anyone who takes this drug

NUTRITIONAL INTERACTIONS

GASTROINTESTINAL DISTRESS: This drug is likely to cause severe gastric upset.

Prevention and Treatment: The tablets should be divided into 3 or 4 pieces and taken after meals to lessen gastric irritation.

EDEMA: It is conceivable that use of oxyphenbutazone will lead to water and salt retention, which will tend to cause swelling (called edema) in your legs, ankles, feet, breasts, and around your eyes. An increase in sodium and water retention may also increase the volume of blood in the body, which places an added strain on the heart and tends to elevate blood pressure. Hence, this drug is usually given with a diuretic to avoid these potential problems.

Prevention and Treatment: While on this drug, you should restrict your consumption of sodium. In particular, those foods listed in the table of Sodium-Rich Foods (see page 306) should be avoided or consumed only in small quantities. You should not add salt to food at the table and should use no more than 1 teaspoon per day in cooking.

Some people are unaware of how much salt their diet contains. We only need 220 mg per day, but the average American, in fact, consumes some 15 pounds of salt a year. This is 3 to 4 teaspoons per day, the equivalent of 6 to 8 grams of sodium. Even if you do not salt your food while preparing or eating it, you consume quantities of salt in foods like anchovies, dill pickles, sardines, green olives, canned soups and vegetables, so-called TV dinners, soy sauce, processed cheeses, many snack foods, cold cuts, and catsup.

In order to be more aware of the sodium content of food products, read the lists of ingredients that appear on the labels of all packaged foods. Sodium can be present in food as either common salt, or sodium chloride, or as any other sodium-containing compound, monsodium glutamate being a common one. If sodium appears as one of the first ingredients on the label, the food contains a significant amount of it. If, on the other hand, it appears very near the end of the list (as in bread), then it need not be a concern.

PARA-AMINOSALICYLIC ACID

DRUG FAMILY: Anti-tubercular

BRAND NAMES: [GENERIC/Brand] AMINOSALICYLATE SODIUM/Pamisyl Sodium; Parasal Sodium; Teebacin; AMINOSALICYLATE POTASSIUM/Teebacin Kalium; AMINOSALICYLATE CALCIUM/Teebacin Calcium; PAS Calcium; AMINOSALICYLATE ACID/Teebacin Acid

HOW TO TAKE PARA-AMINOSALICYLIC ACID: With meals or milk

FOODS TO AVOID: None

POSSIBLE SIDE EFFECTS: Gastrointestinal distress; deficiencies of vitamins B_{12}, B_6, and K, folic acid, iron, and magnesium

ACTION OF PARA-AMINOSALICYLIC ACID: This anti-tubercular drug acts by killing the bacteria that cause the disease.

HIGH-RISK GROUPS: Users of oral contraceptives, premenopausal women, the elderly, heavy drinkers, vegetarians, children, smokers, teenagers

NUTRITIONAL INTERACTIONS

GASTROINTESTINAL DISTRESS: The most common nutritional interaction of paraaminosalicylic acid is gastric irritation. Since it is likely you will experience some sort of discomfort of this kind, you should never take this drug on an empty stomach. It causes

some minor malabsorption problems in everyone who takes it, but some sensitive people have a noticeable fat-malabsorption problem that manifests itself in fatty, unpleasant-smelling diarrhea.

Prevention and Treatment: The drug should always be taken with meals or milk to prevent or minimize gastric irritation.

VITAMIN B_{12} DEFICIENCY: Para-aminosalicylic acid significantly impairs the absorption of vitamin B_{12}, which could conceivably lead to a deficiency if the drug is taken over an extended period. Vitamin B_{12} is needed for the normal development of red blood cells and for the healthy functioning of all cells, in particular those of the bone marrow, nervous system, and intestines.

Pernicious anemia is the most common result of a B_{12} deficiency. It is characterized by listlessness, fatigue (especially following such physical exertion as climbing a flight of stairs), numbness and tingling in the fingers and toes, palpitations, angina, lightheadedness, and a pale complexion. A vitamin B_{12} deficiency can also lead to an irreversible breakdown in the brain membranes, involving loss of coordination, confusion, memory loss, paranoia, apathy, tremors, and hallucinations. In extreme cases, degeneration of the spinal cord can also result.

Since this vitamin can be obtained only from animal food sources, strict vegetarians are at particular risk here. Oral contraceptive users too have a greater chance of experiencing this deficiency, since they often have a poor vitamin B_{12} status to begin with. Heavy consumers of alcohol, as well, frequently lack B_{12}, because alcohol impairs the absorption of the vitamin. Some elderly people have difficulty in absorbing this vitamin. In addition, smokers seem to have an increased need for the vitamin. In any case, anyone who is likely to have a vitamin B_{12} absorption problem should be alert for signs of pernicious anemia while taking this drug.

Prevention and Treatment: A balanced diet containing plenty of vitamin B_{12} sources is advised. Only animal products, including dairy foods and fish and shellfish, contain natural vitamin B_{12}. However, some vegetable matter is supplemented with B_{12}; many soy products, for example, are enriched with vitamin B_{12} to safeguard vegetarians. (See table of Vitamin B_{12}-Rich Foods, page 312.)

Vitamin B_{12} is stored in the liver, so one meal that includes a B_{12}-rich source such as calf's liver will normally fulfill your body's need for this vitamin for 2 to 3 weeks. (One 3-ounce serving of calf's liver contains 100 mcg of vitamin B_{12}.) If none of these products figures prominently in your diet, you should take a 6 mcg supplement each day while on this drug.

People who use major amounts of vitamin C should be aware that vitamin C supplements of more than 500 mg per day can destroy vitamin B_{12} and can lead to a B_{12} deficiency. However, anyone who eats red meat two times a week has a three- to five-year supply of B_{12} in his liver.

Baking soda in cooking will destroy vitamin B_{12} and should be avoided whenever possible. B_{12} also degrades at high temperatures, as when meat is placed on a hot griddle. The pasteurization of milk and the sterilization in boiling water of a bottle of milk also cause the loss of some B_{12}.

FOLIC ACID DEFICIENCY: Since para-aminosalicylic acid impairs folic acid absorption, it is conceivable that a deficiency of this nutrient could occur while you are taking the drug. Often the first sign of a folic acid or folacin deficiency is bleeding and inflamed gums. The symptoms that follow are a sore, smooth tongue; diarrhea; forgetfulness; apathy; irritability; anemia; and reduced resistance to infection. Despite the fact that folacin is found in a variety of foods, folacin deficiency is still the most common vitamin deficiency in the United States.

Folic acid deficiencies in adults are limited almost exclusively to the elderly and women, 30 percent of whom have intakes below the recommended daily allowance, and 5 to 7 percent of whom also have severe anemia. There are several factors that account for this bias, but one of the most obvious reasons is that oral contraceptive use decreases the absorption of folic acid. Constant dieting also limits folacin intake. Alcohol interferes with the body's absorption and use of folic acid as well. Folacin is not stored by the body in any appreciable amounts, so an adequate supply must be consumed on a daily basis. Folic acid is also crucial to the normal metabolism of proteins. It is required for normal cell growth. As a result, a folacin deficiency during pregnancy can lead to birth defects.

Prevention and Treatment: To counteract a deficiency in folic acid, your diet should contain liver, yeast, and leafy vegetables such as spinach, kale, parsley, cauliflower, brussels sprouts, and broccoli. The fruits that are highest in folic acid are oranges and cantaloupes. To a lesser degree, folacin is found in almonds and lima beans, corn, parsnips, green peas, pumpkins, sweet potatoes, bran, peanuts, rye, and whole grain wheat. (See table of Folacin-Rich Foods, page 297.) Approximately one half of the folic acid you consume is absorbed by your body.

Normal cooking temperatures (110 to 120 degrees for 10 minutes) destroy as much as 65 percent of the folacin in your food. Your daily diet, therefore, should include some raw vegetables and fruits. Cooking utensils made out of copper speed up folacin's destruction.

The recommended daily consumption of folacin is 400 mcg. Oral contraceptive users should consume 800 mcg daily.

IRON DEFICIENCY: An iron deficiency is also conceivable while taking para-aminosalicylic acid, because of malabsorption. Iron is especially important to the oxygen-carrying cells of the blood and muscles, which consume two thirds of the iron your body requires. An iron shortage reduces the blood's oxygen-carrying capacity. The result is an anemia signaled by such symptoms as tiredness, general feelings of malaise, irritability, decreased attention span, pale complexion, rapid heart rhythm, headaches, the loss of concentration, and breathlessness on exertion. A mild iron deficiency will also impair the functioning of your immune system.

To be absorbed from any vegetable source, iron must be converted to another form by the action of the hydrochloric acid produced in the stomach. Since the elderly secrete less hydrochloric acid than normal, they absorb iron poorly even under normal circumstances. The mineral is also not present in adequate quantities in the diets of many Americans for their normal needs. For example, 10 percent of American women suffer from an iron deficiency, and up to 30 percent have inadequate iron stores. Other people who are at significant risk of an iron deficiency are women who have had several pregnancies and those whose menstrual periods are heavy.

Another contributing factor to the shortage of iron in many people is the switch away from cast-iron cookware to aluminum, stainless steel, and nonstick surfaces. Iron used to be leached from the iron pots and pans, and became available as dietary iron.

Prevention and Treatment: To counteract an iron deficiency, iron-rich foods should be included in your diet: liver, whole grain products, oysters, dried apricots, prunes, peaches, leafy green vegetables, and, occasionally, lean red meat. (See table of Iron-Rich Foods, page 298.)

A variety of other drugs and foods have an effect on the way your body absorbs (or does not absorb) iron. There are two kinds of iron in food sources: heme iron in meat and ionic iron in vegetables. Up to 30 percent of the iron from meat, fish, and poultry is absorbed, but less than 10 percent is absorbed from eggs, whole grains, nuts, and dried beans. Only 10 percent of ionic iron is absorbed from vegetable sources, with as little as 2 percent being absorbed from spinach. Antacids will interfere with iron absorption in vegetables, as will commercial black and pekoe tea, taken in substantial quantities, because of its tannin content. Coffee also seems to decrease iron absorption, but not to the same degree as tea. Vitamin C supplements or citrus fruit juices increase the absorption of iron from vegetable sources by two to three times if taken simultaneously.

If your diet is rich in high-fiber foods, you will have impaired iron absorption because the fiber will bind to the iron and pass it out in the stool. This is the same action that contributes to the poor absorption of iron from vegetable sources. Foods high in phosphorus (e.g. meat) interfere with iron absorption, which explains why only 30 percent of the iron in meat is captured. (However, meat and fish facilitate iron absorption from vegetables.) For that matter, use of any large quantities of mineral supplements, such as zinc, will impair iron absorption. Because iron can be leached from vegetables if they are cooked in large amounts of water, it is preferable to steam them.

No iron supplements should be taken without a physician's guidance because an accumulation of too much iron can lead in extreme cases to such serious problems as anemia, malfunctioning of the pancreas and the heart, cirrhosis of the liver, a brown cast to the skin, and depression.

MAGNESIUM DEFICIENCY: A magnesium deficiency may also occur while taking para-aminosalicylic acid, though such a deficiency is quite unlikely because the average American diet contains appreciable amounts of magnesium. Clinical signs of magnesium deficiency include muscle weakness, tremors, depression, emotional instability, and irrational behavior. Alcohol also increases the excretion of magnesium.

Prevention and Treatment: A diet containing the four food groups provides the normal amount of magnesium. However, if a magnesium depletion is suspected, your diet should feature foods such as nuts (almonds and cashews are highest), meat, fish, milk, whole grains, and fresh greens, since cooking can wash away some magnesium. (See table of Magnesium-Rich Foods, page 300.) Alcohol provokes magnesium excretion, so its intake should be restricted to 2 drinks per day while you are on para-aminosalicylic acid.

VITAMIN B_6 DEFICIENCY: Para-aminosalicylic acid inactivates vitamin B_6, which could conceivably result in a deficiency. Common symptoms of this deficiency are a sore mouth and tongue, cracks in the lips and corners of the mouth, and patches of itching, scaling skin. A severe vitamin B_6 deficiency may cause depression and confusion.

Vitamin B_6 deficiencies are common among the elderly. Alcoholics, as well, often experience this deficiency, since alcohol interferes with the body's ability to use B_6. In addition, smokers seem to have an increased need for the vitamin. It is estimated that one of every two Americans consumes less than 70 percent of the Recommended Dietary Allowance of B_6.

Prevention and Treatment: To avoid a B_6 deficiency, you should consume a diet featuring such food sources of vitamin B_6 as liver (beef, calf, and pork), herring, salmon, walnuts, peanuts, wheat germ, carrots, peas, potatoes, grapes, bananas, and yeast. (See table of Vitamin B_6(Pyridoxine)-Rich Foods, page 311.) The vitamin is present in significant amounts in meats, fish, fruits, cereals, and vegetables, and to a lesser extent in milk and other dairy products.

Since vitamin B_6 is decomposed at high temperatures, modern food processing often diminishes dietary sources of the vitamin. Consequently, the more processed foods you eat, the more susceptible you will be to a deficiency of this vitamin. The same losses also occur in cooking: meat loses as much as 45 to 80 percent, vegetables 20 to 30 percent.

It has been observed that 15 to 20 percent of oral contraceptive users show direct evidence of vitamin B_6 deficiency. If you are among these people, you should take 25 to 50 mg of the vitamin per day. Smokers should take a 5 mg daily supplement. However, keep in mind that you can take too much vitamin B_6, since people taking over 1 gram per day have been reported to experience a toxic reaction.

VITAMIN K DEFICIENCY: Para-aminosalicylic acid, by virtue of its antibacterial activity, kills the bacteria in the large intestine that make vitamin K. People with an abnormally low dietary intake of vitamin K are at risk of bleeding with unusual ease if they use this drug for a long period of time.

Normally vitamin K helps produce blood-clotting substances in the liver. Without sufficient levels of vitamin K in the diet, however, bleeding may take place in the gastrointestinal tract (causing black or blood-stained stools), in the urinary tract (causing blood in the urine), and in the uterus (causing blood loss at times other than the normal menstrual periods). Excessive blood loss may occur from an injury or surgery as well. Another sign of a deficiency of this vitamin is more frequent and more visible bruising than normal.

Half the vitamin K in humans comes from dietary sources: predominantly green leafy vegetables and to a lesser extent fruit, cereals, dairy products, and meat. The rest of the vitamin K in our bodies is synthesized by the bacteria in the intestines. The daily need for the vitamin is in the range of 70 to 140 mcg. Women who have had several pregnancies or whose menstrual periods are heavy are at high risk. Many of the elderly are at risk of a vitamin K deficiency because they have a problem of poor fat absorption, and vitamin K, a fat-soluble vitamin, must be accompanied by sufficient dietary fat to be properly absorbed.

Prevention and Treatment: A vitamin K deficiency can be countered by a vitamin K supplement of 100 mcg per day, and a diet that includes foods rich in the vitamin, such as kale, spinach, cabbage, cauliflower, leafy green vegetables, liver (especially pork liver), and fish. (See table of Vitamin K-Rich Foods, page 315.)

Vitamin E supplements should not be taken when at risk of a vitamin K shortage, because vitamin E impairs the absorption of K.

PARALDEHYDE

DRUG FAMILY: Anti-alcoholism

HOW TO TAKE PARALDEHYDE: Immediately after meals with a strong-tasting beverage such as orange juice, tea, or milk

FOODS TO AVOID: Alcoholic beverages

POSSIBLE SIDE EFFECTS: Vitamin C deficiency; stomach cramps

ACTION OF PARALDEHYDE: This drug is prescribed in the treatment of withdrawal symptoms associated with abstinence, and as a tranquilizer.

HIGH-RISK GROUPS: Smokers, users of oral contraceptives, the elderly

NUTRITIONAL INTERACTIONS

VITAMIN C DEFICIENCY: Paraldehyde increases the rate at which vitamin C is broken down in the body, making it far less effective and increasing the need for the vitamin. With an adequate vitamin C intake, the body normally maintains a fixed pool of the vitamin, and rapidly excretes any excess in the urine. Ordinarily, 60 to 100 mg of vitamin C per day will fulfill the body's needs, except perhaps in the case of smokers who may need a little more.

However, with an inadequate intake, this reservoir becomes depleted at the rate of up to 3 percent per day. Obvious symptoms of a vitamin C deficiency do not appear until the available vitamin C has been reduced to about one fifth of its optimal level, and this may take as much as two months to occur. The earliest signs of a deficiency are spongy or bleeding gums, slightly swollen wrists and ankles, and capillaries that break under the skin, producing pinpoint hemorrhages around hair follicles on the arms and legs.

Vitamin C is important to the function of your bodily systems in a number of ways. When your body is deficient in vitamin C, your white blood cells are less able to detect and destroy invading bacteria. On the other hand, megadoses of the vitamin (over 2 grams daily) can also impair this ability. Vitamin C also helps your body guard itself against such pollutants as the known cancer-causing agents nitrites and nitrosamines, and protects vitamin A and E from degradation. In addition, it aids in iron absorption, speeds up wound healing, and strengthens blood vessels. Other well-known effects are that, in some people, vitamin C reduces the symptoms of a cold by one third and is important in preventing plaque formation on the teeth, which reduces the likelihood of gum disease and tooth decay.

Prevention and Treatment: Patients taking paraldehyde should be sure to get 100 mg per day of vitamin C. Vitamin C-rich foods include citrus fruits, broccoli, spinach, cabbage, and cantaloupe. (See table of Vitamin C-Rich Foods, page 313.) In preparing foods rich in vitamin C, you should keep in mind that it is readily oxidized (during both food processing and storage when exposed to the air). Copper and iron cooking utensils will speed up the oxidation, and the longer the food is cooked and the higher the temperature, the greater the vitamin loss. Large amounts of water used in cooking will wash out the vitamin. Bruising or cutting the fruit also decreases its vitamin C content.

Supplements can also be taken, although the body tends to eliminate any surplus of C, so large supplements of more than 100 mg a day are unnecessary. In fact, megadoses of the drug can cause nausea, abdominal cramps, and diarrhea, among other undesirable side effects.

OTHER ADVICE: Paraldehyde can irritate the stomach and cause cramps. It also has a disagreeable taste. This drug should be taken immediately after meals. In this way, the stomach will not become irritated, and the taste will not interfere with your appetite. Orange juice, tea, or milk can also mask the taste.

Alcohol increases the potency of the drug and can lead to difficulty in breathing and abnormally low blood pressure.

PENICILLAMINE

DRUG FAMILY: Chelating agent

BRAND NAMES: Cuprimine; Depen

HOW TO TAKE PENICILLAMINE: Usually taken on an empty stomach ½ hour to 1 hour before meals

FOODS TO AVOID: None

POSSIBLE SIDE EFFECTS: Deficiencies of vitamin B_6 and zinc; gastrointestinal disturbances

ACTION OF PENICILLAMINE: Penicillamine is used as a treatment for copper poisoning, lead poisoning, and rheumatoid arthritis. This drug binds to heavy metals like copper, zinc, and lead, and flushes them out of the body in the urine.

HIGH-RISK GROUPS: Anyone who takes this drug

NUTRITIONAL INTERACTIONS

VITAMIN B_6 DEFICIENCY: This drug binds to vitamin B_6 and prevents it from carrying out its normal functions. As a result, it is likely that you will develop a vitamin B_6 deficiency while taking penicillamine.

B_6 deficiency in penicillamine users has been reported to cause anemia characterized by lethargy, inability to concentrate, breathlessness on exertion, a pale complexion, and inflammation of the eye, as well as more common symptoms of a B_6 deficiency such as a sore mouth and tongue, cracks in the lips and corners of the mouth, and patches of itching, scaling skin. A severe vitamin B_6 deficiency may cause depression and confusion.

Vitamin B_6 deficiencies are common among the elderly. Smokers also have lower than normal body levels of this vitamin, and alcoholics, as well, often experience this deficiency, since alcohol interferes with the body's ability to use B_6. It is estimated that one of every two Americans consumes less than 70 percent of the Recommended Dietary Allowance of B_6.

Prevention and Treatment: To avoid B_6 deficiency, you should consume a diet featuring such food sources of vitamin B_6 as liver (beef, calf, and pork), herring, salmon, walnuts, peanuts, wheat germ, carrots, peas, potatoes, grapes, bananas, and yeast. (See table of Vitamin B_6(Pyridoxine)-Rich Foods, page 311.) The vitamin is present in significant amounts in meats, fish, fruits, cereals, and vegetables, and to a lesser extent in milk and other dairy products.

Since vitamin B_6 is decomposed at high temperatures, modern food processing often diminishes dietary sources of the vitamin. Consequently, the more processed foods you eat, the more susceptible you will be to a deficiency of this vitamin. The same losses also occur in cooking: meat loses as much as 45 to 80 percent, vegetables 20 to 30 percent.

If penicillamine is taken at high doses, 75 mg per day or more, a daily supplement of 100 mg of B_6 should be added to the patient's regimen. If it is being taken in lower doses, 25 to 50 mg of B_6 should be added. This quantity of vitamin B_6 cannot be obtained in the diet alone, so a supplement has to be taken.

It has been observed that 15 to 20 percent of oral contraceptive users show direct evidence of a vitamin B_6 deficiency. If you are among these people, you should take 50 mg of vitamin B_6 per day if you are on penicillamine for a short period, and 100 mg daily if you take the drug for longer than a week.

ZINC DEFICIENCY: In elderly patients, taking the drug for extended periods (usually for rheumatoid arthritis) can lead to zinc deficiency, which involves impaired healing of wounds, scaly dry skin on the face and limbs, and anorexia associated with loss of taste. Zinc deficiencies probably account for the drug impairing the sense of taste for sweet and salt, which often leads to a decreased appetite.

Prevention and Treatment: Foods rich in zinc such as red meats, whole wheat bread, and brown rice should be included in the diet. (See table of Zinc-Rich Foods, page 315.) To decrease the effect of the drug on appetite, take it 1 hour before or 3 hours after meals.

OTHER ADVICE: Many patients taking penicillamine experience stomachache, nausea, vomiting, blunting of taste, and diarrhea. All of these effects usually disappear when use of the drug is discontinued.

PENICILLIN

DRUG FAMILY: Antibiotic

BRAND NAMES: [GENERIC/Brand] PENICILLIN (ORAL)/Cyclapen-W; Omnipen; Pathocil; Pentids; Pen.Vee K; Principen; Unipen; Veetids; Wymox; PENICILLIN (REPOSITORY)/ Bicillin C-R; Bicillin C-R 900/300; Bicillin L-A; PENICILLIN V POTASSIUM/Betapen-VK; Penicillin V Potassium; Pen.Vee K; SK-Penicillin VK; V-Cillin K; Veetids

HOW TO TAKE PENICILLIN: On an empty stomach 1 hour before or 2 hours after meals with water

FOODS TO AVOID: The drug should never be taken with fruit juices, sodas, wine, or other acidic beverages

POSSIBLE SIDE EFFECTS: Deficiencies of vitamins K, B_6, and B_{12}, folic acid, and potassium

ACTION OF PENICILLIN: This familiar drug is the one most often chosen for a wide variety of bacterial infections, including respiratory problems, scarlet fever, erysipelas (acute inflamation of the skin and underlying tissues), pneumonia, pharyngitis, and Vincent's gingivitis (trench mouth).

HIGH-RISK GROUPS: The elderly, vegetarians, pregnant women, users of oral contraceptives, heavy drinkers, smokers, lactating women, children, teenagers

NUTRITIONAL INTERACTIONS

VITAMIN K DEFICIENCY: Penicillin may decrease your vitamin K levels by killing the bacteria in the large intestine responsible for its synthesis. It should not result in a deficiency unless your intake of the vitamin is minimal. If foods rich in vitamin K feature in your diet, you are not at risk. (See table of Vitamin K-Rich Foods, page 315.)

FOLIC ACID DEFICIENCY: Penicillin decreases the body's ability to use folacin. Since a large number of premenopausal women and oral contraceptive users have only marginal folacin stores, use of this drug could be sufficient to push them into a folacin deficiency.

Often the first sign of a folic acid or folacin deficiency is inflamed and bleeding gums. The symptoms that follow are a sore, smooth tongue; diarrhea; forgetfulness; apathy; irritability; anemia, and a reduced resistance to infection. Despite the fact that folacin is found in a variety of foods, folacin deficiency is still the most common vitamin deficiency in the United States.

In adults, deficiencies are limited almost exclusively to the elderly and women, 30 percent of whom have intakes below the recommended daily allowance, and 5 to 7 percent of whom also have severe anemia. There are several factors that account for this bias, but one of the most obvious reasons is that oral contraceptive use decreases the absorption of folic acid. Constant dieting also limits folacin intake. Alcohol interferes with the body's absorption and use of folic acid as well. Folacin is not stored by the body in any appreciable amounts, so an adequate supply must be consumed on a daily basis.

Pregnant women should be especially careful, since folate deficiencies can cause fetal abnormalities. Folic acid is also crucial to the normal metabolism of proteins.

Prevention and Treatment: To counteract a deficiency in folic acid, your diet should contain liver, yeast, and leafy vegetables such as spinach, kale, parsley, cauliflower, brussels sprouts, and broccoli. The fruits that are highest in folic acid are oranges and cantaloupes. To a lesser degree, folacin is found in almonds and lima beans, corn, parsnips, green peas, pumpkins, sweet potatoes, bran, peanuts, rye, and whole grain wheat. (See table of Folacin-Rich Foods, page 297.) Approximately one half of the folic acid you consume is absorbed by your body.

Normal cooking temperatures (110 to 120 degrees for 10 minutes) destroy about 65 percent of the folacin in your food. Your daily diet, therefore, should include some raw vegetables and fruits. Cooking utensils made out of copper speed up folacin's destruction.

The recommended daily consumption of folacin is 400 mcg. Lactating women should assume a daily need of 1,200 mcg. Pregnant women and oral contraceptive users should consume 800 mcg daily.

VITAMIN B$_6$ DEFICIENCY: Penicillin inactivates vitamin B$_6$; therefore users of penicillin could conceivably experience a vitamin B$_6$ deficiency. Especially at risk are women who take birth control pills, who tend to have marginal deficiencies. Common symptoms of this deficiency are a sore mouth and tongue, cracks in the lips and corners of the mouth, and patches of itching, scaling skin. A severe vitamin B$_6$ deficiency may cause depression and confusion.

Vitamin B$_6$ deficiencies are common among the elderly. Alcoholics, as well, often experience this deficiency, since alcohol interferes with the body's ability to use B_6. In addition, smokers seem to have an increased need for this vitamin. It is estimated that one of every two Americans consumes less than 70 percent of the Recommended Dietary Allowance of B_6.

Prevention and Treatment: To avoid a B_6 deficiency, you should consume a diet featuring such food sources of vitamin B_6 as liver (beef, calf, and pork), herring, salmon, walnuts, peanuts, wheat germ, carrots, peas, potatoes, grapes, bananas, and yeast. (See table of Vitamin B_6(Pyridoxine)-Rich Foods, page 311.) The vitamin is present in significant amounts in meats, fish, fruits, cereals, and vegetables, and to a lesser extent in milk and other dairy products.

Since vitamin B_6 is decomposed at high temperatures, modern food processing often diminishes dietary sources of the vitamin. Consequently, the more processed foods you eat, the more susceptible you will be to a deficiency of this vitamin. The same losses also occur in cooking: meat loses as much as 45 to 80 percent, vegetables 20 to 30 percent.

It has been observed that 15 to 20 percent of oral contraceptive users show direct evidence of vitamin B_6 deficiency. If you are among these people, you should take 25 to 50 mg of vitamin B_6 per day. Smokers need a 5 mg daily supplement. However, you can take too much vitamin B_6; people using over 1 gram per day have been reported to experience nerve degeneration.

VITAMIN B_{12} DEFICIENCY: Penicillin also leads to malabsorption of vitamin B_{12}. Vitamin B_{12} is needed for the normal development of red blood cells and for the healthy functioning of all cells, in particular those of the bone marrow, nervous system, and intestines. A vitamin B_{12} deficiency should only occur if penicillin is used for an extended period and then only in the high-risk groups.

The most common result of a B_{12} deficiency is pernicious anemia, which is characterized by listlessness, fatigue (especially following such physical exertion as climbing a flight of stairs), numbness and tingling in the fingers and toes, palpitations, angina, light-headedness, and a pale complexion. A vitamin B_{12} deficiency can also lead to an irreversible breakdown in the brain membranes, causing loss of coordination, confusion, memory loss, paranoia, apathy, tremors, and hallucinations. In extreme cases, degeneration of the spinal cord can also result.

Since vitamin B_{12} can be obtained only from animal food sources, strict vegetarians are at particular risk here. Oral contraceptive users, too, have a greater chance of experiencing this deficiency since they often have a poor vitamin B_{12} status to begin with. Heavy consumers of alcohol, as well, frequently lack B_{12}, because alcohol impairs the absorption of the vitamin. Patients with bacterial or parasitic infections of the intestine also have difficulty in absorbing this vitamin, as do some elderly people. In addition, smokers seem to have an increased need for the vitamin. In any case, anyone who is likely to have a vitamin B_{12} absorption problem should be alert for signs of pernicious anemia while taking this drug.

Prevention and Treatment: A balanced diet containing plenty of vitamin B_{12} sources is advised. Only animal products, including dairy foods and fish and shellfish, contain natural vitamin B_{12}. However, some vegetable matter is supplemented with B_{12}; many soy products, for example, are enriched with vitamin B_{12} to safeguard vegetarians. (See table of Vitamin B_{12}-Rich Foods, page 312.)

Vitamin B_{12} is stored in the liver, so one meal that includes a B_{12}-rich source such as calf's liver will normally fulfill your body's need for this vitamin for 2 to 3 weeks. (One 3-ounce serving of calf's liver contains 100 mcg of vitamin B_{12}.) If none of these products figures prominently in your diet, you should take a 6 mcg supplement each day while you are on penicillin.

People who use major amounts of vitamin C should be aware that vitamin C supplements of more than 500 mg per day can destroy B_{12} and contribute to a B_{12} deficiency. However, anyone who eats red meat two times a week has a three- to five-year supply of B_{12} in his liver.

The presence of baking soda in cooking will destroy vitamin B_{12} and should be avoided whenever possible. B_{12} also degrades at high temperatures, as when meat is placed on a hot griddle. The pasteurization of milk and the sterilization in boiling water of a bottle containing milk also cause the loss of some B_{12}.

POTASSIUM AND OTHER DEFICIENCIES: Penicillin may also cause the malabsorption of calcium, magnesium, glucose, carotene (the plant form of vitamin A), and cholesterol. Provided a well-balanced diet based on the four basic food groups is consumed, no problems should occur as a result of these shortages.

However, penicillin increases the excretion of potassium, which can lead to a potassium deficiency, particularly if you are taking thiazide diuretics or cortisone-containing drugs, since these also deplete body potassium. Potassium regulates the amount of water in the cells of the body and is essential for the proper functioning of the kidneys and the heart muscle, and the secretion of stomach juices. The most alarming symptom of a potassium deficiency is an irregular heartbeat, which can led to a heart attack.

Prevention and Treatment: Potassium depletion can be avoided by including such potassium-rich foods in your diet as tomato juice, lentils, dried apricots, asparagus, bananas, peanut butter, chicken, almonds, and milk. (See table of Potassium-Rich Foods, page 302.)

Potassium supplements should never be taken unless prescribed by a physician. They can cause anemia by interfering with the absorption of vitamin B_{12}. Just a few grams can also drastically increase the risk of heart failure. If you experience difficulty in swallowing while taking potassium supplements, consult your physician immediately. If supplements are prescribed, be aware that the absorption of the supplements potassium iodide and potassium chloride is decreased by dairy products, and that both are gastric irritants and should be taken with meals.

Too much salt in your diet can also compromise your body's supply of potassium, as can large amounts (1 to 3 ounces) of licorice candy made from natural extract. Imported licorice usually contains natural licorice extract, whereas domestic brands usually do not. Check the package.

OTHER ADVICE: Penicillin leaves an aftertaste that may decrease appetite. It should be taken between meals.

The absorption of penicillin is delayed when it is taken with food. It is also destroyed when consumed with fruit juice or with other acidic drinks and foods.

PENICILLIN G

DRUG FAMILY: Antibiotic

BRAND NAMES: [GENERIC/Brand] BENZA-THINE/Bicillin C-R; Bicillin C-R 900/300; Bicillin L-A; Permapen; PENICILLIN G PO-TASSIUM/Pentids; Pfizerpen; SK-Penicillin G; PENICILLIN G PROCAINE/Bicillin C-R; Bicillin C-R 900/300; Crysticillin 300 A.S. & Crysticillin 600 A.S.; Pfizerpen-AS; Wycillin; Wycillin & Probenecid; PENICILLIN G SODIUM

HOW TO TAKE PENICILLIN G: With water on an empty stomach 1 hour before or 2 to 3 hours after meals

FOODS TO AVOID: The drug should not be taken with acid-containing beverages like fruit juices, soft drinks, or wine. You should cut down on the amount of salty foods you consume.

POSSIBLE SIDE EFFECTS: Potassium deficiency; hypertension

ACTION OF PENICILLIN G: This anti-bacterial agent is the antibiotic of choice for a wide variety of infectious diseases, including peritonitis, middle-ear infections, pneumonia, arthritis, meningitis, endocarditis, diphtheria, anthrax, rat-bite fever, syphilis, pelvic inflammatory disease, and numerous others.

HIGH-RISK GROUPS: Hypertensives, people taking diuretics

NUTRITIONAL INTERACTIONS

POTASSIUM DEFICIENCY: While you are taking penicillin G, you could conceivably experience a potassium deficiency. Potassium regulates the amount of water in the cells of the body and is essential for the proper functioning of the kidneys and the heart muscle, and the secretion of stomach juices. People with a potassium deficiency may have such symptoms as weakness, a loss of appetite, nausea, vomiting, dryness of the mouth, increased thirst, listlessness, apprehension, and diffuse pain that comes and goes. The most alarming symptom of a potassium deficiency is an irregular heartbeat, which can lead to heart failure.

Low blood serum levels of potassium, called hypokalemia, are associated with laxative abuse, because many laxatives promote an increased loss of potassium in the gastrointestinal tract. This risk is especially high in elderly patients, who often consume diets low in potassium.

Proper potassium levels in your body can also be threatened if penicillin G is taken concurrently with cortisone-containing drugs. Diuretics, commonly prescribed for people with heart disease, also decrease the level of body potassium. Therefore, the risk of a deficiency is significantly increased if a diuretic is taken concurrently with this drug.

Prevention and Treatment: Potassium depletion can be avoided by including such potassium-rich foods in your diet as tomato juice, lentils, dried apricots, asparagus, bananas, peanut butter, chicken, almonds, and milk. (See table of Potassium-Rich Foods, page 302.)

Potassium supplements should never be taken unless prescribed by a physician. They can cause anemia by interfering with the absorption of vitamin B_{12}. Just a few grams can also drastically increase the risk of heart failure. If you experience difficulty in swallowing while taking potassium supplements, consult your physician immediately. If supplements are prescribed, be aware that the absorption of the supplements potassium iodide and potassium chloride is decreased by dairy products, and that both are gastric irritants and should be taken with meals.

Too much salt in your diet can also compromise your body's supply of potassium, as can 1 to 3 ounces per day of natural licorice. Imported licorice usually contains natural licorice extract, whereas domestic brands usually do not. Check the package.

HYPERTENSION: Penicillin G contains considerable amounts of sodium, and may, when given in large doses, elevate blood pressure.

High blood pressure, or hypertension, is a disease that may present no noticeable symptoms for years, but if left untreated it can increase the risk of heart disease and kidney failure. Your susceptibility to high blood pressure can be linked to identifiable factors such as family history, stress, alcoholism, obesity, or diet.

Hypertension affects 60 million Americans—roughly 75 percent of all Americans have hypertension at sixty-five. It increases the work load of the heart and makes the kidneys work harder to regulate elevated blood pressure. One result of untreated high blood pressure can be a two- to threefold increase in the risk of cardiovascular problems, and a sevenfold increase in the likelihood of having a stroke.

Sodium causes water retention in some people, particularly in combination with a low potassium intake. Water retention increases the volume of fluid in the arteries, which is responsible for the elevated blood pressure.

Prevention and Treatment: To minimize the problems of water retention through the use of penicillin G, you should consume natural diuretics, foods rich in potassium, such as citrus fruits, bananas, almonds, dates, dairy products, apricots, and bamboo shoots. (See table of Potassium-Rich Foods, page 302.) As many as 15 percent of all Americans have a genetic susceptibility to the effects of excess sodium; therefore, it is advised that everyone be watchful of his salt intake, particularly those who have already been diagnosed as hypertensive. We only need about 220 mg of sodium each day, but the average American consumes 6 to 8 grams of salt per day, or 3 to 4 teaspoons.

No salt should be added at the table, but up to 1 teaspoon can be added per day during cooking. Pickled foods, such as sauerkraut, and extremely salty foods, such as luncheon meats, snack chips, and processed cheeses, should be eliminated altogether.

You should be aware of the sodium content of food products. Read the list of ingredients that appears on the label of all packaged foods. Sodium can be present in a food as either common salt or sodium chloride, or as any other sodium-containing compound, monosodium glutamate being a common one. If sodium appears as one of the first ingredients on the label, the food contains a significant amount of it. If, on the other hand, it appears very near the end of the list (as in bread), then it need not be a concern. Recent evidence points to a protective value for calcium against the harmful effects of sodium, so eat plenty of calcium-containing foods such as dairy products.

You should limit your intake of sodium to 1 to 3 grams per day, watch your weight, and exercise.

OTHER ADVICE: Penicillin G is best absorbed in a fasting state, so it should be taken 1 hour before or 2 to 3 hours after meals.

PENTAZOCINE HYDROCHLORIDE

DRUG FAMILY: Analgesic

BRAND NAMES: Talwin Compound; Talwin Nx; Talacen

HOW TO TAKE PENTAZOCINE HYDROCHLORIDE: With meals or milk

FOODS TO AVOID: Alcoholic beverages

POSSIBLE SIDE EFFECTS: Diarrhea and constipation

ACTION OF PENTAZOCINE HYDROCHLORIDE: This drug is used to relieve moderate to severe pain. It also is used as a sedative.

HIGH-RISK GROUPS: Anyone who consumes alcohol

NUTRITIONAL INTERACTIONS

GASTROINTESTINAL DISTRESS: This drug could conceivably cause you to experience nausea and other gastrointestinal disturbances. Doses of 15 mg tend to cause diarrhea, while high doses of 30 to 45 mg tend to cause constipation.

Prevention and Treatment: Pentazocine hydrochloride should be taken with milk or meals to reduce the risk of gastrointestinal disturbances.

Should you experience constipation, you should increase the bulk in your diet. This means consuming larger servings of any of the following: dried or fresh fruits, salad vegetables, radishes, oatmeal, and whole grain foods (brown rice, whole wheat breads, and cereals). It is not necessary to purchase products that claim "extra fiber" has been added to them.

Persistent constipation may also be relieved by doubling the amount of fluid consumed each day. Bran, if used, should be added to the diet gradually, and fluid should be increased by at least ¾ cup per teaspoon of bran. (See table of Dietary Fiber-Rich Foods, page 293.)

OTHER ADVICE: Alcohol is likely to increase the depressant effects of the drug on the brain, and impair motor coordination and mental judgment, making it dangerous to drive a car or operate machinery demanding a high degree of coordination. As a result, alcohol should not be taken concurrently with pentazocine.

Smokers are less responsive to the drug and need higher doses to benefit, so you should advise your physician of your smoking habits.

PERPHENAZINE

DRUG FAMILY: Anti-anxiety

BRAND NAMES: Etrafon; Triavil; Trilafon

HOW TO TAKE PERPHENAZINE: As directed by your physician

FOODS TO AVOID: All alcoholic beverages

POSSIBLE SIDE EFFECTS: Constipation and dryness of the mouth

ACTION OF PERPHENAZINE: This potent drug is prescribed as a tranquilizer and as an anti-emetic agent to prevent or relieve nausea and vomiting. It is used in the treatment of people with moderate to severe depression and/or anxiety.

HIGH-RISK GROUPS: Anyone who consumes alcohol

NUTRITIONAL INTERACTIONS

ALCOHOL INTERACTION: Alcohol should not be taken concurrently with perphenazine, since it is likely to lead to abnormally low blood pressure. Severe depression can also result.

CONSTIPATION AND DRYNESS OF THE MOUTH: Constipation is usually safely remedied by an increase in bulk in the diet. This means consuming larger servings of fiber-rich foods. (See table of Dietary Fiber-Rich Foods, page 293.) Both dryness of the mouth and constipation may be relieved by doubling the amount of fluid consumed each day. If bran is used, it should be added to the diet gradually, and fluid should be increased by at least ¾ cup per teaspoon of bran.

PHENACETIN

DRUG FAMILY: Analgesic

BRAND NAMES: A.P.C. with Codeine; Propoxyphene Compound 65; Soma Compound; Soma Compound w/Codeine

HOW TO TAKE PHENACETIN: On an empty stomach 1 hour before or 2 to 3 hours after meals

FOODS TO AVOID: Brussels sprouts, cabbage, and charcoal-broiled beef

POSSIBLE SIDE EFFECTS: Kidney damage

ACTION OF PHENACETIN: This analgesic is used to relieve mild to moderate pain, with or without fever. It does not have significant anti-inflammatory effects and is not useful in the treatment of pain associated with inflammation and swelling, as in rheumatic pain.

HIGH-RISK GROUPS: The elderly

NUTRITIONAL INTERACTIONS

GENERAL ADVICE: Phenacetin is better absorbed on an empty stomach. It should be taken 1 hour before or 2 to 3 hours after meals.

Chronic overdosage of this drug could conceivably lead to kidney damage, so you should carefully obey the dosage instructions you are given.

Brussels sprouts, cabbage, and other vegetables of the genus *Brassica* and charcoal-broiled beef speed up the degradation of this drug and decrease its effectiveness.

PHENAZOPYRIDINE HYDROCHLORIDE

DRUG FAMILY: Analgesic

BRAND NAMES: Azo Gantanol; Azo Gantrisin; Pyridium; Pyridium Plus; Thiosulfil Duo-Pak; Thiosulfil-A Forte; Thiosulfil-A

HOW TO TAKE PHENAZOPYRIDINE HYDRO-CHLORIDE: Immediately after meals

FOODS TO AVOID: None

POSSIBLE SIDE EFFECTS: Dry mouth and gastrointestinal disturbances

ACTION OF PHENAZOPYRIDINE HYDROCHLO-RIDE: This drug relieves the pain, burning, urgency, and frequency of urination arising from irritation of the urinary tract.

HIGH-RISK GROUPS: Anyone who takes this drug

NUTRITIONAL INTERACTIONS

GASTROINTESTINAL DISTRESS: In occasional cases, gastrointestinal disturbances have been reported. The drug does cause dry mouth in roughly one third of those who use it, which can make swallowing more difficult.

Prevention and Treatment: Phenazopyridine hydrochloride should be taken immediately after meals to minimize the chances of these discomforts.

PHENFORMIN (No longer available in the United States)

DRUG FAMILY: Anti-diabetic

BRAND NAME: D.B.I.

HOW TO TAKE PHENFORMIN: With meals or milk

FOODS TO AVOID: All alcoholic beverages and foods containing alcohol

POSSIBLE SIDE EFFECTS: Vitamin B_{12} deficiency, stomach cramps, and diarrhea

ACTION OF PHENFORMIN: This drug acts by stimulating the production of insulin by the pancreas.

HIGH-RISK GROUPS: Vegetarians, the elderly, users of oral contraceptives, heavy drinkers, smokers

NUTRITIONAL INTERACTIONS

ALCOHOL INTERACTIONS: Phenformin impairs your body's ability to break down alcohol completely. The result is likely to be a buildup of an early breakdown product of alcohol called acetaldehyde. If you are susceptible to this reaction, you may experience any or all of the following symptoms: severe headaches, flushing, nausea, vomiting, a dramatic drop in blood pressure, weakness, vertigo, blurred vision, and even convulsions. The reaction occurs 5 to 10 minutes after one's consumption of the alcohol. As little as 1 teaspoon of liquor is sometimes sufficient to bring on the reaction.

Prevention and Treatment: If you are taking this drug, you should avoid all alcoholic beverages, foods with any wine content, and casseroles or desserts that have liquor or vinegar in them.

VITAMIN B_{12} DEFICIENCY: Phenformin decreases the absorption of vitamin B_{12}, and this could lead to a vitamin B_{12} deficiency if the drug is taken over an extended period.

This vitamin is needed for the normal development of red blood cells and for the healthy functioning of all cells, in particular those of the bone marrow, nervous system, and intestines.

The most common result of a B_{12} deficiency is pernicious anemia, which is characterized by listlessness, fatigue (especially following such physical exertion as climbing a flight of stairs), numbness and tingling in the fingers and toes, palpitations, angina, light-headedness, and a pale complexion. A vitamin B_{12} deficiency can also lead to an irreversible breakdown of the brain membranes, causing loss of coordination, confusion, memory loss, paranoia, apathy, tremors, and hallucinations. In extreme cases, degeneration of the spinal cord can also result.

Since vitamin B_{12} can be obtained only from animal food sources, strict vegetarians are at particular risk here. Oral contraceptive users too have a greater chance of experiencing this deficiency since they often have a poor vitamin B_{12} status to begin with, as is the case with some smokers. Heavy consumers of alcohol, as well, frequently lack B_{12} because alcohol impairs the absorption of the vitamin. Some elderly people also have difficulty in absorbing this vitamin. In any case, anyone who is likely to have a vitamin B_{12} absorption problem should be alert for signs of pernicious anemia while taking phenformin.

Prevention and Treatment: A balanced diet containing plenty of vitamin B_{12} sources is advised. Only animal products, including dairy foods and fish and shellfish, contain natural vitamin B_{12}. However, some vegetable products are supplemented with B_{12}; many soy products, for example, are enriched with vitamin B_{12} to safeguard vegetarians. (See table of Vitamin B_{12}-Rich Foods, page 312.)

Vitamin B_{12} is stored in the liver, so one meal that includes a B_{12}-rich source such as calf's liver will normally fulfill your body's need for this vitamin for 2 to 3 weeks. (One 3-ounce serving of calf's liver contains 100 mcg of vitamin B_{12}.) If none of these products figures prominently in your diet, you should take a 6 mcg supplement each day while on phenformin.

People who use major amounts of vitamin C should be aware that vitamin C supplements of more than 500 mg per day can destroy B_{12} and contribute to a B_{12} deficiency. However, anyone who eats red meat two times a week has a three- to five-year supply of B_{12} in his liver.

The presence of baking soda in cooking will destroy vitamin B_{12} and should be avoided whenever possible. B_{12} also degrades at high temperatures, as when meat is placed on a hot griddle. The pasteurization of milk and the sterilization in boiling water of a bottle containing milk also cause the loss of some B_{12}.

GENERAL INSTRUCTIONS: Since this drug is likely to cause stomach cramps and diarrhea on an empty stomach, it should always be taken with meals or milk.

PHENMETRAZINE HYDROCHLORIDE

DRUG FAMILY: Appetite suppressant

BRAND NAME: Preludin

HOW TO TAKE PHENMETRAZINE HYDRO-CHLORIDE: On an empty stomach 1 hour before or 2 to 3 hours after meals

FOODS TO AVOID: None

POSSIBLE SIDE EFFECTS: Nausea, diarrhea, vomiting, stomachache, and a dry and unpleasant-tasting mouth

ACTION OF PHENMETRAZINE HYDROCHLORIDE: This drug is used for the suppression of appetite in treating obesity. Although it is not an amphetamine, it has the same adverse side effects as the amphetamines but to a lesser degree.

HIGH-RISK GROUPS: Anyone who takes this drug

Nutritional Interactions

WEIGHT-REDUCTION PROGRAMS: Phenmetrazine hydrochloride is addictive and should be used only as a short-term aid to weight loss. A reasonable and moderate weight-reduction program should aim at a manageable 1- to 2-pound loss per week. By reducing your intake by 500 calories per day for a weekly total of 3,500 calories without regard to your present weight, you will lose 1 pound per week. Two eggs and a milk shake, 1½ cups of tuna salad, 4 ounces of a roast, 3 frankfurters, 2 cups of ice cream, or 2 pieces of cheesecake all represent approximately 500 calories.

The Weight Watchers exercise and behavior modification program is among those that offer a sensible balance of proper nutrition, exercise, and support in making a dietary change.

OTHER ADVICE: Use of phenmetrazine hydrochloride may result in the development of unwanted side effects, including such gastrointestinal disorders as nausea, diarrhea, vomiting, stomachache, and a dry and unpleasant-tasting mouth.

Food present in the stomach will decrease the absorption of this drug and therefore reduce its effectiveness. To gain the full benefit of this drug, it should always be taken 1 hour before or 3 hours after any meal.

PHENOBARBITAL

DRUG FAMILY: Anti-epileptic; sedative

BRAND NAMES: [GENERIC/Brand] PHENOBARBITAL/Antispasmodic; Antrocol; Arco-Lase Plus; Bronkolixir; Bronkotabs; Chardonna-2; Isuprel Hydrochloride Compound; Levsin/Phenobarbital; Levsinex/Phenobarbital; Mudrane GG; Mudrane; Phazyme-PB; Primatene-P Formula; Pro-Banthine w/ Phenobarbital; Quadrinal; SK-Phenobarbital; Solfoton; T-E-P; Theofedral; Valpin 50; PHENOBARBITAL SODIUM

HOW TO TAKE PHENOBARBITAL: As directed by your physician

FOODS TO AVOID: All alcoholic beverages; large quantities of alkaline foods such as milk, buttermilk, cream, almonds, chestnuts, coconut, all vegetables except corn and lentils, and all fruit except cranberries, prunes, and plums

POSSIBLE SIDE EFFECTS: Deficiencies of folic acid and vitamins B_{12}, D, K, and B_6

ACTION OF PHENOBARBITAL: Phenobarbital depresses the central nervous system. In small doses, it produces a sedative effect; in large doses, it induces sleep. It is also effective as an anti-convulsant and an anti-epileptic.

HIGH-RISK GROUPS: Oral contraceptive users, vegetarians, smokers, the elderly, pregnant women, teenagers, children, anyone who consumes alcohol

NUTRITIONAL INTERACTIONS

FOLIC ACID DEFICIENCY: Phenobarbital impairs the absorption of a number of vitamins, including folic acid. Often the first sign of a folic acid or folacin deficiency is inflamed and bleeding gums. The symptoms that follow are a sore, smooth tongue; diarrhea; forgetfulness; apathy; irritability; anemia; and a reduced resistance to disease. Despite the fact that folacin is found in a variety of foods, folacin deficiency is still the most common vitamin deficiency in the United States.

In adults, deficiencies are limited almost exclusively to the elderly and women, 30 percent of whom have intakes below the recommended daily allowance, and 5 to 7 percent of whom also have severe anemia. There are several factors that account for this bias, but one of the most obvious reasons is that oral contraceptive use decreases the absorption of folic acid. Constant dieting also limits folacin intake, and alcohol interferes with the body's use of folic acid, as well. Folacin is not stored by the body in any appreciable amounts, so an adequate supply must be consumed on a daily basis.

Folic acid is essential for the synthesis of new cells, so a folic acid deficiency during pregnancy may result in birth defects. A reduced resistance to infection will result. Folic acid is also crucial to the normal metabolism of proteins.

Prevention and Treatment: To counteract a deficiency in folic acid, your diet should contain liver, yeast, and leafy vegetables such as spinach, kale, parsley, cauliflower, brussels sprouts, and broccoli. The fruits that are highest in folic acid are oranges and cantaloupes. To a lesser degree, folacin is found in almonds and lima beans, corn, parsnips, green peas, pumpkins, sweet potatoes, bran, peanuts, rye, and whole grain wheat. (See table of Folacin-Rich Foods, page 297.) Approximately one half of the folic acid you consume is absorbed by your body.

Normal cooking temperatures (110 to 120 degrees for 10 minutes) destroy 65 percent of the folic acid in your food. Your daily diet, therefore, should include some raw vegetables and fruits. Cooking utensils made out of copper speed up folacin's destruction.

The recommended daily consumption of folacin is 400 mcg. While taking this drug, pregnant women and oral contraceptive users should consume a supplement of 800 mcg daily. Lactating women require a 1,200 mcg supplement. Everybody else needs a 400 mcg supplement.

VITAMIN B$_{12}$ DEFICIENCY: The absorption of vitamin B$_{12}$ is also impaired by phenobarbital. Vitamin B$_{12}$ is needed for the normal development of red blood cells, and for the healthy functioning of all cells, in particular those of the bone marrow, nervous system, and intestines.

The most common result of a B$_{12}$ deficiency is pernicious anemia, which is characterized by listlessness, fatigue (especially following such physical exertion as climbing a flight of stairs), numbness and tingling in the fingers and toes, palpitations, angina, light-headedness, and a pale complexion. A vitamin B_{12} deficiency can also lead to an irreversible breakdown in the brain membranes, causing loss of coordination, confusion, memory loss, paranoia, apathy, tremors, and hallucinations. In extreme cases, degeneration of the spinal cord can also result.

Since vitamin B_{12} can be obtained only from animal food sources, strict vegetarians are at particular risk here. Oral contraceptive users too have a greater chance of experiencing this deficiency, since they often have a poor vitamin B_{12} status to begin with, as do some smokers. Heavy consumers of alcohol, as well, frequently lack B_{12}, because alcohol impairs the absorption of the vitamin. Patients with bacterial or parasitic infections of the intestine also have difficulty in absorbing this vitamin, as do those who take excessive amounts of antacids at mealtimes, since the antacids tend to break down the vitamin. Many elderly people also have a problem absorbing vitamin B_{12}. In any case, everyone who is likely to have a vitamin B_{12} absorption problem, should be alert for signs of pernicious anemia while on phenobarbital.

Prevention and Treatments: A balanced diet containing plenty of vitamin B_{12} sources is advised. Only animal products, including dairy foods and fish and shellfish, contain natural vitamin B_{12}. However, some vegetable matter is supplemented with B_{12}; many soy products, for example, are enriched with vitamin B_{12} to safeguard vegetarians. (See table of Vitamin B_{12}-Rich Foods, page 312.)

Vitamin B_{12} is stored in the liver, so one meal that includes a B_{12}-rich source such as calf's liver will normally fulfill your body's need for this vitamin for 2 to 3 weeks. (One 3-ounce serving of calf's liver contains 100 mcg of vitamin B_{12}.) If none of these products figures prominently in your diet, you should take a 6 mcg supplement each day while on phenobarbital.

People who use major amounts of vitamin C should be aware that vitamin C supplements of more than 500 mg per day can damage B_{12} and contribute to a B_{12} deficiency. Copper and thiamin also seem to decrease its availability. However, anyone who eats red meat two times a week has a three- to five-year supply of B_{12} in his liver.

The presence of baking soda in cooking will destroy vitamin B_{12} and should be avoided whenever possible. B_{12} also degrades at high temperatures, as when meat is placed on a hot griddle or, in the case of liver, when it is boiled for 5 minutes. The pasteurization of milk and the sterilization in boiling water of a bottle of milk also cause the loss of some B_{12}.

VITAMIN D DEFICIENCY: Phenobarbital accelerates the breakdown of vitamin D, creating a mild deficiency.

Vitamin D is needed for the body to absorb calcium and phosphorus, to promote the development of strong teeth and bones. Whenever calcium blood levels are low, the body will liberate the calcium it needs from the bones, where it is stored. The result will be that the bones are weakened, a condition called osteomalacia. In severe cases the bones are weakened to the degree that they will fracture easily. Prominent symptoms are bone pain in the back, thighs, shoulder region, or ribs; difficulty in walking; and weakness in the muscles of the legs. The condition is reversible once the calcium blood levels are raised.

A prolonged deficiency of vitamin D can also lead to osteoporosis, another condition where the bones are weakened and made brittle. But osteoporosis, an unexplained and rapid loss of calcium from the bones, is irreversible. The common symptoms are backache, a gradual loss of height, and periodontal disease. Fractures of the vertebrae, hip, and wrist occur, sometimes spontaneously.

In children, a vitamin D deficiency can result in a condition known as rickets, in which the bones become bent or malformed. Children under four years of age may also develop pigeon breast, bowlegs, a protruding abdomen due to a weakness of stomach muscles, and poorly formed teeth that tend to decay.

Prevention and Treatment: To avoid a vitamin D deficiency while on phenobarbital, you should take 400 to 800 IU of the vitamin per day as a supplement to a diet of foods rich in D, such as fortified milk, butter, liver, egg yolks, salmon, tuna, and sardines. (See table of Vitamin D-Rich Foods, page 312.)

Vitamin D is initially formed in the skin from exposure to sunlight and activated in the liver and kidneys. The production of vitamin D is dependent upon climatic conditions, air pollution, skin pigmentation (the darker the skin, the lower the production), the area of skin exposed, the duration of exposure to the sun, and the use of sun screens, as well. Adults who are not often exposed to sunlight (e.g. those who are housebound or by custom heavily clothed), require dietary sources of vitamin D to prevent osteomalacia.

Vitamin D is also indispensable to infants, children, and to pregnant or lactating women, whose requirements are high due to bone growth or skeletal mineral replacement. Supplementation for pregnant women is crucial, since vitamin D deficiencies can cause fetal abnormalities. However, no more than 800 IU of the vitamin should be taken by pregnant women, because excessive consumption can cause kidney damage. In nonpregnant adults, 2,000 IU of the vitamin should be taken if osteomalacia is indicated. If your intake of vitamin D exceeds 4,000 IU per day, toxicity of vitamin D poisoning can occur. The symptoms are loss of appetite, headache, excessive thirst, irritability, and kidney stones.

In all of these cases, foods rich in calcium should be included in the diet, especially dairy products. (See table of Calcium-Rich Foods, page 289.) If these foods must be avoided because of an intolerance to lactose, the sugar found in dairy products (some 30 million Americans have such a problem digesting dairy products), a 1,200 to 1,500 mg daily supplement of calcium should be taken. (See Calcium Supplements entry page 51.)

VITAMIN K DEFICIENCY: Phenobarbital also increases the rate at which vitamin K is broken down, so people with an abnormally low dietary intake of vitamin K are at risk of bleeding with unusual ease if they use this drug for a long period of time.

Normally, vitamin K helps produce blood-clotting substances in the liver. Without sufficient levels of vitamin K in the diet, however, bleeding may take place in the gastrointestinal tract (causing black or blood-stained stools), in the urinary tract (causing blood in the urine), and in the uterus (causing blood loss at times other than the normal menstrual periods). Excessive blood loss may occur from an injury or surgery, as well. Another sign of a deficiency of this vitamin is more frequent and more visible bruising than normal.

Half the vitamin K in humans comes from dietary sources: predominantly green leafy vegetables, and to a lesser extent fruit, cereals, dairy products, and meat. The rest of the vitamin K in our bodies is synthesized by the bacteria in the intestines. The daily need for the vitamin is in the range of 70 to 140 mcg.

Pregnant women are at high risk because a vitamin K deficiency can led to hemorrhaging in the fetus. A fetus is more susceptible than an adult, since it does not have a bacterial population in the large intestine to make vitamin K and does not develop the capacity to do so for the first week of life. Women who have had several pregnancies or whose menstrual periods are heavy should also be careful. Many of the elderly are at risk of a vitamin K deficiency because they have a problem of poor fat absorption, and vitamin K, a fat-soluble vitamin, must be accompanied by sufficient dietary fat to be properly absorbed. Finally, anyone suffering from a kidney disease, cancer, or who is on prolonged antibiotic therapy may be at risk.

Prevention and Treatment: A vitamin K deficiency can be countered by a vitamin K supplement of 100 mcg per day and a diet that includes foods rich in the vitamin, such as kale, spinach, cabbage, cauliflower, leafy green vegetables, liver (especially pork liver), and fish. (See table of Vitamin K-Rich Foods, page 315.) Pregnant women on this drug should take 5 mg of vitamin K per day for 3 days prior to anticipated delivery, but only under the guidance of a physician. A newborn baby whose mother has been on phenobarbital should be given 1 mg vitamin K per day, to prevent anemia caused by the destruction of red blood cells. Infant formulas are often fortified with vitamin K.

Vitamin E supplements should not be taken when at risk of a vitamin K shortage, because vitamin E impairs the absorption of K.

VITAMIN B6 DEFICIENCY: People taking phenobarbital will have an increased need for vitamin B_6, so users of this drug may experience a vitamin B_6 deficiency. Common symptoms of this deficiency are a sore mouth and tongue, cracks in the lips and corners of the mouth, and patches of itching, scaling skin. A severe vitamin B_6 deficiency may cause depression and confusion.

Vitamin B_6 deficiencies are common among the elderly. Alcoholics, as well, often experience this deficiency, since alcohol interferes with the body's ability to use B_6. It is estimated that one of every two Americans consumes less that 70 percent of the recommended daily allowance of B_6. Smokers tend to have lower levels than nonsmokers.

Prevention and Treatment: To avoid a B_6 deficiency, you should consume a diet featuring such food sources of vitamin B_6 as liver (beef, calf, and pork), herring, salmon, walnuts, peanuts, wheat germ, carrots, peas, potatoes, grapes, bananas, and yeast. (See table of Vitamin B_6(Pyridoxine)-Rich Foods, page 311.) The vitamin is present in significant amounts in meats, fish, fruits, cereals, and vegetables, and to a lesser extent in milk and other dairy products.

Since vitamin B_6 is decomposed at high temperatures, modern food processing often diminishes dietary sources of the vitamin. Consequently, the more processed foods you eat, the more susceptible you will be to a deficiency of this vitamin. The same losses also occur in cooking: meat loses as much as 45 to 80 percent, vegetables 20 to 30 percent.

It has been observed that 15 to 20 percent of oral contraceptive users show direct evidence of vitamin B_6 deficiency. If you are among these people, you should take a 5 mg supplement of vitamin B_6 per day. However, keep in mind that you can take too much vitamin B_6. People taking over 1 gram per day have been reported to experience a toxic reaction. In addition, if you take more than 400 mg of vitamin B_6, it will decrease the effectiveness of phenobarbital.

ALKALINE URINE: Alkaline urine speeds up the rate of excretion of this drug, making it less effective.

Prevention and Treatment: Foods causing alkaline urine should be eaten only in moderation by people on phenobarbital. Fruits, vegetables, and dairy products tend to be alkaline, and high-protein foods tend to be acidic. Foods causing the production of alkaline urine include milk, buttermilk,

cream, almonds, chestnuts, coconuts, all vegetables except corn and lentils, and all fruits except cranberries, prunes, and plums.

Antacids that neutralize the acid in the stomach will also neutralize the acid in the urine, causing it to turn alkaline. Therefore, you should avoid taking antacids when taking this drug.

OTHER ADVICE: Phenobarbital increases cholesterol and triglyceride levels, thereby increasing the risk of heart disease.

The drug also accelerates the rate of deactivation of drugs. Among those affected are oral contraceptives and digitoxin, both of which are rendered less effective if used concurrently with phenobarbital. Be sure to advise your doctor of the other medications you take.

Alcohol increases the depressant effect of phenobarbital by inhibiting the body's ability to break it down. This can lead to loss of consciousness, coma, and death. Consequently, alcoholic beverages should never be taken by users of this drug.

PHENTERMINE RESIN AND PHENTERMINE HYDROCHLORIDE

DRUG FAMILY: Appetite suppressant

BRAND NAMES: Adipex-P; Fastin; Ionamin; Oby-Trim 30; Teramine

HOW TO TAKE PHENTERMINE: Immediately before breakfast, with a strong-tasting liquid such as fruit juice

FOODS TO AVOID: Those rich in tyramine or dopamine must be restricted, such as aged cheeses, raisins, avocados, liver, bananas, eggplant, sour cream, salami, meat tenderizers, chocolate, yeast, and soy sauce; also, alcoholic beverages, especially Chianti wines, vermouth, and beer.

POSSIBLE SIDE EFFECTS: Dryness of the mouth, diarrhea, constipation, and an unpleasant taste in the mouth

ACTION OF PHENTERMINE: This drug is prescribed as an adjunct to the treatment of obesity. It reduces the appetite.

HIGH-RISK GROUPS: People with a history of abdominal distress

NUTRITIONAL INTERACTIONS

GASTROINTESTINAL DISTRESS: This drug causes dryness of the mouth, diarrhea, constipation, and other gastrointestinal disturbances in some people. It also has an unpleasant taste.

Prevention and Treatment: Phentermine should be taken immediately after breakfast to minimize the likelihood of the diarrhea and dry mouth.

Constipation is usually safely remedied by an increase in the bulk in the diet. This means consuming larger servings of any of the following: dried or fresh fruits, salad vegetables, radishes, oatmeal, and whole grain foods (brown rice, whole wheat breads, and cereals). It is not necessary to purchase products that claim "extra fiber" has been added to them.

Persistent constipation may also be relieved by doubling the amount of fluid consumed each day. Bran, if used, should be added to the diet gradually, and fluid should be increased by at least ¾ cup per teaspoon of bran. (See table of Dietary Fiber-Rich Foods, page 293.)

TYRAMINE-RICH FOODS: In combination with foods rich in tyramine this drug may lead to an excessive rise in blood pressure.

Prevention and Treatment: Tyramine-containing foods must be restricted while you are being treated with this drug. Tyramine is common in many foods, but it is found in the greatest amounts in high-protein foods that have undergone some decomposition, like aged cheese. Tyramine is also found in chicken and beef livers, bananas, eggplant, sour cream, alcoholic beverages, salami, meat tenderizers, chocolate, yeast, and soy sauce. (See table of Tyramine-Rich Foods, page 307.) Raisins and avocados should also be avoided because they contain dopamine, which has the same effect as tyramine.

OTHER ADVICE: If your doctor has prescribed any acidic compounds such as sodium warfarin, iron, thyroid preparations, tetracycline, or thiazide diuretics, they should be taken at least 1 hour before this drug.

Finally, in order to minimize the unpleasant taste, take this drug with pulpy fruit such as applesauce, or a strong-tasting liquid such as fruit juice.

PHENYLBUTAZONE

DRUG FAMILY: Anti-inflammatory

BRAND NAMES: Azolid; Butazolidin

HOW TO TAKE PHENYLBUTAZONE: With meals or milk

FOODS TO AVOID: Restrict your consumption of sodium-rich foods such as canned soups and vegetables, TV dinners, processed cheese, salty snack foods, and foods garnished with monosodium glutamate

POSSIBLE SIDE EFFECTS: Iodine deficiency; edema; upset stomach

ACTION OF PHENYLBUTAZONE: Phenylbutazone is an anti-inflammatory, analgesic, and fever-reducing drug. It is used to relieve acute pain due to degenerative joint disease of the hips and knees, when other treatments fail. Gouty arthritis, rheumatoid arthritis, painful shoulder, and spinal immobility are often treated with this drug.

Phenylbutazone is rarely used for long periods of time because of its extreme toxicity.

HIGH-RISK GROUPS: The elderly, heart patients, hypertensives, teenagers

NUTRITIONAL INTERACTIONS

IODINE DEFICIENCY: Frequent use of phenylbutazone will inhibit the absorption of iodine by the thyroid gland, which could conceivably lead to an underproduction of thyroid hormone or a condition called hypothyroidism. Since the thyroid controls the rate at which the body works, this iodine deficiency can cause a sluggish thyroid, resulting in a feeling of lassitude, a lack of energy, and weight gain. Growing children, and pregnant and nursing women are at special risk in the event of an iodine deficiency because it will lead to retarded growth of the children, unborn infants, and nursing infants.

Prevention and Treatment: To avoid the threat of hypothyroidism while taking phenylbutazone, it is recommended you eat a diet containing foods rich in iodine. (See table of Iodine-Rich Foods, page 298.) Note, however, that certain foods such as cabbage, peanuts, and soybeans (or soy products) contribute to hypothyroidism, since they contain substances called goitrogens that prevent, the thyroid's intake of iodine and thus the manufacture of thyroid hormone.

EDEMA: This drug should not be taken if you already suffer from hypertension, since it is likely to lead to water and salt retention, which will tend to cause swelling (called edema) in your legs, ankles, feet, breasts, and around your eyes. An increase in sodium and water retention may also increase the volume of blood in the body, which places an added strain on the heart and tends to elevate blood pressure. Hence, this drug is usually given with a diuretic to avoid these potential problems.

High sodium retention causes some women to experience irritability, depression, and headaches, in particular before the onset of their menstrual periods.

Prevention and Treatment: While taking this drug, you should restrict your consumption of salt. In particular, those foods listed in the table of Sodium-Rich Foods (see page 306) should be avoided or consumed in small quantities. You should not add salt at the table and should restrict the salt added in cooking to no more than 1 teaspoon per day.

Many people are unaware of how much salt their diet contains. The average American, in fact, consumes some 6 to 8 grams of sodium per day, which is equivalent to 3 to 4 teaspoons of table salt (sodium chloride). Even if you do not salt your food while preparing or eating it, you consume considerable quantities of salt in commercially processed foods like canned soups and vegetables, so-called TV dinners, processed cheeses, many snack foods, and catsup. You also consume salt that is naturally present, though generally in lesser quantities, in vegetables and animal foods, and small amounts in drinking water.

While taking phenylbutazone, you would be well advised to restrict your salt intake to no more than 2 grams per day. This means using no more than 1 teaspoon per day during cooking, adding no salt to your food at the table, and avoiding extremely salty foods such as sauerkraut, anchovies, sardines, cold cuts, snack chips, and processed cheeses.

OTHER ADVICE: It is also likely that you will experience stomach irritation while you are on phenylbutazone, so it should be taken with meals or milk.

PHENYLEPHRINE HYDROCHLORIDE

DRUG FAMILY: Decongestant

BRAND NAMES: Anatuss; Bromphen; Codimal DH; Codimal DM; Codimal PH; Colrex; Comhist LA; Congespirin; Coryban-D; Dallergy; Dimetapp; Donatussin DC; Dristan Advanced Formula; Dura Tap-PD; Dura-Vent/DA; E.N.T.; Entex; Extendryl; Histalet Forte; Histaspan-D; Histor-D; Hycomine Compound; Korigesic; Naldecon; Neo-Synephrine Hydrochloride; Neo-tep; P-V-Tussin; Pediacof; Phenergan VC; Protid; Quelidrine; Ru-Tuss; S-T Forte; Singlet; Tamine S.R.; Tussar DM; Tympagesic

HOW TO TAKE PHENYLEPHRINE HYDROCHLORIDE: Shortly after meals or with milk

FOODS TO AVOID: Alcoholic beverages

POSSIBLE SIDE EFFECTS: Nausea and other gastrointestinal disturbances

ACTION OF PHENYLEPHRINE HYDROCHLORIDE: This drug is a nasal decongestant used to relieve seasonal allergies.

HIGH-RISK GROUPS: People with a history of gastrointestinal distress, anyone who consumes alcohol

NUTRITIONAL INTERACTIONS

GASTROINTESTINAL DISTRESS: This drug could conceivably cause nausea and other gastrointestinal disturbances.

Prevention and Treatment: Take phenylephrine hydrochloride shortly after meals or with milk.

OTHER ADVICE: This drug is an antihistamine and as such, tends to make you drowsy and impairs your coordination. Alcohol taken concurrently increases these effects. As a result, work performance and driving skills are impaired. Consequently, you should not consume alcohol while taking this drug.

PHENYLPROPANOLAMINE HYDROCHLORIDE

DRUG FAMILY: Decongestant

BRAND NAMES: Anatuss; Appedrine, Maximum Strength; Bayer Children's Cold Tablets; Bayer Cough Syrup for Children; Bromphen Compound; Codimal; Comtrex;

Conex; Conex with Codeine; Congespirin; Control; Coryban-D; Children's CoTylenol; Cremacoat 3; Cremacoat 4; Dehist; Dexatrim; Dieutrim; Dimetapp; Dorcol; Dristan Advanced Formula; Drize; Dura Tap-PD; Dura-Vent; Dura-Vent/A; E.N.T.; Entex; Entex LA; 4-Way Cold; Fiogesic; Head & Chest; Help; Histalet Forte; Hycomine; Korigesic; Kronohist Kronocaps; Naldecon; Naldecon-CX; Naldecon-DX; Naldecon-EX; Nolamine; Ornade; Phenate; Poly-Histine; Poly-Histine-D; Prolamine; Propagest; Protid; Resaid T.D.; Rescaps-D T.D.; Rhindecon; Rhindecon-G; Rhinolar; Rhinolar-EX; Rhinolar-EX 12; Robitussin; Ru-Tuss; Ru-Tuss II; Ru-Tuss with Hydrocodone; Sinubid; Sinulin; Tamine S.R.; Tavist-D; Triaminic; Triaminic TR; Triaminic-DM; Triaminic-12; Triaminicol; Tuss-Ornade

HOW TO TAKE PHENYLPROPANOLAMINE HYDRO-CHLORIDE: With food or milk

FOODS TO AVOID: Alcoholic beverages

POSSIBLE SIDE EFFECTS: Nausea and other gastrointestinal disturbances; reduced appetite

ACTION OF PHENYLPROPANOLAMINE HYDRO-CHLORIDE: This nasal decongestant is prescribed to relieve congestion of the nose, throat, and sinuses caused by allergic disorders and infections. It is also used to suppress the appetite in weight management.

HIGH-RISK GROUPS: Anyone who takes this drug

NUTRITIONAL INTERACTIONS

GASTROINTESTINAL DISTRESS: This drug can cause nausea and other gastrointestinal disturbances.

Prevention and Treatment: Take phenylpropanolamine hydrochloride with food or milk.

WEIGHT LOSS: This drug tends to reduce the appetite and can lead to unwanted weight loss.

Prevention and Treatment: Body weight should be monitored to avoid unwanted weight loss.

OTHER ADVICE: This drug is an antihistamine and as such tends to make you drowsy and impairs your coordination. Alcohol taken concurrently makes these effects more pronounced. As a result, work performance and driving skills are impaired. Consequently, you should not consume alcohol while you are on phenylpropanolamine.

PHENYLTOLOXAMINE CITRATE

DRUG FAMILY: Antihistamine

BRAND NAMES: Comhist LA; Comhist; Magsal; Naldecon; Percogesic; Poly-Histine-D; Sinubid

HOW TO TAKE PHENYLTOLOXAMINE CITRATE: With meals

FOODS TO AVOID: Alcoholic beverages and alkaline foods

POSSIBLE SIDE EFFECTS: Loss of appetite, nausea, vomiting, stomach cramps, constipation, diarrhea, increased urination, and dryness of the mouth

ACTION OF PHENYLTOLOXAMINE CITRATE: This drug is used in the treatment of motion sickness and as a nasal decongestant.

HIGH-RISK GROUPS: Heavy drinkers, people with a history of gastrointestinal distress

NUTRITIONAL INTERACTIONS

GASTROINTESTINAL DISTRESS: One conceivable side effect you may experience while taking phenyltoloxamine citrate is gastrointestinal distress, which may include a loss of appetite, nausea, vomiting, stomach cramps, constipation, diarrhea, increased urination, and dryness of the mouth.

Prevention and Treatment: These drugs should be taken with meals to avoid the gastric symptoms. To prevent dehydration due to excess urination, drink at least 6 to 8 glasses of water, or its equivalent in other nonalcoholic fluids, per day.

Body weight should also be monitored to avoid unwanted weight loss.

ALKALINE URINE: Since phenyltoloxamine citrate is alkaline, it is excreted at a normal rate only if your urine is acidic. However, if the quantity of alkaline foods in your diet is high, your urine will lose its acidity, and the excretion of this drug will be slowed. A hazardous buildup could conceivably result, leading to drowsiness, restlessness, dizziness, weakness, dry mouth, anorexia, nausea, vomiting, headache, nervousness, blurring of vision, excess urination, an inability to urinate, heartburn, and dermatitis.

Prevention and Treatment: Fruits, vegetables, and dairy products tend to be alkaline, and high-protein foods tend to be acidic. Foods causing the production of alkaline urine include milk, buttermilk, cream, almonds, chestnuts, coconuts, all vegetables except corn and lentils, and all fruits except cranberries, prunes, and plums.

Antacids that neutralize the acid in the stomach will also neutralize the acid in the urine, causing it to turn alkaline. Therefore, you should avoid antacids when taking this drug.

ALCOHOL INTERACTION: Alcohol is likely to heighten the danger of a loss of coordination. Dizziness, lassitude, uncoordination, fatigue, blurred vision, nervousness, or double vision may also occur, as well as an exacerbation of the gastric effects.

Alcohol in any form should not be consumed concurrently with phenyltoloxamine citrate.

PHENYTOIN

DRUG FAMILY: Anti-epileptic

BRAND NAMES: Dilantin Infatabs; Dilantin-30 Pediatric/Dilantin-125 Suspension; Dilantin Kapseals; Dilantin Parenteral; Dilantin with Phenobarbital; Phenytoin Sodium

HOW TO TAKE PHENYTOIN: With food or milk

FOODS TO AVOID: Alcoholic beverages

POSSIBLE SIDE EFFECTS: Deficiencies of vitamins D and K and folic acid; megadoses of vitamin B_6 decrease the drug's potency.

ACTION OF PHENYTOIN: This is an anti-epileptic drug that prevents the development of seizures.

HIGH-RISK GROUPS: Pregnant women, lactating women, teenagers, users of oral contraceptives, children, the elderly, vegetarians, anyone who consumes alcohol

NUTRITIONAL INTERACTIONS

VITAMIN D DEFICIENCY: Phenytoin can accelerate the breakdown of vitamin D and impair its activation in the liver, and is likely to cause a deficiency.

Vitamin D is needed for the body to absorb calcium and phosphorus, to promote the development of strong teeth and bones. Whenever calcium blood levels are low, the body will liberate the calcium it needs from the bones, where it is stored. The result will be that the bones are weakened, in severe cases to the degree that they will fracture easily. Prominent symptoms of this condition, called osteomalacia, are pain in the back, thighs, shoulder region, or ribs; difficulty in walking; and weakness in the muscles of the legs. The condition is reversible once the calcium blood levels are raised.

A chronic loss of bone calcium is believed to cause osteoporosis, another condition in which the bones are weakened and made brittle. Osteoporosis, however, is irreversible. The common symptoms are backache, a gradual loss of height, and periodontal disease. Fractures of the vertebrae, hip, and wrist occur, sometimes spontaneously.

In children, a vitamin D deficiency can result in a condition known as rickets in which the bones become bent or malformed. Children under four years of age may also develop pigeon breast, bowlegs, a protruding abdomen due to a weakness of the stomach muscles, and poorly formed teeth that tend to decay.

Prevention and Treatment: To avoid a vitamin D deficiency while on phenytoin, you should take 400 to 800 IU of vitamin D per day as a supplement to a diet of foods rich in vitamin D, such as fortified milk, butter, liver, egg yolks, salmon, tuna, and sardines. (See table of Vitamin D-Rich Foods, page 313.)

This vitamin is formed initially in your skin from exposure to sunlight, then activated in the liver and kidneys. As a result, the production of vitamin D is dependent upon climatic conditions, air pollution, skin pigmentation (the darker the skin, the lower the production), the area of skin exposed, the duration of exposure to the sun, and the use of sun screens, as well. Adults who are not often exposed to sunlight (e.g. those who are housebound or by custom heavily clothed), require dietary sources of vitamin D to prevent osteomalacia.

Vitamin D is indispensable to infants, children, and pregnant or lactating women, whose requirements are high due to bone growth or skeletal mineral replacement. Supplementation for pregnant women is crucial, since vitamin D deficiencies can cause fetal abnormalities. However, no more than 800 IU of the vitamin should be taken by pregnant women because excessive consumption can cause kidney damage. In nonpregnant adults, 2,000 IU of the vitamin should be taken if osteomalacia is indicated. If your intake of vitamin D exceeds 4,000 IU per day, toxicity or vitamin D poisoning can occur. The symptoms are loss of appetite, headache, excessive thirst, irritability, and kidney stones.

In all of these cases, foods rich in calcium should be included in the diet, especially dairy products. (See table of Calcium-Rich Foods, page 289.) If these foods must be avoided because of an intolerance to lactose, the sugar found in dairy products (some 30 million Americans have such a problem digesting dairy products), a 1,200 to 1,500 mg daily supplement of calcium should be taken. (See Calcium Supplements entry, page 51.)

FOLIC ACID DEFICIENCY: Phenytoin also impairs folacin status by decreasing its absorption and decreasing its potency in the body. A complication from prolonged use of this drug is likely to be megaloblastic anemia, which reduces the oxygen-carrying capacity of the blood, and may result from an extreme deficiency of folacin. Pregnant women should be especially careful since folate deficiencies can cause fetal abnormalities.

Often the first sign of a folic acid or folacin deficiency is inflamed and bleeding gums. The symptoms that follow are a sore, smooth tongue; diarrhea; weight loss; swollen ankles; and a reduced resistance to infection. Despite the fact that folacin is found in a variety of foods, folacin deficiency is still the most common vitamin deficiency in the United States.

In adults, deficiencies are limited almost exclusively to the elderly and women, 30 percent of whom have intakes below the recommended daily allowance, and 5 to 7 percent of whom have such a severe deficiency that anemia can be diagnosed. There are several factors that account for this phenomenon. One of the most obvious reasons is that oral contraceptive use decreases the absorption of folic acid. Constant dieting also limits folacin intake. Alcohol interferes with the body's absorption and use of folic acid. Folacin is not stored by the body in any appreciable amounts, so an adequate supply must be consumed on a daily basis.

Prevention and Treatment: To counteract a deficiency in folic acid, your diet should contain liver, yeast, and leafy vegetables such as spinach, kale, parsley, cauliflower, brussels sprouts, and broccoli. The fruits that are highest in folic acid are oranges and cantaloupes. To a lesser degree, folacin is found in almonds and lima beans, corn, parsnips, green peas, pumpkins, sweet potatoes, bran, peanuts, rye, and whole grain wheat. (See table of Folacin-Rich Foods, page 297.) Approximately one half of the folic acid you consume is absorbed by your body.

Typical cooking temperatures (110 to 120 degrees for 10 minutes) break down some 65 percent of the folacin in your food. Your daily diet, therefore, should include some raw vegetables and fruits. Cooking utensils made out of copper speed up folacin's destruction.

The recommended daily consumption of folacin is 400 mcg. Lacatating women should assume a daily need of 1,200 mcg. Pregnant women and oral contraceptive users should consume 800 mcg daily. People taking phenytoin should take a 0.4 to 1.0 mg supplement of folic acid daily.

VITAMIN K DEFICIENCY: Phenytoin also leads to inefficient use of vitamin K, since the drug accelerates the rate at which the vitamin is broken down. People with an abnormally low dietary intake of vitamin K could conceivably be at risk of bleeding with unusual ease if they use phenytoin for a long period of time.

Normally, vitamin K helps produce blood-clotting substances in the liver. Without sufficient levels of vitamin K in the diet, however, bleeding may take place in the gastrointestinal tract (causing black or blood-stained stools), in the urinary tract (causing blood in the urine), and in the uterus (causing blood loss at times other than the normal menstrual periods). Excessive blood loss may occur from an injury or surgery. Another sign of a deficiency of this vitamin is more frequent and more visible bruising than normal.

Half the vitamin K in humans comes from dietary sources: predominantly green leafy vegetables, and to a lesser extent fruit, cereals, dairy products, and meat. The rest of the vitamin K in our bodies is synthesized by the bacteria in the intestines. The daily need for the vitamin is in the range of 70 to 140 mcg.

Pregnant women are at high risk because a vitamin K deficiency can lead to hemorrhaging in the fetus. A fetus is more susceptible than an adult, since it does not have a bacterial population in the large intestine to make vitamin K and does not develop the capacity to do so for the first week of life. Women who have had several pregnancies or whose menstrual periods are heavy should also be careful. Many of the elderly are at risk of a vitamin K deficiency because they have a problem of poor fat absorption, and vitamin K, a fat-soluble vitamin, must be accompanied by sufficient dietary fat to be properly absorbed.

Prevention and Treatment: A vitamin K deficiency can be countered by a vitamin K supplement of 100 mcg per day, and a diet that includes foods rich in the vitamin, such as kale, spinach, cabbage, cauliflower, leafy green vegetables, liver (especially pork liver), and fish. (See table of Vitamin K-Rich Foods, page 315.) Pregnant women on phenytoin should take 5 mg of Vitamin K per day for 3 days prior to anticipated delivery, but only under the guidance of a physician. A newborn baby whose mother has been on this drug should be given 1 mg per day for a few days, since the child risks anemia caused by the destruction of his red blood cells.

Vitamin E supplements should not be taken when at risk of a vitamin K shortage, because vitamin E impairs the absorption of K.

GENERAL INSTRUCTIONS: Phenytoin should be taken with foods or milk in order to avoid gastrointestinal disturbance.

Women on oral contraceptives also should know that phenytoin actually decreases the effectiveness of the oral contraceptives.

Aspirin will increase the effects of phenytoin, while alcohol will decrease its effects. Therefore, if you are taking phenytoin you should use aspirin and alcohol only in moderation and inform your doctor, since he will need to adjust your daily dose appropriately.

Women taking large doses of vitamin B_6 will need higher doses of phenytoin, since over 400 mg of vitamin B_6 has a significant impeding effect on the drug's activity.

PIROXICAM

DRUG FAMILY: Anti-inflammatory

BRAND NAME: Feldene

HOW TO TAKE PIROXICAM: With milk or meals

FOODS TO AVOID: Restrict your consumption of foods rich in sodium, such as anchovies, dill pickles, sardines, green olives, canned soups and vegetables, TV dinners, soy sauce, processed cheeses, salty snack foods, cold cuts, and catsup.

POSSIBLE SIDE EFFECTS: Stomachache, nausea, gastric and duodenal ulcers, and gastrointestinal bleeding; edema

ACTION OF PIROXICAM: This drug reduces inflammation, pain, and fever, and is used for the relief of symptoms of osteoarthritis and rheumatoid arthritis.

HIGH-RISK GROUPS: Hypertensives, heart patients, people with a history of abdominal distress

NUTRITIONAL INTERACTIONS

GASTROINTESTINAL DISTRESS: Some 20 percent of all patients taking piroxicam are reported to experience gastrointestinal problems such as stomachache and nausea. Gastric and duodenal ulcers, and gastrointestinal bleeding, have also been reported as side effects in some patients. Symptoms of the latter are black, sticky stools.

Prevention and Treatment: This drug should always be taken with milk or food to reduce the risk of gastrointestinal disturbances. Consult your physician if you experience signs of gastrointestinal bleeding.

EDEMA: Piroxicam is likely to lead to water and salt retention, which will tend to cause swelling (called edema) in your legs, ankles, feet, and breasts, and around your eyes. An increase in sodium and water retention may also increase the volume of blood in the body, which places an added strain on the heart and tends to elevate blood pressure.

Hence, this drug is usually given with a diuretic to avoid these potential problems.

Prevention and Treatment: While taking this drug, you should restrict your consumption of sodium. In particular, those foods listed in the table of Sodium-Rich Foods (see page 306) should be avoided or consumed in small quantities. You should not add salt at the table and should use no more than 1 teaspoon per day in cooking.

The amount of sodium is in the average American's diet comes as a surprise to most people. We consume 6 to 8 grams per day, which amounts to 3 to 4 teaspoons. This adds up to a per capita consumption of some 15 pounds of salt a year. Even if you do not salt your food while preparing or eating it, you consume quantities of salt in foods such as anchovies, dill pickles, sardines, green olives, canned soups and vegetables, so-called TV dinners, soy sauce, processed cheeses, many snack foods, cold cuts, and catsup. Sodium is also consumed as additives, such as monosodium glutamate, widely used in the preparation of processed foods.

You can always tell how much sodium is in a processed food by looking at the label. If sodium features high on the list of ingredients, then it is present in significant quantities, and if it is at the bottom of the list, it means that there is little in the food.

POTASSIUM-BASED SALINE CATHARTICS

DRUG FAMILY: Laxative

BRAND NAME: Potassium Sodium Tartrate

HOW TO TAKE SALINE CATHARTICS: Preferably at bedtime and definitely not within 2 hours of taking a meal

FOODS TO AVOID: None

POSSIBLE SIDE EFFECTS: Calcium deficiency; increased excretion of sodium, potassium, protein, and fat

ACTION OF SALINE CATHARTICS: By increasing the action of the muscles lining the intestines, these laxatives reduce the time required for food to pass through the intestinal tract. Saline cathartics, including potassium salts, act partly by drawing water into the colon to increase the bulk of the stools. They also act by releasing cholecystokinin, a hormone, into the small intestine, which causes bile to be secreted into the intestine. Bile contains a lot of sodium, and this increases the amount of water drawn into the colon and adds bulk to the stool.

HIGH-RISK GROUPS: The elderly

Nutritional Interactions

CALCIUM DEFICIENCY: If taken chronically or with food, saline cathartics will decrease the absorption of calcium and could conceivably lead to a deficiency. Whenever calcium blood levels are low, the body will liberate the necessary amounts of calcium from the bones, where it is stored, thereby weakening them and making them more susceptible to fractures. A condition called osteomalacia can result. This is more likely after middle age, since in older people the body uses dietary calcium less efficiently.

Osteomalacia, a weakening of the bones as a consequence of uniform and steady calcium loss, affects millions of older Americans, but also many younger people. In fact, one out of every four postmenopausal women suffers from this problem. Prominent symptoms are bone pain in the back, thighs, shoulder region, or ribs; difficulty in walking; and weakness in the muscles of the legs. The condition is reversible once calcium blood levels are raised.

A prolonged dietary deficiency of calcium is also believed to cause osteoporosis, another condition in which the bones are made weak and brittle. However, osteoporosis, an unexplained and rapid loss of calcium from the bones, is irreversible. Here the first symptoms are backache, a gradual loss of height, and periodontal disease. In cases of osteoporosis, fractures of the vertebrae, hip, and wrist occur frequently, sometimes spontaneously.

About 7 percent of women fifty years of age and older have osteoporosis, and certain observers believe that the incidence of this disease is on the rise; between 15 and 20 million Americans are said to have osteoporosis today. In some 30 percent of people over sixty-five, the disease is severe enough to result in fractures. By age eighty, virtually all women experience some degree of osteoporosis; early menopause is a strong predictor of the disease. One out of five cases of the disease is found in men, but generally men get it at a later age and less severely than women.

Prevention and Treatment: The Recommended Dietary Allowance of calcium is 800 mg, and all women should consume at least 1,200 mg of calcium per day. The average intake in the United States, however, is only 450 to 550 mg. For the elderly, and women who have already reached menopause or are about to, this should be increased to 1,500 mg by the consumption of foods rich in calcium, particularly milk and dairy products (including yogurt and hard cheeses) and, to a lesser extent, almonds. Three 8-ounce glasses of milk, for example, provide 1,500 mg of calcium. (See table of Calcium-Rich Foods, page 289.)

If you cannot eat many foods rich in calcium because of an intolerance to lactose, the sugar found in dairy products (a problem for an estimated 30 million Americans), a 1,000 mg daily supplement of calcium should be taken. The best-absorbed supplement is calcium carbonate. (See Calcium Supplements entry, page 51.) If magnesium is included in the supplement, the calcium is slightly better absorbed, and any tendency to constipation is reduced. The supplement should be taken in two 500 mg doses, one of which should be consumed before bedtime because most of the calcium loss from your body occurs while you sleep.

Remember that vitamin C assists calcium absorption, while cigarette smoking increases calcium loss from the body, as does excessive alcohol consumption. Foods that can decrease the absorption of calcium should be temporarily restricted, such as kale, rhubarb, spinach, cocoa, chocolate, beet greens, tea, and coffee. A deficiency might arise also if the ratio of phosphorus to calcium in your diet is very high; processed foods, especially carbonated beverages, are particularly high in phosphorus. The ideal ratio is essentially 1 to 1, as in dairy products; when the ratio is 15 or 20 to 1, as in meat, very little calcium is absorbed. High-fiber foods may contribute to a calcium deficiency, since fiber binds to

calcium and passes it out in the stool. Excess fat and protein in the diet also hinder absorption.

Given that there is little calcium in strict vegetarian diets (those that avoid dairy products as well as meat), vegetarians are at greater risk of a calcium deficiency. People who take magnesium- or aluminum-based antacids are also more prone to calcium deficiencies, because both magnesium and aluminum in excess impair calcium absorption.

It is recommended that, besides a change in dietary habits and the use of calcium supplements, anyone at risk of this deficiency adopt an exercise regimen that causes the bones to support the weight of the body, to strengthen the bones and to counteract the loss of bone density. A regular walking or jogging program, for example, can help prevent the bone degeneration of the spine, hips, and legs. Note, however, that swimming, though good for the heart as an aerobic exercise, is not especially beneficial for bone buildup.

OTHER NUTRITIONAL DEFICIENCIES: All the saline cathartics produce small increases in the excretion of sodium, potassium nitrogen, and fat, no matter when they are taken, though the effect is usually only a modest one. But this could be intensified if the laxative is administered with or shortly after eating.

Prevention and Treatment: None of the saline cathartics should be taken with meals, or within 2 hours of a meal.

POTASSIUM SUPPLEMENTS

DRUG FAMILY: Mineral supplements

BRAND NAMES: [GENERIC/Brand] POTASSIUM CHLORIDE/Infalyte; K-Lor; K-Lyte/Cl & K-Lyte/Cl 50; K-Tab; Kaochlor 10%; Kaochlor S-F 10%; Kaon Cl-10; Kaon-Cl; Kato; Kay Ciel; Klor-Con/25; Klor-Con; Klor-Con 20%; Klor 10%; Klorvess; Klorvess 10%; Klotrix; Kolyum; Micro-K; Potage; Potassium Chloride Concentrate; Rum-K; Slow-K; POTASSIUM GLUCONATE/Bi-K; Kaon; Kolyum; Twin-K; Twin-K-Cl; POTASSIUM IODIDE/Iodo-Niacin; Isuprel Hydrochloride Compound; Mudrane; Mudrane-2; Pediacof; Pima; Quadrinal; SSKI

HOW TO TAKE POTASSIUM SUPPLEMENTS: With food

FOODS TO AVOID: Dairy products must not be eaten within 2 hours of taking potassium chloride or potassium iodide

POSSIBLE SIDE EFFECTS: Vitamin B_{12} deficiency; upset stomach

ACTION OF POTASSIUM SUPPLEMENTS: Most often, potassium supplements are prescribed for people who are taking diuretics that deplete body potassium.

HIGH-RISK GROUPS: Vegetarians, heavy drinkers, the elderly, users of oral contraceptives, smokers

NUTRITIONAL INTERACTIONS

POTASSIUM ABSORPTION: The absorption of potassium chloride and potassium iodide compounds is decreased by dairy products.

Prevention and Treatment: Potassium iodide or potassium chloride must not be taken within 2 hours of eating dairy products.

VITAMIN B_{12} DEFICIENCY: All potassium compounds impair the absorption of vitamin B_{12} and can cause a deficiency in the high-risk groups. Vitamin B_{12} is needed for the normal development of red blood cells and for the healthy functioning of all cells, in particular those of the bone marrow, nervous system, and intestines.

The most common result of a B_{12} deficiency is pernicious anemia, which is characterized by listlessness, fatigue (especially following such physical exertion as climbing a flight of stairs), numbness and tingling in the fingers and toes, palpitations, angina, light-headedness, and pale complexion. A vitamin B_{12} deficiency can also lead to an irreversible breakdown of the brain membranes, causing loss of coordination, confusion, memory loss, paranoia, apathy, tremors, and hallucinations. In extreme cases, degeneration of the spinal cord can also result.

Since vitamin B_{12} can be obtained only from animal food sources, strict vegetarians are at particular risk here. Oral contraceptive users too have a greater chance of experiencing this deficiency since they often have a poor vitamin B_{12} status to begin with, as do smokers. Heavy consumers of alcohol, as well, frequently lack B_{12} because alcohol impairs the absorption of the vitamin. Patients with bacterial or parasitic infections of the intestine also have difficulty in absorbing this vitamin, as do those who take excessive amounts of antacids at mealtimes and many elderly people. In any case, anyone who is likely to have a vitamin B_{12} absorption problem should be alert for signs of pernicious anemia while taking this drug.

Prevention and Treatment: A balanced diet containing plenty of vitamin B_{12} sources is advised, and if insufficient quantities are included in the diet, a daily supplement of 6 mcg of the vitamin should be taken.

Only animal products, including dairy foods and fish and shellfish, contain natural vitamin B_{12}. However, some vegetable foods are supplemented with vitamin B_{12}; many soy products, for example, are enriched with B_{12} to safeguard vegetarians. (See table of Vitamin B_{12}-Rich Foods, page 312.)

Vitamin B_{12} is stored in the liver, so one meal that includes a B_{12}-rich source such as calf's liver will normally fulfill your body's need for this vitamin for 2 to 3 weeks. (One 3-ounce serving of calf's liver contains 100 mcg of vitamin B_{12}.)

People who use major amounts of vitamin C should be aware that vitamin C supplements of more than 500 mg per day can damage B_{12} and contribute to a B_{12} deficiency. However, anyone who eats red meat two times a week has a three- to five-year supply of B_{12} in his liver.

The presence of baking soda in cooking will destroy vitamin B_{12} and should be avoided whenever possible. B_{12} also degrades at high temperatures, as when meat is placed on a hot griddle. The pasteurization of milk and the sterilization in boiling water of a bottle of milk also cause the loss of some B_{12}.

GASTROINTESTINAL DISTRESS: It is conceivable that you will experience some gastric irritation while you are taking potassium supplements.

Prevention and Treatment: These supplements should be taken with meals to minimize the likelihood of these discomforts. Users of the supplements should also be aware that alcohol can intensify the gastrointestinal symptoms.

PRIMIDONE

DRUG FAMILY: Anti-epileptic

BRAND NAME: Mysoline

HOW TO TAKE PRIMIDONE: As directed by your physician

FOODS TO AVOID: Alcoholic beverages

POSSIBLE SIDE EFFECTS: Deficiencies of vitamins K and D, and folic acid

ACTION OF PRIMIDONE: This drug is a suitable treatment for most types of epilepsy.

HIGH-RISK GROUPS: Anyone who consumes alcohol, the elderly, children, users of oral contraceptives, pregnant women, lactating women, teenagers

NUTRITIONAL INTERACTIONS

VITAMIN K DEFICIENCY: Use of primidone is likely to lead to a rapid rate of degradation of vitamin K. The risk is of bleeding with unusual ease.

Vitamin K normally assists in the production of blood-clotting substances in the liver. Without sufficient levels of vitamin K in the diet, however, bleeding may take place in the gastrointestinal tract (causing black or blood-stained stools), in the urinary tract (causing blood in the urine), and in the uterus (causing blood loss at times other than the normal menstrual periods). Excessive blood loss may also occur after an injury or surgery. Another sign of a deficiency of this vitamin is more frequent and more visible bruising than normal.

Half the vitamin K in humans comes from dietary sources: predominantly green leafy vegetables, and to a lesser extent fruit, cereals, dairy products, and meat. The rest of the vitamin K in our bodies is synthesized by the bacteria in the intestines. The daily need for the vitamin is in the range of 70 to 140 mcg.

Pregnant women are at high risk because a vitamin K deficiency can lead to hemorrhaging in the fetus. A fetus is more susceptible than an adult, since it does not have a bacterial population in the large intestine to make vitamin K and does not develop the capacity to do so for the first week of life. Women who have had several pregnancies or whose menstrual periods are heavy should also be careful.

Many of the elderly are at risk of a vitamin K deficiency because they have a problem of poor fat absorption, and vitamin K, a fat-soluble vitamin, must be accompanied by sufficient dietary fat to be properly absorbed. Finally, anyone suffering from a kidney disease or cancer, or who is on prolonged antibiotic therapy, may be at risk.

Prevention and Treatment: A vitamin K deficiency can be countered by a vitamin K supplement of 100 mcg per day and a diet that includes foods rich in the vitamin, such as kale, spinach, cabbage, cauliflower, leafy green vegetables, liver (especially pork liver), and fish. (See table of Vitamin K-Rich Foods, page 315.) Pregnant women on this drug should take 5 mg of vitamin K per day for 3 days prior to anticipated delivery, but only under the guidance of a physician. A newborn baby whose mother has been on primidone should be given 1 mg per day to avoid anemia caused by the destruction of red blood cells. Infant formulas are often fortified with vitamin K.

Vitamin E supplements should not be taken when at risk of a vitamin K shortage, because vitamin E impairs the absorption of K.

FOLIC ACID DEFICIENCY: Primidone use leads to the depletion of the body's folacin (folic acid), and it is conceivable that a deficiency will result. Often the first sign of a folic acid or folacin deficiency is inflamed and bleeding gums. The symptoms that follow are a sore, smooth tongue; diarrhea; forgetfulness; apathy; irritability; anemia; and a reduced resistance to infection.

Despite the fact that folacin is found in a variety of foods, folacin deficiency is still the most common vitamin deficiency in the United States. In adults, deficiencies are limited almost exclusively to the elderly and women, 30 percent of whom have intakes below the recommended daily allowance, and 5 to 7 percent of whom also have severe anemia. There are several factors that account for this bias, but one of the most obvious reasons is that oral contraceptive use decreases the absorption of folic acid. Constant dieting also limits folacin intake, and alcohol interferes with the body's use of folic acid, as well. Folacin is not stored by the body in any appreciable amounts, so an adequate supply must be consumed on a daily basis.

Folic acid is crucial to the normal metabolism of protein. Folacin is also essential to the production of new cells in the body. A deficiency of this vitamin during pregnancy can lead to birth defects.

Prevention and Treatment: To counteract a deficiency in folic acid, your diet should contain liver, yeast, and leafy vegetables such as spinach, kale, parsley, cauliflower, brussels sprouts, and broccoli. The fruits that are highest in folic acid are oranges and cantaloupes. To a lesser degree, folacin is found in almonds and lima beans, corn, parsnips, green peas, pumpkins, sweet potatoes, bran, peanuts, rye, and whole grain wheat. (See table of Folacin-Rich Foods, page 297.) Approximately one half of the folic acid you consume is absorbed by your body.

Because normal cooking temperatures (110 to 120 degrees for 10 minutes) destroy up to 65 percent of dietary folacin, your daily diet should include some raw vegetables and fruits. Cooking utensils made out of copper speed up folacin's destruction.

The recommended daily consumption of folacin is 400 mcg. Lactating women should assume a daily need of 1,200 mcg. Pregnant women and oral contraceptive users should consume 800 mcg daily.

VITAMIN D DEFICIENCY: Primidone also speeds up the degradation of vitamin D. The result could conceivably be a deficiency of this critical vitamin.

Vitamin D is needed for the body to absorb calcium and phosphorus, to promote the development of strong teeth and bones. Whenever calcium blood levels are low, the body will liberate the calcium it needs from the bones, where it is stored. The result will be that the bones are weakened, in severe cases to the degree that they will fracture easily. Prominent symptoms of osteomalacia, as the condition is called, are bone pain in the back, thighs, shoulder region, or ribs; difficulty in walking; and weakness in the muscles of the legs. The condition is reversible once the calcium blood levels are raised.

A prolonged calcium deficiency may cause osteoporosis, another condition where the bones are weakened and made brittle. Osteoporosis, an unexplained and rapid loss of calcium from the bones, is irreversible. The common symptoms are backache, a gradual loss of height, and periodontal disease. Fractures of the vertebrae, hip, and wrist occur, sometimes spontaneously.

In children, a vitamin D deficiency can result in a condition known as rickets, in which the bones become bent or malformed. Children under four years of age may also develop pigeon breast, bowlegs, a protruding abdomen due to a weakness of the stomach muscles, and poorly formed teeth that tend to decay.

Prevention and Treatment: To avoid a vitamin D deficiency while taking this drug, you should take 400 to 800 IU of vitamin D per day as a supplement to a diet of foods rich in vitamin D, such as fortified milk, butter, liver, egg yolks, salmon, tuna, and sardines. (See table of Vitamin D-Rich Foods, page 313.)

Exposure to sunlight results in vitamin D being formed in the skin, and it is activated in the liver and kidneys. The production of vitamin D is dependent upon climatic conditions, air pollution, skin pigmentation (the darker the skin, the lower the production), the area of skin exposed, the duration of exposure to the sun, and the use of sun screens, as well. Adults who are not often exposed to sunlight (e.g. those who are housebound or by custom heavily clothed), require dietary sources of vitamin D to prevent osteomalacia.

Vitamin D is indispensable to infants, children, and pregnant or lactating women, whose requirements are high due to bone growth or skeletal mineral replacement. Supplementation for pregnant women is crucial since vitamin D deficiencies can cause fetal abnormalities. However, no more than 800 IU of the vitamin should be taken by pregnant women, because excessive consumption can cause fetal kidney damage. In nonpregnant adults, 2,000 IU of the vitamin should be taken if osteomalacia is indicated. If your intake of vitamin D exceeds 4,000 IU per day, toxicity or vitamin D poisoning can occur. The symptoms are loss of appetite, headache, excessive thirst, irritability, and kidney stones.

In all of these cases, foods rich in calcium should be included in the diet, especially dairy products. (See table of Calcium-Rich Foods, page 289.) If these foods must be avoided because of an intolerance to lactose, the sugar found in diary products (some 30 million Americans have such a problem digesting dairy products), a 1,200 to 1,500 mg daily supplement of calcium should be taken. (See Calcium Supplements entry, page 51.)

OTHER ADVICE: Alcohol decreases the body's ability to break down primidone and intensifies its sedative effect. If enough is consumed, it can lead to loss of consciousness and coma. Consequently, it is ill advised to drink alcohol while taking this drug.

PROBENECID

DRUG FAMILY: Anti-gout

BRAND NAMES: Ampicillin-Probenecid; Benemid; ColBENEMID; Col-Probenecid; Polycillin-PRB; Principen with Probenecid; Probenecid w/Colchicine; SK-Probenecid; Wycillin & Probenecid

HOW TO TAKE PROBENECID: Immediately after meals

FOODS TO AVOID: Do not eat large quantities of acidic foods such as meat, fish, poultry, eggs, cheese, peanut butter, bacon, Brazil nuts, filberts, peanuts, walnuts, bread, crackers, pasta, cookies, and cakes. Moderate your intake of coffee, tea, and cola beverages. Do not drink herbal teas. Limit your consumption of alcohol, especially beer, and sweet foods.

POSSIBLE SIDE EFFECTS: Kidney stones, upset stomach

ACTION OF PROBENECID: This drug is prescribed for patients with gout, to reduce the level of uric acid in the blood and body tissues that causes gout. It increases the rate of excretion of uric acid via the kidneys.

Gout is an arthritis-type disease that is the result of deposits of uric acid crystals in the joints. It usually occurs in single joints, most often the big toe, in painful episodes that last only a few days but are likely to recur. Middle-aged men are chiefly afflicted.

Your doctor is likely to recommend a special diet low in purine-rich foods in addition to prescribing this or another of the anti-gout medications. That diet is a crucial part of the treatment, since the purines in foods are broken down by your body to form uric acid. (See table of Purine-Rich Foods, page 303.)

HIGH-RISK GROUPS: Anyone who takes this drug

NUTRITIONAL INTERACTION

KIDNEY STONES AND OTHER COMPLICATIONS: Probenecid may conceivably lead to the production of kidney stones. The odds of this are increased when there are foods in your diet, such as those rich in purines, that cause acidic urine. Normally, purine-rich foods are excreted as uric acid, but this drug may cause an unusual buildup of this acid in the kidneys, leading to the formation of uric acid crystals, one form of kidney stones. Difficulty in urinating and blood in the urine may signal the development of kidney stones.

Prevention and Treatment: To prevent the formation of kidney stones, you should drink no less than 8 glasses or 5 to 6 pints of liquid every 24 hours, particularly at night when the urine becomes concentrated. To keep your urine alkaline, or nonacidic, consume a diet rich in alkaline foods such as milk, cream, buttermilk, almonds, chestnuts, coconut, all vegetables except corn and lentils, and all fruits except cranberries, prunes, and plums. You should also cut down on foods that make the urine acidic, including meat, fish, poultry, eggs, cheese, peanut butter, bacon, Brazil nuts, filberts, peanuts, walnuts, bread, crackers, macaroni, spaghetti, noodles, cakes, and cookies.

OTHER ADVICE: Do not consume large quantities of coffee, tea, or cola beverages, because they are likely to reduce the effectiveness of the drug.

Probenecid should be taken after eating to reduce stomach irritation. It should not be used if you have a history of peptic ulcers. This drug may also decrease the absorption of protein. Avoid herbal teas; they contain phenylbutazone, which raises blood uric acid levels.

You should also avoid alcohol, especially beer, and simple sugars (see table of Simple and Complex Carbohydrates, page 305), because they can raise the blood level of uric acid and impair the drug's ability to manage chronic gout.

If obese, the gout sufferer should also achieve ideal body weight by gradual weight reduction (1 to 2 pounds per week). All sufferers should decrease their animal fat intake and increase their complex carbohydrate intake.

PROCAINAMIDE AND PROCAINAMIDE HYDROCHLORIDE

DRUG FAMILY: Heart drugs

BRAND NAMES: Procan SR; Pronestyl; Pronestyl-SR

HOW TO TAKE PROCAINAMIDE: With food

FOODS TO AVOID: Moderate your intake of alkaline foods, including milk, buttermilk, cream, almonds, chestnuts, coconut, all vegetables except corn and lentils, and all fruits except cranberries, prunes, and plums

POSSIBLE SIDE EFFECTS: Loss of appetite, vomiting, and diarrhea

ACTION OF PROCAINAMIDE: This is prescribed for patients with irregular heart rates.

HIGH-RISK GROUPS: Anyone who takes this drug

NUTRITIONAL INTERACTIONS

GASTROINTESTINAL DISTRESS: Use of procainamide can lead to a loss of appetite, vomiting, and diarrhea.
Prevention and Treatment: You should take procainamide with food. If the above symptoms persist, you should inform your doctor so that he can switch you to a different drug.

ALKALINE URINE: Alkaline urine prevents the body from excreting the drug via the kidneys and can lead to a toxic buildup in the body, causing extremely low blood pressure and a rapid heart rate.
Prevention and Treatment: Foods causing the production of alkaline urine should be taken in moderation. These include milk, buttermilk, cream, almonds, chestnuts, coconuts, all vegetables except corn and lentils, and all fruits except cranberries, prunes, and plums.

Antacids that neutralize the acid in the stomach will also neutralize the acid in the urine, causing it to turn alkaline. Therefore, you should avoid taking antacids while you are on procainamide.

PROCARBAZINE

DRUG FAMILY: Anti-cancer

BRAND NAME: Matulane

HOW TO TAKE PROCARBAZINE: As directed by your physician

FOODS TO AVOID: Those rich in tyramine or dopamine must be restricted, such as aged cheeses, raisins, avocados, liver, bananas, eggplant, sour cream, salami, meat tenderizers, chocolate, yeast, and soy sauce; also, all alcoholic beverages.

POSSIBLE SIDE EFFECTS: Nausea, vomiting, impaired taste; mouth sores; poor appetite

ACTION OF PROCARBAZINE: This drug is used in the treatment of Hodgkin's disease.

HIGH-RISK GROUPS: Anyone who takes this drug

NUTRITIONAL INTERACTIONS

TYRAMINE-RICH FOODS: Procarbazine is a weak monoamine-oxidase inhibitor, which means that its use will conceivably lead to an increase in your blood pressure.

Tyramine, a food substance, may further exacerbate this potential side effect of procarbazine. The ingested tyramine is usually converted in the liver to an inactive form through the action of monoamine oxidase (MAO). However, drugs in the MAO-inhibitor class leave tyramine in its active form. As a result, the tyramine remains in the blood and can increase blood pressure to dangerous levels. In some people, migraine headaches also result.

Prevention and Treatment: Tyramine-containing foods must be restricted while you are being treated with this drug. Tyramine is common in many foods, but it is found in the greatest amounts in high-protein foods that have undergone some decomposition, like aged cheese. Tyramine is also found in chicken and beef livers, bananas, eggplant, sour cream, alcoholic beverages, salami, meat tenderizers, chocolate, yeast, and soy sauce. (See table of Tyramine-Rich Foods, page 317.) Raisins and avocados should also be avoided, because they contain dopamine, which has the same effect as tyramine.

ALCOHOL INTERACTION: The ingestion of alcohol while taking procarbazine is likely to cause you to experience intense warmth and a reddening of the face, headache, breathing difficulties, gastrointestinal disturbances, and confusion. This is due to the buildup of acetaldehyde in your blood, as procarbazine prevents your body from detoxifying acetaldehyde, a breakdown product of alcohol.

Prevention and Treatment: Consequently, no alcohol should be consumed while you are taking procarbazine.

GASTROINTESTINAL DISTRESS: Procarbazine is likely to cause nausea, vomiting, impaired taste, mouth sores, and anorexia.

Prevention and Treatment: Nausea and vomiting may be controlled by taking several basic steps. First, you should eat smaller meals and limit your intake of high-fat foods. Second, when you experience nausea, you should slowly sip clear beverages like ginger ale. Sucking a Popsicle may also alleviate the condition. You should lie down, loosen your clothes, and get fresh air as well.

If you find that you vomit frequently, you should take plenty of liquids to prevent dehydration.

PROCHLORPERAZINE

DRUG FAMILY: Anti-anxiety, anti-psychotic

BRAND NAMES: Combid; Compazine; Prochlor-Iso

HOW TO TAKE PROCHLORPERAZINE: With meals

FOODS TO AVOID: Alcoholic beverages; only moderate amounts of alkaline foods should be consumed, such as milk, buttermilk, cream, almonds, chestnuts, coconut, all vegetables except corn and lentils, and all fruits except cranberries, prunes, and plums.

POSSIBLE SIDE EFFECTS: Upset stomach; increased appetite

ACTION OF PROCHLORPERAZINE: This drug is used in managing moderate to severe anxiety, tension, and psychotic disorders. It is also used in the control of severe nausea and vomiting.

HIGH-RISK GROUPS: Anyone who takes this drug

NUTRITIONAL INTERACTIONS

ALCOHOL INTERACTION: The effect of prochlorperazine is likely to be enhanced by alcohol. Central nervous system depression may be increased, in some case with severe respiratory failure. Prochlorperazine can also enhance the effects of alcohol in inhibiting driving skills, with a consequent increase in the chances of motor accidents.

Prevention and Treatment: Alcohol should not be consumed concurrently with this drug.

ALKALINE URINE: Because prochlorperazine is alkaline, it is excreted at a normal rate only if your urine is acidic. However, if the quantity of alkaline foods in your diet is high, your urine will lose its acidity, and the excretion of this drug will be slowed. A hazardous buildup could conceivably result. The symptoms of such a buildup or overdose are drowsiness, dizziness, loss of control of movements, muscular spasms, rapid heart rate, low blood pressure (especially on standing), and jitters.

Prevention and Treatment: Fruits, vegetables, and dairy products tend to be alkaline, and high-protein foods tend to be acidic. Foods causing the production of alkaline urine include milk, buttermilk, cream, almonds, chestnuts, coconuts, all vegetables except corn and lentils, and all fruits except cranberries, prunes, and plums.

Antacids that neutralize the acid in the stomach will also neutralize the acid in the urine, causing it to turn alkaline. Therefore, you should avoid taking antacids while you are on prochlorperazine.

GASTROINTESTINAL DISTRESS: This drug could conceivably cause you to experience gastric irritation and should not be taken on an empty stomach.

However, prochlorperazine also increases appetite and leads to weight gain in some people.

Prevention and Treatment: This drug should always be taken with a meal to prevent stomach irritation. You should also carefully monitor your weight to ensure that the drug does not cause an obesity problem, with its associated health risks.

PROCYCLIDINE HYDROCHLORIDE

DRUG FAMILY: Anti-Parkinsonism

BRAND NAME: Kemadrin

HOW TO TAKE PROCYCLIDINE HYDROCHLORIDE: During or after meals, or with milk

FOODS TO AVOID: None

POSSIBLE SIDE EFFECTS: Stomachache, nausea, vomiting, constipation, and a dry mouth

ACTION OF PROCYCLIDINE HYDROCHLORIDE: This drug is used to treat patients with Parkinson's disease and is most effective in the treatment of the symptoms of rigidity (rather than the tremor) accompany the ailment.

HIGH-RISK GROUPS: The elderly

NUTRITIONAL INTERACTIONS

GASTROINTESTINAL DISTRESS: This drug is a gastric irritant, and its use could conceivably lead to abdominal pain, nausea, and vomiting.

Other potential side effects are dry mouth and constipation.

Prevention and Treatment: Procyclidine hydrochloride should always be taken during or after meals, or with milk, to reduce the gastric symptoms.

At least 8 glasses of fluid should be consumed daily to reduce the dry mouth sensation. Sucking mints or chewing gum can also help alleviate the problem.

Constipation is usually safely remedied by an increase in the bulk in the diet. This means consuming larger servings of any of the following: dried or fresh fruits, salad vegetables, radishes, oatmeal, and whole grain foods (brown rice, whole wheat breads, and cereals). It is not necessary to purchase products that claim "extra fiber" has been added to them.

Persistent constipation may also be relieved by doubling the amount of fluid consumed each day. Bran, if used, should be added to the diet gradually, and fluid should be increased by at least ¾ cup per teaspoon of bran. (See table of Dietary Fiber-Rich Foods, page 293.)

PROPANTHELINE BROMIDE

DRUG FAMILY: Anti-muscarinic

BRAND NAMES: Pro-Banthine; SK-Propantheline Bromide

HOW TO TAKE PROPANTHELINE BROMIDE: On an empty stomach one-half hour before eating

FOODS TO AVOID: Moderate your intake of alkaline foods such as milk, buttermilk, cream, almonds, chestnuts, coconut, all vegetables except corn and lentils, and all fruits except cranberries, prunes, and plums.

POSSIBLE SIDE EFFECTS: Dry mouth

ACTION OF PROPANTHELINE BROMIDE: Propantheline bromide is an anti-muscarinic drug that relaxes smooth muscles and reduces glandular secretion. It interferes with the transmission of nerve impulses to smooth muscles, causing them to relax. Various glands are also affected, their rate of secretion being reduced. This results in less gastrointestinal motility and gastric secretion. This drug is used as an adjunctive therapy for peptic ulcers, to control diarrhea, as a bladder relaxant, and in the treatment of vertigo.

HIGH-RISK GROUPS: Anyone who takes this drug

NUTRITIONAL INTERACTIONS

ALKALINE URINE: The action of propantheline is prolonged by alkaline urine. If the quantity of alkaline foods in your diet is high, your urine will lose its acidity, and the excretion of this drug will be slowed. A hazardous buildup could conceivably result.

The symptoms of such a buildup or overdose are blurred vision, urinary retention, rapid heart rate, palpitations, the temporary loss of your sense of taste, headache, nervousness, mental confusion, drowsiness, weakness, dizziness, insomnia, nausea, constipation, a bloated feeling, impotence, and allergic reactions.

Prevention and Treatment: Fruits, vegetables, and dairy products tend to be alkaline, and high-protein foods tend to be acidic. Foods causing the production of alkaline urine include milk, buttermilk, cream, almonds, chestnuts, coconuts, all vegetables except corn and lentils, and all fruits except cranberries, prunes, and plums.

Antacids that neutralize the acid in the stomach will also neutralize the acid in the urine, causing it to turn alkaline. Therefore, you should avoid antacids when taking this drug.

OTHER ADVICE: Significant doses of propantheline increase the absorption of digoxin, so be sure your doctor is aware that you are taking both drugs.

This drug can also cause a dry mouth sensation, so drink at least 6 to 8 glasses of fluid per day.

Propantheline should be taken one-half hour before meals, since it is best absorbed, and therefore most effective, on an empty stomach.

PROPOXYPHENE HYDROCHLORIDE AND PROPOXYPHENE NAPSYLATE

DRUG FAMILY: Analgesic

BRAND NAMES: Darvon; Darvon Compound; Darvon Compound-65; Darvon with A.S.A.; Propox 65 w/APAP; Propoxyphene & Apap 65/650; Propoxyphene Compound 65; SK-65 APAP; SK-65; Wygesic; Darvocet-N 50; Darvocet-N 100; Darvon-N; Darvon-N with A.S.A.

HOW TO TAKE PROPOXYPHENE: With meals or milk

FOODS TO AVOID: Alcoholic beverages

POSSIBLE SIDE EFFECTS: Nausea, diarrhea, vomiting, and stomachache

ACTION OF PROPOXYPHENE: These analgesics are prescribed for the relief of mild to moderate pain.

HIGH-RISK GROUPS: People with a history of abdominal distress, anyone who consumes alcohol

NUTRITIONAL INTERACTIONS

GENERAL ADVICE: The chronic and extensive use of these drugs could conceivably result in the development of unwanted side effects, including such gastrointestinal disorders as nausea, diarrhea, vomiting, and stomachache. This can be limited by taking the drugs with meals or milk.

ALCOHOL INTERACTION: Alcohol increases the depressant effects of these drugs on the central nervous system, making the user very drowsy. If large quantities of alcohol are consumed, coma and even death may result. In consequence, alcohol should not be taken at the same time as these drugs.

PROPRANOLOL HYDROCHLORIDE

DRUG FAMILY: Anti-hypertensive

BRAND NAMES: Inderal; Inderal LA; Inderide

HOW TO TAKE PROPRANOLOL HYDROCHLORIDE: With milk or food

FOODS TO AVOID: Alcoholic beverages

POSSIBLE SIDE EFFECTS: Nausea, vomiting, mild diarrhea, and constipation

ACTION OF PROPRANOLOL HYDROCHLORIDE: This drug is used in the management of hypertension, angina pectoris, and irregular heart rate, and in the prevention of common migraine headache

HIGH-RISK GROUPS: Anyone who takes this drug

NUTRITIONAL INTERACTIONS

GASTROINTESTINAL DISTRESS: When first placed on propranolol, you are likely to suffer from such gastrointestinal disturbances as nausea, vomiting, mild diarrhea, and constipation. These unpleasant side effects usually subside after a few days of the therapy.

OTHER ADVICE: Alcohol may increase the blood-pressure-lowering effect of the drug and exaggerate its mild sedative action.

PSEUDOEPHEDRINE SULFATE

DRUG FAMILY: Decongestant

BRAND NAMES: Trinalin; Drixoral

HOW TO TAKE PSEUDOEPHEDRINE SULFATE: With meals

FOODS TO AVOID: Alcoholic beverages

POSSIBLE SIDE EFFECTS: Gastrointestinal distress and a poor appetite

ACTION OF PSEUDOEPHEDRINE SULFATE: This decongestant is used to treat allergies.

HIGH-RISK GROUPS: People with a history of abdominal distress, anyone who consumes alcohol

NUTRITIONAL INTERACTIONS

GASTROINTESTINAL DISTRESS: You may find that when you take pseudoephedrine sulfate, you experience gastrointestinal distress or anorexia.

Prevention and Treatment: Take this drug with meals, to avoid gastrointestinal discomfort. You should also monitor your body weight carefully to avoid unwanted weight loss due to decreased appetite.

ALCOHOL INTERACTION: Alcohol tends to intensify the effects of this central nervous system depressant, making the user drowsy, and impairing his ability to concentrate and

his coordination. This makes efficient working difficult and driving dangerous. Consequently, people taking this drug should not drink concurrently.

PYRIMETHAMINE

DRUG FAMILY: Anti-malarial

BRAND NAMES: Daraprim; Fansidar

HOW TO TAKE PYRIMETHAMINE: With meals

FOODS TO AVOID: None

POSSIBLE SIDE EFFECTS: Folic acid deficiency; nausea, stomachache

ACTION OF PYRIMETHAMINE: Used as a preventive measure to protect a patient from contracting malaria, abnormally high numbers of red cells in the blood (polycythemia vera), and meningeal leukemia

HIGH-RISK GROUPS: Users of oral contraceptives, heavy drinkers, pregnant women, children, the elderly, teenagers

NUTRITIONAL INTERACTIONS

FOLIC ACID DEFICIENCY: Pyrimethamine is a potent folacin antagonist, since it prevents folacin from being converted to its active form. If the drug is taken over an extended period or in doses in excess of 25 mg daily, then a deficiency of the vitamin is likely.

Most often, the first sign of a folic acid or folacin deficiency is inflamed and bleeding gums. Other symptoms that follow may be a sore, smooth tongue; diarrhea; forgetfulness; apathy; irritability; anemia; and a reduced resistance to infection. Despite the fact that folacin is found in a variety of foods, folacin deficiency is still the most common vitamin deficiency in the United States.

Studies show that in adults, deficiencies are limited almost exclusively to the elderly and women, 30 percent of whom have intakes below the recommended daily allowance, and 5 to 7 percent of whom also have severe anemia. There are several factors that account for this bias, but one of the most obvious reasons is that oral contraceptive use decreases the absorption of folic acid. Constant dieting also limits folacin intake, and alcohol interferes with the body's use of folic acid, as well. Folacin is not stored by the body in any appreciable amounts, so an adequate supply must be consumed on a daily basis.

This nutrient is essential for the synthesis of new cells; thus, a folic acid deficiency can cause birth defects if pyrimethamine is taken by pregnant women. As a result, this drug should only be used by them if they take folacin supplements at the same time. Pyrimethamine will also impair growth in children if used over an extended period. Folic acid is also crucial to the normal metabolism of proteins.

Prevention and Treatment: To counteract a deficiency in folic acid, your diet should contain liver, yeast, and such leafy vegetables as spinach, kale, parsley, cauliflower, brussels sprouts, and broccoli. The fruits that are highest in folic acid are oranges and cantaloupes. To a lesser degree, folacin is found in almonds and lima beans, corn, parsnips, green peas, pumpkins, sweet potatoes, bran, peanuts, rye, and whole grain wheat. (See table of Folacin-Rich Foods, page 297.) Approximately one half of the folic acid you consume is absorbed by your body.

Normal cooking temperatures (110 to 120 degrees for 10 minutes) destroy up to 65 percent of the folacin in your food. Your daily diet, therefore, should include some raw vegetables and fruits. Cooking utensils made out of copper speed up folacin's destruction.

The recommended daily consumption of folacin is 400 mcg. Lactating women should assume a daily need of 1,200 mcg. Pregnant women and oral contraceptive users should consume 800 mcg daily.

If you are taking doses of pyrimethamine greater than 25 mg per day, you should also take a supplement of 800 mcg of folic acid per day. This means that a person needs 1,200 mcg per day, and a pregnant woman requires about 1,600 mcg daily.

OTHER ADVICE: This drug causes nausea and stomach pain, which may be avoided by taking it with meals.

QUINACRINE

DRUG FAMILY: Anti-protozoal infection compound

BRAND NAMES: Atabrine Hydrochloride; Quinacrine Hydrochloride

HOW TO TAKE QUINACRINE: After meals

FOODS TO AVOID: Large amounts of alkaline foods such as milk, buttermilk, cream, almonds, chestnuts, coconuts, all vegetables except corn and lentils, and all fruits except cranberries, prunes, and plums; any alcoholic beverages or foods containing alcohol

POSSIBLE SIDE EFFECTS: Nausea, vomiting, and diarrhea

ACTION OF QUINACRINE: This drug is prescribed for giardiasis, a parasitic infection of the small intestine.

HIGH-RISK GROUPS: Anyone who takes this drug

NUTRITIONAL INTERACTIONS

ALKALINE URINE: Because quinacrine is alkaline, it is excreted at a normal rate only if your urine is acidic. However, if the quantity of alkaline foods in your diet is high, your urine will lose its acidity, the excretion of this drug will be slowed, and a hazardous buildup of the drug will likely result.

The symptoms of such a buildup, or overdose, are dizziness, headache, yellow staining of the skin, vomiting, dermatitis, blood abnormalities, blue or black pigmentation of the nails, problems with vision, and even psychosis.

Prevention and Treatment: Fruits, vegetables, and dairy products tend to be alkaline, and high-protein foods tend to be acidic. Foods causing the production of alkaline urine include milk, buttermilk, cream, almonds, chestnuts, coconuts, all vegetables except corn and lentils, and all fruits except cranberries, prunes, and plums.

Antacids that neutralize the acid in the stomach will also neutralize the acid in the urine, causing it to turn alkaline. Therefore, you should avoid antacids when taking this drug.

ALCOHOL INTERACTION: Quinacrine prevents the complete breakdown of alcohol, which is likely to lead to a buildup of acetaldehyde (a breakdown product of alcohol), causing such uncomfortable symptoms as headache, flushing, breathing difficulties, gastrointestinal disturbances, and confusion.

Prevention and Treatment: Do not drink alcohol while taking this medication. Even the small amounts found in desserts and sauces can be sufficient to bring on the symptoms.

GASTROINTESTINAL DISTURBANCES: This drug irritates the gastrointestinal tract and can cause nausea, vomiting, and diarrhea.

Prevention and Treatment: In order to reduce the risk of these unpleasant side effects, quinacrine should always be taken after meals.

QUINIDINE GLUCONATE

DRUG FAMILY: Heart drug

BRAND NAMES: Duraquin; Quinaglute

HOW TO TAKE QUINIDINE GLUCONATE: With meals

FOODS TO AVOID: Large amounts of alkaline foods such as milk, buttermilk, cream, almonds, chestnuts, coconut, all vegetables except corn and lentils, and all fruits except cranberries, prunes, and plums

POSSIBLE SIDE EFFECTS: Diarrhea, nausea, vomiting, stomachache

ACTION OF QUINIDINE SULFATE: This drug is used to control irregular heartbeats.

HIGH-RISK GROUPS: The elderly

NUTRITIONAL INTERACTIONS

GASTROINTESTINAL DISTRESS AND OTHER SIDE EFFECTS: One out of three people who take quinidine gluconate experiences side effects, especially at the beginning of the therapy. The main problem is that of gastrointestinal disturbances such as diarrhea, nausea, vomiting, and abdominal pain.

Prevention and Treatment: Quinidine should always be taken with meals.

ALKALINE URINE: The concurrent consumption of antacids and/or the consumption of foods causing alkaline urine will slow down the rate at which this drug will be excreted. A toxic buildup of quinidine in your system could conceivably result. One symptom of such a buildup or overdose is low blood pressure, causing faintness or light-headedness upon standing up, or in some instances fainting spells. Irregular heartbeat, the very condition the drug is taken to correct, can also occur. A ringing in the ears, loss of hearing, and slightly distorted vision may occur as well, and the gastrointestinal disturbances may also be exacerbated.

Under normal circumstances, the elderly excrete quinidine less readily than younger users, so the problem is especially likely in older users.

Prevention and Treatment: Foods causing the production of alkaline urine, such as milk, buttermilk, cream, almonds, chestnuts, coconuts, all vegetables except corn and lentils, and all fruits except cranberries, prunes, and plums, should be severely limited.

Antacids should not be used while you are on quinidine gluconate. If they are taken with it, they will delay its absorption. Taken at other times, they will reduce the rate at which quinidine is excreted, permitting toxic levels to build up.

QUININE SULFATE

DRUG FAMILY: Antibiotic

BRAND NAMES: Quinamm; Quindan; Quinine; Quiphile

HOW TO TAKE QUININE SULFATE: After meals

FOODS TO AVOID: Large amounts of alkaline foods such as milk, buttermilk, cream, almonds, chestnuts, coconuts, all vegetables except corn and lentils, and all fruit except cranberries, plums, and prunes; any food or beverage that contains alcohol

POSSIBLE SIDE EFFECTS: Stomachache, nausea, vomiting, and diarrhea

ACTION OF QUININE SULFATE: This drug is used in treating malaria and nocturnal leg cramps.

HIGH-RISK GROUPS: Anyone who takes this drug

NUTRITIONAL INTERACTIONS

ALKALINE URINE: Because quinine sulfate is alkaline, it is excreted at a normal rate only if your urine is acidic. However, if the quantity of alkaline foods in your diet is high, your urine will lose its acidity, the excretion of this drug will be slowed, and a hazardous buildup will likely result. The symptoms of such a buildup or overdose are a ringing in the ears, headache, nausea, and distorted vision.

Prevention and Treatment: Fruits, vegetables, and dairy products tend to be alkaline, and high-protein foods tend to be acidic. Foods causing the production of alkaline urine include milk, buttermilk, cream, almonds, chestnuts, coconuts, all vegetables except corn and lentils, and all fruits except cranberries, prunes, and plums.

Antacids that neutralize the acid in the stomach will also neutralize the acid in the urine, causing it to turn alkaline. Therefore, you should avoid antacids when taking this drug.

ALCOHOL INTERACTION: Quinine sulfate prevents the complete breakdown of alcohol, which is likely to lead to a buildup of acetaldehyde (a breakdown product of alcohol) and cause such uncomfortable symptoms as headache, flushing, breathing difficulties, gastrointestinal disturbances, and confusion.

Prevention and Treatment: You should not drink alcohol while taking this medication. Even the small amounts found in desserts and sauces can be sufficient to bring on the symptoms.

GASTROINTESTINAL DISTURBANCES: Quinine sulfate irritates the gastrointestinal tract and causes stomachache, nausea, vomiting, and diarrhea.

Prevention and Treatment: In order to reduce the likelihood of these discomforts, quinine sulfate should be taken after meals.

RESERPINE

DRUG FAMILY: Vasodilator

BRAND NAMES: Chloroserpine; Chlorothiazide w/Reserpine; Demi-Regroton; Diupres; Diutensen-R; H-H-R; Hydrochlorothiazide, Hydralazine Hydrochloride, Reserpine; Hydrochlorothiazide/Reserpine; Hydrochlorothiazide w/Reserpine; Hydro-Fluserpine; Hydromox R; Hydropres; Hydroserpine; Metatensin; Naquival; Regroton; Renese-R; SK-Reserpine; Salutensin/Salutensin-Demi; Ser-Ap-Es; Serpasil; Serpasil-Apresoline; Serpasil-Esidrix; Unipres

HOW TO TAKE RESERPINE: With milk or meals

FOODS TO AVOID: Large amounts of tyramine- or dopamine-containing foods like aged cheese, raisins, avocados, liver, bananas, eggplant, sour cream, alcoholic beverages, salami, meat tenderizers, chocolate, yeast, and soy sauce; licorice candy made from natural extract; foods rich in sodium like pickled foods, and salty foods such as cold cuts, snack chips, and processed cheeses. Alcohol should be avoided altogether.

POSSIBLE SIDE EFFECTS: Gastrointestinal distress

ACTION OF RESERPINE: This drug is used in the treatment of high blood pressure.

HIGH-RISK GROUPS: Anyone who takes this drug

NUTRITIONAL INTERACTIONS

GASTROINTESTINAL DISTRESS: Reserpine is likely to cause upset stomach and should not be used by patients with peptic ulcers or intestinal colitis.

Prevention and Treatment: This drug should always be taken with milk or meals.

TYRAMINE-RICH FOODS: Consumption of foods containing tyramine, a food substance, tends to increase blood pressure and decrease the effectiveness of the drug.

Prevention and Treatment: Tyramine-containing foods must be restricted while you are being treated with this drug. Tyramine is common in many foods, but it is found in the greatest amounts in high-protein foods that have undergone some decomposition, like aged cheese. Tyramine is also found in chicken and beef livers, bananas, eggplant, sour cream, alcoholic beverages, salami, meat tenderizers, chocolate, yeast, and soy sauce. (See table of Tyramine-Rich Foods, page 307.) Raisins and avocados should also be avoided, because they contain dopamine, which has the same effect as tyramine.

POTENCY: The effectiveness of the drug may be decreased by other food substances that tend to cause increased blood pressure, such as licorice candy and foods containing a lot of salt.

Prevention and Treatment: An ounce or more of licorice candy per day (licorice, that is, that contains natural licorice extract) can cause sodium and water retention, and as a result high blood pressure. Hence, licorice should be avoided when you are on this drug.

Sodium causes water retention in some people, particularly in combination with a low potassium intake. Water retention increases the volume of fluid in the arteries, which is responsible for the elevated blood pressure. To limit the problem of water retention, your diet should contain natural diuretics, foods rich in potassium, such as citrus fruits, bananas, almonds, dates, dairy products, apricots, and bamboo shoots. (See table of Potassium-Rich Foods, page 302.) As many as 15 percent of all Americans have a genetic susceptibility to the effects of excess sodium. We only need about 220 mg of sodium each day, but the average American consumes 6 to 8 grams, or 3 to 4 teaspoons, of salt per day.

No salt should be added at the table, but up to 1 teaspoon per day can be added during cooking. Pickled foods, such as sauerkraut, and extremely salty foods, such as luncheon meats, snack chips, and processed cheeses, should be eliminated altogether.

To sharpen your awareness of the sodium content of food products, read the list of ingredients that appears on the label of all packaged foods. Sodium can be present in a food as either common salt (sodium chloride) or as any other sodium-containing compound, monosodium glutamate being a common one. If sodium appears as one of the first ingredients on the label, the food contains a significant amount of it. If, on the other hand, it appears very near the end of the list (as in bread), then it need not be a concern. Recent evidence points to a protective value for calcium against the harmful effects of sodium, so eat plenty of calcium-containing foods such as dairy products.

You should limit your intake of sodium to 2 to 3 grams per day, watch your weight, and exercise.

ALCOHOL INTERACTION: Alcohol should not be taken by patients using reserpine. Alcohol has a potent vasodilation effect, which enhances the effects of the drug. A glass (6 ounces) of sherry or 10 ounces of table wine will significantly dilate the blood vessels for 4 hours and tend to lower blood pressure.

RIFAMPIN

DRUG FAMILY: Antibiotic; anti-tubercular

BRAND NAMES: Rifadin; Rifamate; Rimactane

HOW TO TAKE RIFAMPIN: Ideally, on an empty stomach 1 hour before or 2 hours after a meal. If stomach problems result, however, the drug may be taken with food.

FOODS TO AVOID: Alcoholic beverages

POSSIBLE SIDE EFFECTS: Gastrointestinal problems; liver damage; reduced effectiveness of oral contraceptives

ACTION OF RIFAMPIN: This antibiotic is used in conjunction with isoniazid in the treatment of tuberculosis. It is also used to protect at-risk populations against meningococcal disease.

HIGH-RISK GROUPS: The elderly, heavy drinkers, users of oral contraceptives

NUTRITIONAL INTERACTIONS

GASTROINTESTINAL DISTRESS: Rifampin is best absorbed on an empty stomach, although it often causes gastrointestinal problems.

Prevention and Treatment: The drug should ideally be taken on an empty stomach, 1 hour before and more than 2 hours after a meal. However, if stomach problems result, it may be taken with meals. The normal 600 mg daily dose still maintains levels high enough to destroy the tuberculosis mycobacterium.

OTHER ADVICE: Women taking oral contraceptives should be aware that this drug decreases the effectiveness of the contraceptive by speeding up its degradation in the body. If breakthrough bleeding should occur, you should check with your physician to ensure that your contraceptive contains adequate estrogen to cancel out the effects of the rifampin.

Rifampin has also been known to cause liver damage, particularly in the elderly and in alcoholics. Consequently, you should alert your physician to your alcohol consumption, and he in turn should monitor your condition carefully.

SCOPOLAMINE HYDROBROMIDE

DRUG FAMILY: Gastrointestinal

BRAND NAMES: Donnatal; Ru-Tuss

HOW TO TAKE SCOPOLAMINE HYDROBROMIDE: One to 2 hours before or after meals

FOODS TO AVOID: None

POSSIBLE SIDE EFFECTS: Constipation, dry mouth

ACTION OF SCOPOLAMINE HYDROBROMIDE: This drug is used in the treatment of duodenal ulcer, irritable bowel syndrome, and colitis. It decreases the rate of contraction of the muscles in the intestine and so prevents spasms. It also decreases salivary secretion and the secretion of digestive enzymes and acid in the stomach.

Scopolamine hydrobromide is a mild sedative as well.

HIGH-RISK GROUPS: The elderly

NUTRITIONAL INTERACTIONS

CONSTIPATION: By decreasing the secretion of acid and digestive enzymes in the stomach, the drug impairs the digestive process, especially in the elderly, who tend to have reduced acid secretion to begin with. Its anti-spasmodic actions reduce the rate of muscular contraction in the intestines and decrease the rate at which food passes down the intestine. As a result, use of the drug can lead to constipation. It also decreases salivation, causing a dry mouth, which makes swallowing difficult.

Prevention and Treatment: This drug should be taken 1 to 2 hours before or after meals. Plenty of fluids should be taken to combat the dry mouth.

Constipation is usually safely remedied by an increase in the bulk in the diet. This means consuming larger servings of any of the following: dried or fresh fruits (such as unpeeled apples or pears), salad vegetables, radishes, oatmeal, and whole grain foods (brown rice, whole wheat breads, and cereals). It is not necessary to purchase products that claim "extra fiber" has been added to them.

Persistent constipation may also be relieved by doubling the amount of fluid consumed each day. Bran, if used, should be added to the diet gradually, and fluid should be increased by at least ¾ cup per teaspoon of bran. (See table of Dietary Fiber-Rich Foods, page 293.)

SODIUM-BASED SALINE CATHARTICS

DRUG FAMILY: Laxative

BRAND NAMES: [GENERIC/Brand] SODIUM PHOSPHATE/Fleet Enema; Fleet Phospho-Soda; Fleet Prep Kits; SODIUM SULFATE/ GoLYTELY

HOW TO TAKE SALINE CATHARTICS: Ideally at bedtime, but they can be taken at other times provided it is not within 2 hours of a meal

FOODS TO AVOID: None

POSSIBLE SIDE EFFECTS: Hypertension in patients with kidney or heart disease; decreased absorption of potassium, protein, sugar, fat, and vitamin D

ACTION OF SODIUM-BASED SALINE CATHARTICS: These drugs act as laxatives by increasing the activity of the muscles lining the intestines, and so reducing the time required for food to pass through the intestinal tract. Saline cathartics, including sodium salts, act partly by drawing water into the colon to increase the bulk of the stools.

They also act by releasing cholecystokinin, a hormone, into the small intestine, which is responsible for causing bile to be secreted into the intestine. Because bile contains sodium, this further increases the amount of water in the colon and adds bulk to the stool. It also accelerates the rate at which the muscles in the intestine contract and shortens the time needed to push stools downward.

HIGH-RISK GROUPS: The elderly, hypertensives, heart patients

NUTRITIONAL INTERACTIONS

CARDIAC AND KIDNEY COMPLICATIONS:
Sodium-based saline cathartics should not
be used by people with heart disease, since
the sodium in these drugs is likely to cause
the blood to increase in volume, thereby
forcing the kidneys to excrete the excess of
both the sodium and the water. Should the
kidneys fail to excrete all of this sodium and
water, as is common in the elderly, the heart
must work harder to pump the extra fluid
around the body, which leads to higher blood
pressure, and possibly kidney or heart failure.

Prevention and Treatment: Most people
are unaware of how much sodium their diet
contains. The average American consumes
15 pounds of salt (sodium chloride) annually,
or 3 to 4 teaspoons per day. Each teaspoon
contains 2 grams of sodium. One third of
our salt intake is found naturally in the foods
we eat, one third is added in processing,
and one third is added at the table.

If sodium-containing compounds are used
frequently, a low-salt diet should be followed. This means that no salt should be
added to your food at the table, but up to
1 teaspoon can be added per day during
cooking. Obviously salty foods such as anchovies, snack chips, green olives, dill pickles, sauerkraut, sardines, canned soups and
vegetables, TV dinners, processed cheeses,
cold cuts, soy sauce, and catsup should be
avoided. (See table of Sodium-Rich Foods,
page 306.)

NUTRITIONAL DEFICIENCIES: All the saline cathartics cause decreases in the absorption of
potassium, protein, glucose, fat, vitamin D,
and calcium, no matter when they are taken,

though the effect is usually only a modest
one. But this could be intensified if they are
administered with or shortly after food.

Prevention and Treatment: None of the
saline cathartics should be taken with meals
or within 2 hours of a meal.

SODIUM BICARBONATE

DRUG FAMILY: Antacids

BRAND NAMES: Alka-Seltzer; Citrocarbonate
Antacid

HOW TO TAKE SODIUM BICARBONATE: Between
meals and at bedtime

FOODS TO AVOID: Large amounts of acid-
containing foods such as soft drinks, fruit
juices, and wine; caffeine-containing foods
such as coffee, tea, cola, and chocolate; milk
and milk products

POSSIBLE SIDE EFFECTS: Hypertension; poor
appetite, nausea, vomiting; headaches; feelings of weakness; impaired vision, poor absorption of most nutrients; kidney damage

ACTION OF SODIUM BICARBONATE: Used to reduce the acidity of the stomach.

HIGH-RISK GROUPS: Hypertensives, the elderly, young women

NUTRITIONAL INTERACTIONS

HYPERTENSION: Because of the considerable
amount of sodium contained in sodium bicarbonate (1,042 mg per dose), continuous
use is likely, in susceptible individuals, to
contribute to hypertension—a disease that
may present no noticeable symptoms for
years but which, if left untreated, can in-

crease the risk of heart disease and kidney failure. Your susceptibility to high blood pressure can be linked to identifiable factors such as family history, stress, alcoholism, obesity, and diet.

Hypertension, or high blood pressure, is a disorder that affects 60 million Americans. Roughly 75 percent of all Americans have hypertension at sixty-five. It increases the work load of the heart and makes the kidneys work harder to regulate elevated blood pressure. One result of untreated high blood pressure can be a two- to threefold increase in the risk of cardiovascular problems, and a sevenfold increase in the likelihood of having a stroke.

Sodium causes water retention in some people, particularly in combination with a low potassium intake. Water retention increases the volume of fluid in the arteries, which is responsible for the elevated blood pressure. Hence, patients with hypertension should not use this drug.

People who do not have clinically diagnosable hypertension but who tend to retain water, such as many pregnant women and some women during their menstrual cycle, also should not use this medication.

Prevention and Treatment: To avoid the problems of water retention through the use of sodium bicarbonate, your diet should contain natural diuretics, foods rich in potassium, such as citrus fruits, bananas, almonds, dates, dairy products, apricots, and bamboo shoots. (See table of Potassium-Rich Foods, page 302.) As many as 15 percent of all Americans have a genetic susceptibility to the effects of excess sodium; therefore, it is advised that everyone be watchful of his salt intake, particularly those who have al-

ready been diagnosed as hypertensive. We only need about 220 mg of sodium each day, but the average American consumes 6 to 8 grams, or 3 to 4 teaspoons, of salt per day.

Do not add salt at the table, but up to 1 teaspoon per day can be added during cooking. Pickled foods, such as sauerkraut, and extremely salty foods, such as luncheon meats, snack chips, and processed cheeses, should be eliminated altogether.

You should be conscious of the sodium content of food products you eat. You might try reading the ingredients list that appears on the label of all packaged foods. Sodium can be present in a food as either common salt or sodium chloride, or as any other sodium-containing compound, monosodium glutamate being a common one. If sodium appears as one of the first ingredients on the lable, the food contains a significant amount of it. If, on the other hand, it appears very near the end of the list (as in bread), then it need not be a concern.

You should limit your intake of sodium to 1 to 3 grams per day, watch your weight, and exercise.

OTHER ADVICE: Sodium bicarbonate is extremely potent, and for the occasional user it is a good product. However, prolonged use, in addition to concerns over hypertension, can conceivably result in the same problems as occur from an overdose of calcium antacids, namely, anorexia, nausea, vomiting, headaches, weakness, and impaired vision. This is especially likely if excessive sodium bicarbonate is taken by somebody who consumes a lot of milk or dairy products. The array of symptoms is sometimes called milk-alkali syndrome.

Malnutrition can result from excessive self-medication with antacids, as a result of malabsorption of nutrients. It should be emphasized that nutrient depletion from antacid use is gradual, and evidence of malnutrition does not make its appearance until nutrient stores are exhausted. If you are a regular user of sodium bicarbonate, you should take a one-a-day vitamin supplement to safeguard against nutrient deficiencies.

People taking antacids therapeutically should avoid large amounts of acid-containing foods, such as fruit juices and foods containing caffeine, which irritate the stomach wall.

SODIUM MECLOFENAMATE

DRUG FAMILY: Anti-inflammatory

BRAND NAME: Meclomen

HOW TO TAKE SODIUM MECLOFENAMATE: With milk or meals

FOODS TO AVOID: None

POSSIBLE SIDE EFFECTS: Diarrhea, nausea, vomiting, stomachache, poor digestion; aspirin reduces the drug's effectiveness.

ACTION OF SODIUM MECLOFENAMATE: A nonsteroidal anti-inflammatory drug, sodium meclofenamate is used to treat the signs and symptoms of acute and chronic rheumatoid arthritis, and osteoarthritis.

HIGH-RISK GROUPS: Anyone who takes this drug.

NUTRITIONAL INTERACTIONS

GASTROINTESTINAL DISTRESS: According to studies, 10 to 33 percent of all people taking sodium meclofenamate experience diarrhea, 11 percent suffer from nausea with or without vomiting, and 10 percent suffer from abdominal pain, poor digestion, and other abdominal discomfort.

Prevention and Treatment: To reduce the chances of experiencing these problems, this drug should always be taken with milk or at mealtimes.

OTHER ADVICE: Since aspirin decreases the effectiveness of meclofenamate compounds, the two medications should not be taken concurrently.

SODIUM NAFCILLIN

DRUG FAMILY: Antibiotic

BRAND NAMES: Nafcil; Unipen

HOW TO TAKE SODIUM NAFCILLIN: On an empty stomach between meals, and not within 1 hour before or 2 hours after meals

FOODS TO AVOID: The drug should not be taken with acid-containing beverages such as fruit juice, soft drinks, and wine

POSSIBLE SIDE EFFECTS: Nausea, vomiting, and diarrhea

ACTION OF SODIUM NAFCILLIN: This antibiotic is used to treat pencillin-resistant strains of *Staphylococcus aureus*.

HIGH-RISK GROUPS: Anyone who takes this drug

NUTRITIONAL INTERACTIONS

GENERAL ADVICE: This drug is best absorbed on an empty stomach, when there is not a lot of acid in the stomach. Consequently, it should not be taken within 1 hour before or within 2 hours after a meal, and never with acid-containing beverages like fruit juices, soft drinks, and wine.

As with all penicillins, this drug sometimes causes nausea, vomiting, and diarrhea.

SODIUM POLYSTYRENE SULFONATE

DRUG FAMILY: Detoxification

BRAND NAME: Kayexalate

HOW TO TAKE SODIUM POLYSTYRENE SULFONATE: As a suspension in a little water or syrup

FOODS TO AVOID: None

POSSIBLE SIDE EFFECTS: Potassium deficiency; constipation, nausea, vomiting, and diarrhea; aluminum hydroxide antacids taken at the same time may make the constipation much worse.

ACTION OF SODIUM POLYSTYRENE SULFONATE: This drug is a resin that exchanges sodium for potassium. Potassium chloride is often administered to replace body potassium lost due to the use of diuretics, but an overdose of potassium can be life-threatening. This resin is used in cases of potassium toxicity.

HIGH-RISK GROUPS: Hypertensives, heart patients, the elderly

NUTRITIONAL INTERACTIONS

POTASSIUM DEFICIENCY: A potassium deficiency is likely to result from the use of this drug. Clearly, the balance of potassium in the body is an important consideration, and symptoms of both a deficiency and a toxic buildup should be watched for carefully.

Potassium is the mineral that regulates the amount of water in the cells of the body and is essential for the proper functioning of the kidneys and the heart muscle, and the secretion of stomach juices. The most alarming symptom of a potassium deficiency is an irregular heartbeat, which can lead to heart failure. Potassium toxicity usually does not show any symptoms before it causes cardiac arrest. However, other symptoms of this condition include weakness in the arms and legs, paralysis, listlessness, mental confusion, low blood pressure, and difficulty in swallowing.

Low blood serum levels of potassium, called hypokalemia, are associated with laxative abuse, because many laxatives promote an increased loss of potassium in the gastrointestinal tract. This risk is especially high in elderly patients, who consume diets low in potassium.

People who take the laxatives phenolphthalein, bisacodyl, and senna on a daily basis have been reported to have a much greater chance of experiencing serious hypokalemia. These people, and others with a potassium deficiency, may have such symptoms as weakness, a loss of appetite, nausea, vomiting, listlessness, apprehension, and diffuse pain that comes and goes.

Proper potassium levels in your body can also be threatened if this drug is taken concurrently with cortisone-containing drugs.

Prevention and Treatment: Potassium depletion can be avoided by including such potassium-rich foods in your diet as tomato juice, lentils, dried apricots, asparagus, bananas, peanut butter, chicken, almonds, and milk. (See table of Potassium-Rich Foods, page 302.)

Diuretics, commonly prescribed for people with heart disease, decrease the level of body potassium. Therefore, the risk of a deficiency is significantly increased if diuretics are taken concurrently with sodium polystyrene sulfonate.

OTHER ADVICE: Use of this drug may cause gastrointestinal disturbances, particularly if high doses are given.

This drug should not be taken with aluminum hydroxide antacids, since intestinal blockage may result. Severe constipation can occur, especially in the elderly. If constipation does result, 10 to 20 ml of 70 percent syrup of sorbitol should be taken every 2 hours or as needed to produce one or two watery stools daily.

SPIRONOLACTONE

DRUG FAMILY: Diuretic

BRAND NAMES: Aldactazide; Aldactone; Spironazide; Spironolactone w/Hydrochlorothiazide

HOW TO TAKE SPIRONOLACTONE: With food or milk

FOODS TO AVOID: Foods rich in potassium should not be eaten to excess; they include tomato juice, lentils, dried apricots, asparagus, bananas, peanut butter, chicken, almonds, and milk.

POSSIBLE SIDE EFFECTS: Potassium toxicity; calcium deficiency; sodium depletion; decreased effectiveness of oral contraceptives; minor gastrointestinal disturbances

ACTION OF SPIRONOLACTONE: This drug increases the excretion of sodium and water by the kidneys.

HIGH-RISK GROUPS: Kidney patients, low-salt dieters, smokers, the elderly, vegetarians, teenagers

NUTRITIONAL INTERACTIONS

POTASSIUM TOXICITY: Spironolactone reduces the normal excretion of potassium, so in some people, particularly those with diseased kidneys that cannot excrete potassium very effectively, potassium levels could conceivably build up in the body, leading to potassium toxicity (hyperkalemia).

Prevention and Treatment: While you are on spironolactone, you should not be taking potassium supplements, nor should a diet rich in potassium be consumed. Potassium-rich foods include tomato juice, lentils, dried apricots, asparagus, bananas, peanut butter, chicken, almonds, and milk. (See table of Potassium-Rich Foods, page 302.)

CALCIUM DEFICIENCY: Spironolactone could also conceivably lead to a calcium deficiency, since it causes increased excretion of this mineral from the body. Whenever calcium blood levels are low, the body will liberate the necessary amounts of calcium from the bones, where it is stored, thereby weakening them and making them more susceptible to fractures.

A condition called osteomalacia can result. This is more likely after middle age, since in older people the body uses dietary calcium less efficiency. Osteomalacia is a weakening of the bones as a consequence of uniform and steady calcium loss. This disease affects millions of older Americans, but also many younger people. In fact, one out of every four postmenopausal women suffers from this problem. Prominent symptoms are bone pain in the back, thighs, shoulder region or ribs; difficulty in walking; and weakness in the muscles of the legs. The condition is reversible once calcium blood levels are raised.

Prolonged calcium deficiencies may also lead to osteoporosis, another condition in which the bones are made weak and brittle. However, osteoporosis, an unexplained and rapid loss of calcium from the bones, is irreversible. Here the first symptoms are backache, a gradual loss of height, and periodontal disease. In cases of osteoporosis, fractures of the vertebrae, hip, and wrist occur frequently, sometimes spontaneously.

By age eighty, virtually all women experience some degree of osteoporosis; early menopause is a strong predictor of the disease. Approximately 7 percent of women fifty years of age and older have osteoporosis, and certain observers believe that the incidence of this disease is on the rise; between 15 and 20 million Americans are said to have osteoporosis today. In some 30 percent of people over sixty-five, the disease is severe enough to result in fractures. One out of five cases of the disease is found in men, but generally men get it at a later age and less severely than women.

If spironolactone is given to children, a condition known as rickets can occur. Again, the effect is on the bones, which become bent or malformed. Children under four years of age may develop pigeon breast, bowlegs, a protruding abdomen due to a weakness of the stomach muscles, and poorly formed teeth that tend to decay.

Prevention and Treatment: The Recommended Dietary Allowance of calcium is 800 mg, and all women should consume at least 1,200 mg of calcium per day. The average intake in the United States, however, is only 450 to 550 mg. For the elderly, and women who have already reached menopause or are about to, this should be increased to 1,500 mg by the consumption of foods rich in calcium, particularly milk and dairy products (including yogurt and hard cheeses) and, to a lesser extent, almonds. Three 8-ounce glasses of milk, for example, provide 1,500 mg of calcium. (See table of Calcium-Rich Foods, page 289.)

If calcium foods must be avoided because of an intolerance to lactose, the sugar found in dairy products (a problem for an estimated 30 million Americans), a 1,000 mg daily supplement of calcium should be taken. The best-absorbed supplement is calcium carbonate. (See Calcium Supplements entry, page 51.) If magnesium is included in the supplement, the calcium is slightly better absorbed and any tendency to constipation is reduced. The supplement should be taken in two 500 mg doses, one of which should be consumed before bedtime, because most of the calcium loss from your body occurs while you sleep.

Vitamin C assists calcium absorption, while cigarette smoking tends to deplete body calcium, as does excessive alcohol consumption. Foods that can decrease the absorption of calcium should be temporarily restricted, such as kale, rhubarb, spinach, cocoa and chocolate, beet greens, tea, and coffee. A deficiency might arise also if the ratio of phosphorus to calcium in your diet is very high; processed foods, especially most carbonated beverages, are particularly high in phosphorus. The ideal ratio is essentially 1 to 1, as in dairy products; when the ratio is 15 or 20 to 1, as in meat, very little calcium is absorbed. High-fiber foods may contribute to a calcium deficiency, since fiber binds to calcium and passes it out in the stool. Excess fat and protein in the diet also hinder absorption.

Since there is little calcium in strict vegetarian diets (those that avoid dairy products as well as meat), vegetarians are at greater risk of a calcium deficiency. People who take magnesium- or aluminum-based antacids are also more prone to calcium deficiencies, because both magnesium and aluminum in excess impair calcium absorption.

Besides a change in dietary habits and the use of calcium supplements, it is recommended that anyone at risk of this deficiency adopt an exercise regimen that causes the bones to support the weight of the body, to strengthen the bones and to counteract the loss of bone density. A regular walking or jogging program, for example, can help prevent the bone degeneration of the spine, hips, and legs. Note, however, that swimming, though good for the heart as an aerobic exercise, is not especially beneficial for bone buildup.

It has been observed that oral contraceptives seem to help calcium absorption, and that during pregnancy the body absorbs calcium more effectively, making the mother's bones actually stronger, despite the calcium needs of the fetus.

OTHER ADVICE: Spironolactone is often taken by women who suffer from edema, or bloating due to water retention. However, as the drug speeds up the degradation of sex hormones, leading to breast tenderness and menstrual irregularities in many people, it also could decrease the effectiveness of oral contraceptives.

Excess excretion of sodium occurs in people taking spironolactone, and this can led to a sodium depletion. The symptoms of such a depletion are anorexia, nausea, vomiting, and muscle weakness. Patients taking spironolactone should not be on a sodium-restricted diet.

Spironolactone causes cramping and diarrhea in a few people, and is best taken with food to reduce the risk of these side effects.

SULFASALAZINE

DRUG FAMILY: Antibiotic

BRAND NAME: Azulfidine

HOW TO TAKE SULFASALAZINE: With or directly after meals

FOODS TO AVOID: Alcoholic beverages should be limited

POSSIBLE SIDE EFFECTS: Folic acid deficiency, stomach cramps, increased intoxicating effect of alcohol

ACTION OF SULFASALAZINE: This drug is prescribed for treating ulcerative colitis and Crohn's disease.

HIGH-RISK GROUPS: Users of oral contraceptives, anyone who consumes alcohol, teenagers, the elderly, children

NUTRITIONAL INTERACTIONS

FOLIC ACID DEFICIENCY: Sulfasalazine decreases the absorption of folic acid, particularly in patients with inflammatory bowel disease. The result is likely to be a folic acid deficiency.

The first sign of a folic acid or folacin deficiency frequently is inflamed and bleeding gums. The symptoms that follow are a sore, smooth tongue; diarrhea; forgetfulness; apathy; irritability; anemia; and a reduced resistance to infection. Despite the fact that folacin is found in a variety of foods, folacin deficiency is still the most common vitamin deficiency in the United States.

In adults, deficiencies are limited almost exclusively to the elderly and women, 30 percent of whom have intakes below the recommended daily allowance, and 5 to 7 percent of whom also have severe anemia. There are several factors that account for this bias, but one of the most obvious reasons is that oral contraceptive use decreases the absorption of folic acid. Constant dieting also limits folacin intake. Alcohol interferes with the body's absorption and utilization of folic acid, as well. Folacin is not stored by the body in any appreciable amounts, so an adequate supply must be consumed on a daily basis.

Folic acid is crucial to the normal metabolism of proteins. Since folic acid is also important for normal cell growth, a deficiency of this vitamin during pregnancy can lead to birth defects.

Prevention and Treatment: To counteract a deficiency in folic acid, your diet should contain liver, yeast, and leafy vegetables such as spinach, kale, parsley, cauliflower, brussels sprouts, and broccoli. The fruits that are highest in folic acid are oranges and cantaloupes. To a lesser degree, folacin is found in almonds and lima beans, corn, parsnips, green peas, pumpkins, sweet potatoes, bran, peanuts, rye, and whole grain wheat. (See table of Folacin-Rich Foods, page 297.) Approximately one half of the folic acid you consume is absorbed by your body.

Normal cooking temperatures (110 to 120 degrees for 10 minutes) reduce the amount of useful folacin in your food by as much as 65 percent. Your daily diet, therefore, should include some raw vegetables and fruits. Cooking utensils made out of copper speed up folacin's destruction.

The recommended daily consumption of folacin is 400 mcg. Oral contraceptive users should consume 800 mcg daily.

STOMACH CRAMPS: This drug is a gastric irritant and can cause stomach cramps.

Prevention and Treatment: To avoid the discomfort of stomach cramps, you should always take this drug with or directly after meals.

OTHER ADVICE: Sulfasalazine increases the intoxicating effects of alcohol; thus, heavy drinking should be avoided.

SULFISOXAZOLE AND SULFAMETHOXAZOLE

DRUG FAMILY: Antibiotic

BRAND NAMES: [GENERIC/Brand] SULFISOX-AZOLE/Azo Gantrisin; Gantrisin; Pediazole; SK-Soxazole; SULFAMETHOXAZOLE/Azo Gantanol; Bactrim DS; Bactrim; Cotrim; Cotrim D.S.; Gantanol DS; Gantanol; Septra DS; Septra; Sulfamethoxazole & Trimethoprim; Sulfamethoxazole w/Trimethoprim DS; Sulfamethoxasole w/Trimethoprim SS; Sulfatrim & Sulfatrim D/S

HOW TO TAKE SULFISOXAZOLE AND SULFAMETHOXAZOLE: After meals

FOODS TO AVOID: Alcoholic beverages should be restricted

POSSIBLE SIDE EFFECTS: Deficiencies of magnesium, vitamins B_{12} and K, folic acid, and calcium; kidney damage; upset stomach, loss of appetite, nausea, vomiting, and diarrhea; increase in the intoxicating effects of alcohol

ACTION OF SULFISOXAZOLE AND SULFAMETHOXAZOLE: These drugs are prescribed as anti-bacterial agents for the treatment of ear infections in children, and for bronchitis and urinary tract infections in adults.

HIGH-RISK GROUPS: Vegetarians, oral contraceptive users, the elderly, children, anyone who consumes alcohol regularly, smokers, teenagers

NUTRITIONAL INTERACTIONS

MAGNESIUM DEFICIENCY: These drugs impair the absorption of magnesium. Heavy drinkers who excrete large amounts of magnesium could conceivably become magnesium deficient, even though magnesium deficiencies are not common since the average American diet contains appreciable amounts of the mineral.

Clinical signs of magnesium deficiency include muscle weakness, tremors, depression, emotional instability, and irrational behavior.

Prevention and Treatment: A diet containing the four food groups provides the normal amount of magnesium. However, if magnesium depletion is suspected, your diet should feature foods such as nuts (almonds and cashews are highest), meat, fish, milk, whole grains, and fresh greens, since cooking can wash away some magnesium. (See table of Magnesium-Rich Foods, page 300.)

VITAMIN B_{12} DEFICIENCY: Sulfisoxazole and sulfamethoxazole impair the absorption of vitamin B_{12}, though it is unlikely that this will cause deficiencies in most people.

However, strict vegetarians, who take no dairy products as well as animal food and who are normally in a marginal vitamin B_{12} status, could be at risk of a deficiency. Some elderly people also tend to absorb vitamin B_{12} inefficiently, as do heavy drinkers. Vitamin B_{12} is needed for the normal development of red blood cells and for the healthy functioning of all cells, in particular those of the bone marrow, nervous system, and intestines.

The most common result of a B_{12} deficiency is pernicious anemia, which is characterized by listlessness, fatigue (especially following such physical exertion as climbing a flight of stairs), numbness and tingling in the fingers and toes, palpitations, angina, light-headedness, and a pale complexion. A vitamin B_{12} deficiency can also lead to an irreversible breakdown in the brain membranes, causing a loss of coordination, confusion, memory loss, paranoia, apathy, tremors, and hallucinations. In extreme cases, degeneration of the spinal cord can also result.

Since vitamin B_{12} can be obtained only from animal food sources, strict vegetarians are at particular risk here. Oral contraceptive users too have a greater chance of experiencing this deficiency since they often have a poor vitamin B_{12} status to begin with, as do many smokers. Heavy consumers of alcohol, as well, frequently lack B_{12} because alcohol impairs the absorption of the vitamin. Patients with bacterial or parasitic infections of the intestine also have difficulty in absorbing this vitamin. In any case, anyone who is likely to have a vitamin B_{12} absorption problem should be alert for signs of pernicious anemia while taking sulfisoxazole or sulfamethoxazole.

Prevention and Treatment A balanced diet containing plenty of vitamin B_{12} sources is advised. Only animal products, including dairy foods and fish and shellfish, contain natural vitamin B_{12}; many soy products, for example, are enriched with vitamin B_{12} to safeguard vegetarians. (See table of Vitamin B_{12}-Rich Foods, page 312.)

Vitamin B_{12} is stored in the liver, so one meal that includes a B_{12}-rich source such as calf's liver will normally fulfill your body's need for this vitamin for 2 to 3 weeks. (One 3-ounce serving of calf's liver contains 100 mcg of vitamin B_{12}.) If none of these products figures prominently in your diet, you should take a 6 mcg supplement each day while on sulfisoxazole or sulfamethoxazole.

People who use major amounts of vitamin C should be aware that vitamin C supplements of more than 500 mg per day can damage B_{12} and contribute to a B_{12} deficiency. However, anyone who eats red meat two times a week has a three- to five-year supply of B_{12} in his liver.

The presence of baking soda in cooking will destroy vitamin B_{12} and should be avoided whenever possible. B_{12} also degrades at high temperatures, as when meat is placed on a hot griddle or, in the case of liver, when it is broiled for 5 minutes. The pasteurization of milk and the sterilization in boiling water of a bottle of milk also cause the loss of some B_{12}.

FOLIC ACID DEFICIENCY: Sulfisoxazole and sulfamethoxazole impair the use of folacin and can cause a folacin deficiency. Folic acid is essential for the synthesis of new cells and for the normal metabolism of proteins.

Often the first sign of a folic acid or folacin deficiency is inflamed and bleeding gums. The symptoms that follow are a sore, smooth tongue; diarrhea; forgetfulness; apathy; irritability; and anemia. Despite the fact that folacin is found in a variety of foods, this deficiency is still the most common vitamin deficiency in the United States.

A folic acid deficiency also results in fewer white blood cells than normal in the body, so there is a reduced resistance to infection. Folacin is required for the body to make new cells; hence, a deficiency during pregnancy can result in birth defects. This deficiency is also especially likely in women who take oral contraceptives.

Prevention and Treatment: To counteract a deficiency in folic acid, your diet should contain liver, yeast, and leafy vegetables such as spinach, kale, parsley, cauliflower, brussels sprouts, and broccoli. The fruits that are highest in folic acid are oranges and cantaloupes. To a lesser degree, folacin is found in almonds and lima beans, corn, parsnips, green peas, pumpkins, sweet potatoes, bran, peanuts, rye, and whole grain wheat. (See table of Folacin-Rich Foods, page 297.) Approximately one half of the folic acid you consume is absorbed by your body.

OTHER POTENTIAL DEFICIENCIES: Sulfisoxazole and sulfamethoxazole could also lead to deficiencies of calcium and vitamin K, though these deficiencies are quite unlikely.

These drugs are antagonists of vitamin B_6; therefore users may experience a vitamin B_6 deficiency. Symptoms frequently are a sore mouth and tongue, cracked lips, cracks in the corners of the mouth, and patches of itching, scaling skin. If severe, a vitamin B_6 deficiency may cause depression and confusion. A vitamin B_6 inadequacy is also common among the elderly. Alcoholics, as well, often experience this deficiency, since alcohol interferes with the body's utilization of B_6. It is estimated that one of every two Americans consumes less than 70 percent of the Recommended Dietary Allowance of B_6. Contraceptive users are also at high risk in this respect, and smokers are at greater risk than nonsmokers.

To avoid a B_6 deficiency, you should consume a diet featuring such B_6 sources as liver (beef, calf, and pork), herring, salmon, walnuts, peanuts, wheat germ, carrots, peas, potatoes, grapes, bananas, and yeast. The vitamin is present in significant amounts in meats, fish, fruits, cereals, and vegetables, and to a lesser extent in milk and other dairy products. Since vitamin B_6 is decomposed at high temperatures, modern food processing often diminishes dietary sources of the vitamin.

It has been observed that 15 to 20 percent of oral contraceptive users show direct evidence of vitamin B_6 deficiency. If you are among these people, you should take a 5 mg supplement of vitamin B_6 per day.

OTHER ADVICE: These drugs are gastric irritants and can cause loss of appetite, nausea, vomiting, stomachache, and diarrhea. They should be taken after meals to reduce these effects. However, when these drugs are taken with foods at mealtimes, their absorption is delayed, and the drugs will take longer to work. Patients on sulfisoxazole or sulfamethoxazole should also drink plenty of fluids to ensure that the drug is not precipitated in the kidneys, which can cause damage. At least 6 to 8 ounces of fluids should be consumed each day. The drug also increases the intoxicating effects of alcohol.

SULFINPYRAZONE

DRUG FAMILY: Anti-gout

BRAND NAME: Anturane

HOW TO TAKE SULFINPYRAZONE: With meals or milk

FOODS TO AVOID: Purine-rich foods such as anchovies, liver, meat extracts, sardines, sweetbreads, and brains; herbal teas; alcoholic beverages, especially beer; large amounts of sweet foods such as cookies, cakes, and candy

POSSIBLE SIDE EFFECTS: Kidney stones; stomachache and diarrhea; decreased effectiveness of oral contraceptives

ACTION OF SULFINPYRAZONE: This drug is prescribed for patients with gout. It increases the excretion of uric acid and hence reduces the level of uric acid in the blood and body tissues.

Gout is an arthritis-type disease that is caused by deposits of uric acid crystals in the joints. It generally occurs in single joints, usually the big toe, in painful episodes that last only a few days but are likely to recur. Middle-aged men are those primarily afflicted.

Your doctor is likely to recommend a special diet low in purine-rich foods in addition to prescribing sulfinpyrazone or another of the anti-gout medications. That diet is a crucial part of the treatment, since the purines in foods are broken down by your body to produce uric acid. (See table of Purine-Rich Foods, page 303.)

HIGH-RISK GROUPS: Anyone who takes this drug

NUTRITIONAL INTERACTIONS

KIDNEY STONES AND OTHER COMPLICATIONS: Sulfinpyrazone could conceivably lead to the production of kidney stones. When purine foods are a part of the diet, they are normally excreted as uric acid. However, this drug may cause such large quantities of uric acid to pass through the kidneys, that it may be deposited in uric acid crystals, a form of kidney stones. A difficulty in urinating and blood in the urine may signal the development of kidney stones.

Prevention and Treatment: To prevent the formation of kidney stones, it is advised you drink no less than 8 glasses, or 5 to 6 pints of liquid, every 24 hours, particularly at night when the urine becomes concentrated.

OTHER ADVICE: Sulfinpyrazone is also a gastric irritant that is likely to lead to abdominal pain and possibly diarrhea. The drug should be taken with meals or milk to avoid stomach distress.

Since some herbal teas contain phenylbutazone, which raises uric acid levels, avoid herbal teas. Avoid alcohol, especially beer, and simple sugars (see table of Simple and Complex Carbohydrates, page 305) because they can raise the blood level of uric acid and impair the drug's ability to manage chronic gout.

Sulfinpyrazone may decrease the effectiveness of oral contraceptives and increase the frequency of breakthrough bleeding—that is, bleeding on days other than those of menstruation.

If obese, gout sufferers would also do well to achieve ideal body weight by gradual weight reduction (1 to 2 pounds per week). All sufferers should decrease their animal fat intake and increase their consumption of complex carbohydrates.

SULINDAC

DRUG FAMILY: Anti-inflammatory

BRAND NAME: Clinoril

HOW TO TAKE SULINDAC: With food

FOODS TO AVOID: Alcoholic beverages and herbal teas

POSSIBLE SIDE EFFECTS: Stomachache, nausea, and constipation

ACTION OF SULINDAC: This nonsteroidal anti-inflammatory drug is also a painkiller and reduces fever. It is used in the relief of osteoarthritis, rheumatoid arthritis, acute gouty arthritis, and ankylosing spondylitis.

HIGH-RISK GROUPS: People with a history of abdominal distress

NUTRITIONAL INTERACTIONS

GASTROINTESTINAL DISTRESS: Studies have revealed that 20 percent of patients taking sulindac experience mild gastrointestinal side effects. Stomach pain and nausea are the most frequent, followed by constipation.
Prevention and Treatment: This drug should always be taken with food. Constipation is usually safely remedied by an increase in the bulk in the diet. This means consuming larger servings of any of the following: dried or fresh fruits (especially unpeeled apples or pears), salad vegetables, radishes, oatmeal, and whole grain foods (brown rice, whole wheat breads, and cereals). It is not necessary to purchase products that claim "extra fiber" has been added to them.

Persistent constipation may also be relieved by doubling the amount of fluid consumed each day. Bran, if used, should be added to the diet gradually, and fluid should be increased by at least ¾ cup per teaspoon of bran. (See table of Dietary Fiber-Rich Foods, page 293.)

OTHER ADVICE: Alcohol tends to increase the severity of the gastrointestinal side effects and is best avoided. Herbal teas containing phenylbutazone can make an arthritic condition worse and should be avoided.

TERBUTALINE

DRUG FAMILY: Anti-asthmatic

BRAND NAMES: Brethine; Bricanyl

HOW TO TAKE TERBUTALINE: With or just after meals

FOODS TO AVOID: None

POSSIBLE SIDE EFFECTS: Nausea and vomiting

ACTION OF TERBUTALINE: This drug is prescribed to dilate the airways in the lungs. It is used in the treatment of asthma, bronchitis, and emphysema.

HIGH-RISK GROUP: Anyone who takes this drug

NUTRITIONAL INTERACTIONS

GASTROINTESTINAL DISTRESS: Terbutaline could conceivably cause you to experience nausea and vomiting.
Prevention and Treatment: This drug should be taken with food to reduce the likelihood of gastrointestinal disturbances.

TETRACYCLINE

DRUG FAMILY: Antibiotic

BRAND NAMES: [GENERIC/Brand] DEMECLO-CYCLINE/Declomycin; DOXYCYCLINE/Doxycycline; DOXYCYCLINE CALCIUM/Vibramycin Calcium; DOXYCYCLINE HYCLATE/Doxy-Lemmon; Vibramycin Hyclate; Vibra-Tabs; DOXYCYCLINE MONOHYDRATE/Vibramycin Monohydrate; METHACYCLINE HYDROCHLORIDE/Rondomycin; MINOCYCLINE HYDROCHLORIDE/Minocin; OXYTETRACYCLINE/Oxymycin; Terramycin; Urobiotic-250; OXYTETRACYCLINE HYDROCHLORIDE/Terra-Cortril; Terramycin; TETRACYCLINE/Mysteclin-F; SK-Tetracycline; Sumycin; TETRACYCLINE HYDROCHLORIDE/Achromycin; Achromycin V; Topicycline

HOW TO TAKE TETRACYCLINE: Preferably on an empty stomach, 1 hour before or 2 hours after meals; if severe gastric reactions occur, however, the drug may be taken with meals provided that they do not contain any dairy products.

FOODS TO AVOID: Dairy products should be avoided 1 hour before and 1 hour after taking tetracycline. Do not eat foods rich in iron, such as red meat and dark green vegetables, at the same time as you take the drug.

POSSIBLE SIDE EFFECTS: Deficiencies of riboflavin, folic acid, calcium, iron, magnesium, zinc, and vitamins C, B_6, and B_{12}; protein and fat malabsorption; loss of appetite, nausea, vomiting, and diarrhea

ACTION OF TETRACYCLINE: This broad-based antibiotic is frequently prescribed for infections caused by all bacteria except streptococci.

HIGH-RISK GROUPS: Heavy drinkers, pregnant women, the elderly, users of oral contraceptives, premenopausal women, children, smokers, teenagers, anyone who consumes alcohol regularly, vegetarians

NUTRITIONAL INTERACTIONS

RIBOFLAVIN DEFICIENCY: Tetracycline increases the excretion of riboflavin (vitamin B_2) and is likely to lead to a deficiency. This may also exacerbate an existing vitamin B_2 deficiency in oral contraceptive users and in the elderly.

The symptom most likely to appear will be a dermatitis around the lips and nostrils, cracks in the corners of the mouth, and a sore tongue. Discomfort in eating and swallowing is the end result of this. The eyes may burn, itch, be more sensitive than usual to light, and tend to be bloodshot. However, be aware that any B vitamin deficiency can cause many of the same symptoms.

Riboflavin helps the body transform protein, fats, and carbohydrates into the energy needed to maintain body tissues and to protect the body against common skin and eye disorders.

Prevention and Treatment: Good sources of riboflavin should be included in the diet. (See table of Vitamin B_2(Riboflavin)-Rich Foods, page 310.)

Milk usually contributes about 50 percent of our riboflavin intake; meat about 25 percent; and dark green leafy vegetables, enriched cereals, and breads the rest. The need for riboflavin provides a major reason for including milk in some form in every day's meals; no other food that is commonly eaten can make such a substantial contribution to meeting our daily riboflavin needs. People who don't use milk products can substitute a generous serving of dark green leafy vegetables, because a cup of greens such as collards provides about the same amount of riboflavin as a cup of milk.

Among the meats, liver is the richest source, but all lean meats, as well as eggs, can provide some riboflavin. Riboflavin is light-sensitive; it can be destroyed by the ultraviolet rays of the sun or fluorescent lamps. For this reason, milk is seldom sold, and should not be stored, in transparent glass containers. Cardboard or plastic containers protect the riboflavin in the milk from ultraviolet rays.

A 5 mg supplement of riboflavin should be taken by people taking this drug for more than a few days.

VITAMIN C DEFICIENCY: Tetracycline increases your body's excretion of vitamin C and is likely to lead to a vitamin C deficiency if the drug is taken for more than a few days. Tetracycline will also exacerbate any marginal deficiency already present in smokers and oral contraceptive users. With an adequate vitamin C intake, the body normally maintains a fixed pool of the vitamin and rapidly excretes any excess in the urine. Ordinarily, 60 mg of vitamin C per day is sufficient to provide for the body's needs.

With an inadequate intake, however, the reservoir becomes depleted at the rate of up to 3 percent per day, and even more quickly in users of this drug. Obvious symptoms of a vitamin C deficiency do not appear until the available vitamin C has been reduced to about one fifth of its optimal level, and this may take two months to occur.

The earliest signs of a deficiency are spongy or bleeding gums, slightly swollen wrists and ankles, and capillaries that break under the skin, producing pinpoint hemorrhages around the hair follicles on the arms and legs.

The functioning of your bodily systems requires vitamin C in a number of ways. When your body is deficient in vitamin C, your white blood cells are less able to detect and destroy invading bacteria. On the other hand, megadoses of the vitamin (over 2 grams daily) can also impair this ability. Vitamin C also helps your body guard itself against such pollutants as known cancer-causing agents nitrites and nitrosamines, and protects vitamins A and E from degradation. Vitamin C also aids in iron absorption, speeds up wound healing, and strengthens blood vessels. Other well-known effects are that, in some people, vitamin C reduces the symptoms of a cold by one third and is important in preventing plaque formation on the teeth, which reduces the likelihood of gum disease and tooth decay.

Prevention and Treatment: Patients taking tetracycline should be sure to get 100 mg per day of vitamin C. Vitamin C-rich foods include citrus fruits, broccoli, spinach, cabbage, and bananas. (See table of Vitamin C-Rich Foods, page 313.) In preparing foods rich in vitamin C, you should keep in mind that it is readily oxidized (when exposed to the air during both food processing and storage). Copper and iron cooking utensils will speed up the oxidization; also, the longer the food is cooked and the higher the temperature, the greater the vitamin loss. Large amounts of water used in cooking will wash out the vitamin. Vitamin C is also destroyed when you cut or bruise fruit and vegetables.

Supplements can be taken, although the body tends to eliminate any surplus of C, so supplements of more than 100 mg a day are unnecessary. In fact, megadoses of the vitamin can cause nausea, abdominal cramps, and diarrhea, among other undesirable side effects.

FOLIC ACID DEFICIENCY: Tetracycline increases the excretion of folic acid. This could conceivably lead to a deficiency if the drug is taken for more than a few days, particularly in heavy drinkers, oral contraceptive users, and pregnant women. In pregnant women, the potential for this deficiency should be of particular concern since a deficiency can lead to growth abnormalities in the fetus. Folic acid is also crucial to the normal metabolism of proteins.

The first sign of a folic acid deficiency often is inflamed and bleeding gums. The symptoms that follow are a sore, smooth tongue; diarrhea; forgetfulness; apathy; irritability; and anemia. A folacin deficiency will also reduce your resistance to infection. Despite the fact that folacin is found in a variety of foods, folacin deficiency is still the most common vitamin deficiency in the United States.

In adults, deficiencies are limited almost exclusively to the elderly and women, 30 percent of whom have intakes below the recommended daily allowance, and 5 to 7 percent of whom also have severe anemia. There are several factors that account for this bias, but one of the most obvious reasons is that oral contraceptive use decreases the absorption of folic acid. Constant dieting also limits folacin intake. Alcohol interferes with the body's absorption and use of folic acid, as well. Folacin is not stored by the body in any appreciable amounts, so an adequate supply must be consumed on a daily basis.

Prevention and Treatment: To counteract a deficiency in folic acid, your diet should contain liver, yeast, and such leafy vegetables as spinach, kale, parsley, cauliflower, brussels sprouts, and broccoli. The fruits that are highest in folic acid are oranges and cantaloupes. To a lesser degree, folacin is found in almonds and lima beans, corn, parsnips, green peas, pumpkins, sweet potatoes, bran, peanuts, rye, and whole grain wheat. (See table of Folacin-Rich Foods, page 297.) Approximately one half of the folic acid you consume is absorbed by your body.

Normal cooking temperatures (110 to 120 degrees for 10 minutes) cause the breakdown of as much as 65 percent of the folacin in food. Therefore, you should include some raw vegetables and fruits in your diet. Cooking utensils made out of copper speed up folacin's destruction.

The recommended daily consumption of folacin is 400 mcg. Lactating women should assume a daily need of 1,200 mcg. Pregnant women and oral contraceptive users should consume 800 mcg daily.

CALCIUM DEFICIENCY: It is conceivable that long-term use of tetracycline will contribute to a calcium deficiency, since the drug impairs the absorption of calcium. In addition, dairy products, which are the best sources of dietary calcium, reduce the efficiency with which minocycline hydrochloride and doxycycline are absorbed, and prevent the absorption of the other tetracyclines and so are best limited while taking this drug.

Whenever calcium blood levels are low, the body will liberate the necessary amounts of calcium from the bones, where it is stored, thereby weakening them and making them more susceptible to fractures. A condition called osteomalacia can result. This is more likely after middle age, since in older people the body uses dietary calcium less efficiently.

Osteomalacia is a weakening of the bones as a consequence of uniform and steady calcium loss. This disease affects millions of older Americans, but also many younger people. In fact, one out of every four postmenopausal women suffers from this problem. Prominent symptoms are pain in the back, thighs, shoulder region, or ribs; difficulty in walking; and weakness in the muscles of the legs. The condition is reversible once calcium blood levels are raised.

A chronic shortage of dietary calcium may also lead to osteoporosis, another condition in which the bones are made weak and brittle. However, osteoporosis, an unexplained and rapid loss of calcium from the bones, is irreversible. Here the first symptoms are backache, a gradual loss of height, and periodontal disease.

In cases of osteoporosis, fractures of the vertebrae, hip, and wrist occur frequently, sometimes spontaneously. Approximately 7 percent of women fifty years of age and older have osteoporosis, and certain observers believe that the incidence of this disease is on the rise; between 15 and 20 million Americans are said to have osteoporosis today. In some 30 percent of people over sixty-five, the disease is severe enough to result in fractures. By age eighty, virtually all women experience some degree of osteoporosis; early menopause is a strong predictor of the disease. One out of five cases of the disease is found in men, but generally men get it at a later age and less severely than women.

Incidentally, tetracycline causes discoloration of the teeth in children. Treatment of pregnant women with the drug also causes discoloration of their offspring's teeth.

Prevention and Treatment: The Recommended Dietary Allowance for calcium is 800 mg, and all women should consume at least 1,200 mg of calcium per day. The average intake in the United States, however, is only 450 to 550 mg. For the elderly, and women who have already reached menopause or are about to, this should be increased to 1,500 mg. Children should be given an 800 mg supplement. The best dietary sources of calcium are dairy products, but since these cannot be consumed in significant quantities by people taking tetracycline, other calcium-containing foods must be emphasized, such as nuts. (See table of Calcium-Rich Foods, page 289.)

The best-absorbed supplement is calcium carbonate. (See Calcium Supplements entry, page 51.) In any case, an 800 to 1,500 mg supplement of calcium should be taken by everybody who is on tetracycline for extended periods of time. The supplement should not be taken within an hour of taking the antibiotic.

If magnesium is included in the supplement, the calcium is slightly better absorbed and any tendency to constipation is reduced. The supplement should be taken in 2 equal doses, 1 of which should be consumed before bedtime because most of the calcium loss from your body occurs while you sleep.

Consider that vitamin C assists calcium absorption, while cigarette smoking increases the rate of loss of bone calcium, as does excessive alcohol consumption. Foods that can decrease the absorption of calcium should be temporarily restricted, such as kale, rhubarb, spinach, cocoa, chocolate, beet greens, tea, and coffee. A deficiency might arise also if the ratio of phosphorus to calcium in your diet is very high; processed foods, particularly carbonated beverages, are high in phosphorus. The ideal ratio is essentially 1 to 1, as in dairy products; when the ratio is 15 or 20 to 1, as in meat, very little calcium is absorbed. High-fiber foods may contribute to a calcium deficiency, since fiber binds to calcium and passes it out in the stool. Excess fat and protein in the diet also hinder absorption.

Since there is little calcium in strict vegetarian diets (those that avoid dairy products as well as meat), vegetarians are at greater risk of a calcium deficiency. People who take magnesium- or aluminum-based antacids are also more prone to calcium deficiencies, because both magnesium and aluminum in excess impair calcium absorption.

Besides a change in dietary habits and the use of calcium supplements, it is recommended that anyone at risk of this deficiency adopt an exercise regimen that causes the bones to support the weight of the body, to strengthen the bones and to counteract the loss of bone density. A regular walking or jogging program, for example, can help prevent the bone degeneration of the spine, hips, and legs. Note, however, that swimming, though good for the heart as an aerobic exercise, is not especially beneficial for bone buildup.

It has been observed that oral contraceptives seem to help calcium absorption, and that during pregnancy the body absorbs cal-cium more effectively, making the mother's bones actually stronger despite the calcium needs of the fetus.

PROTEIN AND FAT MALABSORPTION: Tetracycline can cause a decreased absorption of fat and protein, and impair your body's ability to make protein, which is a continuous process. These results do not affect most people, but there is some evidence that suggests that diuretics exacerbate the problem of protein synthesis, and it has been suggested that they should not be used at the same time as any of the tetracycline drugs.

Prevention and Treatment: Your diet should contain plenty of protein. This means ample fish, meat, egg white, soy products, nuts, beans, peas, and lentils. (See table of Protein-Rich Foods, page 304.) At the same time, limit dietary intake of fatty foods such as dairy products, nuts, meat, and fatty fish.

IRON DEFICIENCY: Tetracycline impairs iron absorption, and iron impairs tetracycline absorption. Consequently, an iron deficiency while you are on tetracycline is conceivable if the drug is taken over a period of time.

Ideally, tetracycline should not be taken at mealtimes, since food in general decreases the drug's absorption. However, tetracycline tends to upset the stomach, and so taking it with meals can help you avoid this problem. One solution is to take one of the two varieties of tetracycline, doxycycline and minocycline, that are less affected by the presence of food in the stomach. It is also advised not to eat foods rich in iron, such as red meats and dark green vegetables, at the same time as you take the drug.

Iron is especially important to the oxygen-carrying cells of the blood and muscles, which account for two thirds of the iron your body requires. An iron shortage reduces the blood's oxygen-carrying capacity. The result is an anemia signaled by such symptoms as tiredness, general feelings of malaise, irritability, decreased attention span, pale complexion, rapid heart rhythm, headaches, loss of concentration, and breathlessness on exertion. A mild iron deficiency will also impair the functioning of your immune system.

In order to absorb iron from vegetable sources, the iron must be converted to another form by the action of the hydrochloric acid produced in the stomach. Some elderly people secrete less hydrochloric acid than normal, so they absorb iron poorly even under normal circumstances. The diets of many Americans lack adequate quantities of this mineral for their normal needs. For example, 10 percent of American women suffer from an iron deficiency, and up to 30 percent have inadequate iron stores. Other people who are at significant risk of an iron deficiency are women who have had several pregnancies and those whose menstrual periods are heavy.

The shortage of iron in many diets is due not only to the selection of foods that are poor sources of iron, but also to the switch away from cast-iron cookware to aluminum, stainless steel, and nonstick surfaces. Iron used to be leached from the iron pots and pans by the acid in foods, and became available as dietary iron.

Prevention and Treatment: To counteract an iron deficiency, iron-rich foods should be included in your diet: liver, whole grain products, oysters, dried apricots, prunes, peaches, leafy green vegetables, and lean red meat. (See table of Iron-Rich Foods, page 299.)

Other foods and drugs have a considerable impact on the way your body absorbs (or does not absorb) iron. There are two kinds of iron in food sources: heme iron in meat and ionic iron in vegetables. Up to 30 percent of the iron from meat, fish, and poultry is absorbed, but less than 10 percent is absorbed from eggs, whole grains, nuts, and dried beans. Only 10 percent of ionic iron is absorbed from vegetable sources, with as little as 2 percent being absorbed from spinach. Antacids will interfere with iron absorption from vegetables, as will commercial black and pekoe tea, taken in substantial quantities, because of its tannin content. Coffee also seems to decrease iron absorption, but not to the same degree as tea. Vitamin C supplements or citrus fruit juices increase the absorption of iron from vegetable sources by two to three times if taken simultaneously.

If your diet is rich in high-fiber foods, you will have impaired iron absorption because the fiber will bind to the iron and pass it out in the stool. This same action contributes to the poor absorption of iron from vegetable sources. Foods high in phosphorus (e.g. meat) interfere with iron absorption, which explains why only 30 percent of the iron in meat is captured. (However, meat and fish facilitate iron absorption from vegetables.) For that matter, any use of large quantities of mineral supplements, such as zinc, will impair iron absorption. Because iron can be leached from vegetables if they are cooked in large amounts of water, it is preferable to steam them.

Iron supplements should not be taken without a physician's recommendation, because an accumulation of too much iron can lead in extreme cases to such serious problems as anemia, malfunctioning of the pancreas and the heart, cirrhosis of the liver, a brown cast to the skin, and depression. Any iron supplement should not be taken within an hour of taking tetracycline.

MAGNESIUM DEFICIENCY: Magnesium deficiencies are not common because the average American diet contains appreciable amounts of magnesium. The higher than normal level of magnesium excretion resulting from taking tetracycline drugs for extended lengths of time increases the chances of such a deficiency, but it is still highly unlikely except in heavy drinkers.

Nevertheless, be alert for such clinical signs of magnesium deficiency as muscle weakness, tremors, depression, emotional instability, and irrational behavior.

Prevention and Treatment: A diet containing the four food groups provides the normal amount of magnesium. However, if a magnesium depletion is suspected, your diet should feature foods such as nuts (almonds and cashews are highest), meat, fish, milk, whole grains, and fresh greens, since cooking can wash away some magnesium. (See table of Magnesium-Rich Foods, page 300.) Alcohol provokes magnesium excretion, so its intake should be restricted to 2 drinks per day when taking this drug.

ZINC DEFICIENCY: Zinc absorption is decreased by tetracycline. A consequent deficiency is unlikely, but for heavy drinkers, pregnant women (in whom a deficiency can lead to fetal growth retardation), and users of oral contraceptives the chances are somewhat higher. A shortage of zinc in your system may result in impaired healing of wounds and ulcers, scaly dermatitis of the face and limbs, and anorexia associated with the loss of taste.

Prevention and Treatment: Patients using tetracycline should be sure to get the Recommended Dietary Allowance of zinc. Animal foods are good sources, with the richest being oysters, herring, milk, and egg yolks. Among plant foods, whole grains are richest in zinc, but it is not as well absorbed from them as from meat. Fiber and phytic acid in the cereal grains hinder its absorption. The recommended intake of 15 mg per day for adults is usually met easily by the diet of the average middle-class person, but deficiencies are more likely if animal protein is underemphasized. As a rule of thumb, two small servings of animal protein a day will provide sufficient zinc. Supplements should not be necessary, provided good sources of the nutrients are included in the diet.

VITAMIN B$_6$ DEFICIENCY: Tetracycline inactivates vitamin B$_6$ and could conceivably cause a deficiency after a few days of use, particularly in heavy drinkers and oral contraceptive users. It is estimated that one of every two Americans consumes less than 70 percent of the Recommended Dietary Allowance of B$_6$.

Common symptoms of this deficiency are a sore mouth and tongue, cracks in the lips and corners of the mouth, and patches of itching, scaling skin. A severe vitamin B$_6$ deficiency may cause depression and confusion.

Prevention and Treatment: To avoid a B_6 deficiency, you should consume a diet featuring food sources of the vitamin: liver (beef, calf, and pork), herring, salmon, walnuts, peanuts, wheat germ, carrots, peas, potatoes, grapes, bananas, and yeast. (See table of Vitamin B_6(Pyridoxine)-Rich Foods, page 311.) The vitamin is present in significant amounts in meats, fish, fruits, cereals, and vegetables, and to a lesser extent in milk and other dairy products.

Since vitamin B_6 is decomposed at high temperatures, modern food processing often diminishes the food content of this vitamin. Consequently, the more processed foods you eat, the more susceptible you will be to a deficiency of this vitamin. The same losses also occur in cooking: meat loses as much as 45 to 80 percent, vegetables 20 to 30 percent.

Some 15 to 20 percent of oral contraceptive users have been observed to have vitamin B_6 deficiencies. If you are among these people, you should take a 5 mg supplement of vitamin B_6 per day. Smokers tend to have lower body levels of this vitamin than nonsmokers and should take a 5 mg supplement while on tetracycline. However, keep in mind that you can take too much vitamin B_6; people taking over 1 gram per day have been reported to experience nerve degeneration.

OTHER ADVICE: Antacids decrease the absorption of tetracycline and should not be taken at the same time. Calcium-, magnesium-, and aluminum-based antacids are particularly bad in this respect. If you experience a severe gastric reaction to the drug, the antacid that may give you relief is sodium bicarbonate. It still impairs the drug's absorption, but not to the same degree as the others do.

Minocin and the Vibramycins are not affected by antacid use.

People taking anti-coagulants are at risk of a vitamin K deficiency, and vegetarians could suffer from a vitamin B_{12} deficiency. Therefore, elderly patients and vegetarians who consume only vegetable matter should take a 6 mcg supplement of vitamin B_{12}.

Dairy products inactivate tetracycline and should not be consumed in abundance by people taking this drug.

Except for minocycline hydrochloride and doxycycline, which can be taken with or without meals, the tetracyclines should be taken on an empty stomach, 1 hour before or 2 hours after meals. The presence of food in the stomach, especially dairy products, significantly reduces the absorption of the drug, and makes it less effective. However, if a severe gastric reaction occurs with the drug, it should be taken with a nondairy meal.

THEOPHYLLINE

DRUG FAMILY: Anti-asthmatic

BRAND NAMES: Accurbron; Aerolate; Aquaphyllin; Bronkaid; Bronkodyl; Bronkolixir; Bronkotabs; Constant-T; Elixicon; Elixophyllin; Isuprel Hydrochloride; LABID; Lodrane; Marax; Mudrane GG; Primatene; Quibron; Respbid; Slo-bid; Slo-Phyllin; Somophyllin-CRT; Somophyllin-T; Sustaire; Synophylate; Synophylate-GG; T.E.H.; T-E-P; Tedral; Theobid; Theoclear L.A.; Theo-

Dur; Theofedral; Theolair; Theo-24; Theon; Theo-Organidin; Theophyl; Theophyl-SR; Theophyl-225; Theospan-SR; Theostat 80; Theostat; Theovent; Theozine; Uniphyl

HOW TO TAKE THEOPHYLLINE: On an empty stomach, with a large glass of water, 1 hour before or 2 to 3 hours after meals; if severe gastrointestinal upsets occur on taking the drug, it should be taken with a meal rich in protein but low in carbohydrates.

FOODS TO AVOID: Large quantities of carbohydrate-rich foods and drinks, and caffeine-containing beverages and foods such as coffee, tea, cola, and chocolate; charcoal-broiled beef

POSSIBLE SIDE EFFECTS: Stomachache and vomiting; nervousness

ACTION OF THEOPHYLLINE: These drugs make it easier for lung patients to breathe. They are prescribed for the relief of symptoms of asthma, bronchitis, and emphysema.

HIGH-RISK GROUPS: Anyone who takes this drug

NUTRITIONAL INTERACTIONS

GASTROINTESTINAL DISTRESS: Theophylline is likely to cause gastrointestinal disturbances, such as stomach pain and vomiting. However, it is optimally absorbed if taken on an empty stomach with a large volume of water, rather than with food.

Prevention and Treatment: If gastrointestinal upsets occur, it is likely the discomfort can be reduced or eliminated by taking the drug after eating.

POTENCY: Carbohydrate-rich foods or drinks decrease its effectiveness, and so should not be consumed at the same time as the theophylline is taken.

Prevention and Treatment: In order to minimize both the gastrointestinal effects and any reduction in potency, theophylline can be taken following a protein-rich meal.

OTHER ADVICE: Theophylline makes some people very nervous. In such individuals, large quantities of caffeine-containing beverages and foods could increase this side effect. Consequently, it is best to avoid large amounts of coffee, tea, cola, and chocolate.

Charcoal-broiled beef speeds up the rate of breakdown of theophylline and decreases its effectiveness; thus, it is advised that you do not eat it when taking the drug.

THIAZIDES

DRUG FAMILY: Diuretics

BRAND NAMES: [GENERIC/Brand] QUINETHAZONE/Hydromox; METOLAZONE/Diulo; Zaroxolyn; CHLORTHALIDONE/Hygroton; CHLOROTHIAZIDE/Diuril; HYDROCHLOROTHIAZIDE/Esidrix; HydroDIURIL; Oretic; HYDROFLUMETHIAZIDE/Saluron; BENDROFLUMETHIAZIDE/Naturetin; BENZTHIAZIDE/Exna; TRICHLORMETHIAZIDE/Metahydrin; Naqua; METHYCLOTHIAZIDE/Enduron; POLYTHIAZIDE/Renese; CYCLOTHIAZIDE/Anhydron

HOW TO TAKE THIAZIDES: With meals or milk

FOODS TO AVOID: Large amounts of licorice candy made from natural extract; when consuming alcoholic beverages, you should be very careful to avoid reducing your blood pressure below normal.

POSSIBLE SIDE EFFECTS: Deficiencies of potassium, zinc, and magnesium; depletion of body calcium and sodium; reduced appetite, nausea, vomiting, diarrhea, indigestion; dizziness upon standing; gout; hyperglycemia

ACTION OF THIAZIDES: These drugs increase the excretion of water, and also of sodium, chloride, potassium, and bicarbonate.

HIGH-RISK GROUPS: The elderly; heavy drinkers, vegetarians

NUTRITIONAL INTERACTIONS

POTASSIUM DEFICIENCY: These drugs reduce the amount of water in the body, and also cause your body to excrete minerals and other substances as well. One likely side effect is a potassium deficiency. Potassium regulates the amount of water in the cells of the body and is essential for the proper functioning of the kidneys and the heart muscle, and the secretion of stomach juices. The most alarming symptom of a potassium deficiency is an irregular heartbeat, which can lead to heart failure.

Low blood serum levels of potassium, called hypokalemia, are associated with laxative abuse, because many laxatives reduce potassium absorption in the gastrointestinal tract. This risk is especially high in elderly patients, who often consume diets low in potassium.

People with a potassium deficiency may have such symptoms as weakness, loss of appetite, nausea, vomiting, dryness of the mouth, increased thirst, listlessness, apprehension, and diffuse pain that comes and goes.

Proper potassium levels in your body can also be threatened if this drug is taken concurrently with cortisone-containing drugs.

Prevention and Treatment: Potassium depletion can be avoided by including such potassium-rich foods in your diet as tomato juice, lentils, dried apricots, asparagus, bananas, peanut butter, chicken, almonds, and milk. (See table of Potassium-Rich Foods, page 302.)

Potassium supplements should never be taken unless prescribed by a physician. They can cause anemia by interfering with the absorption of vitamin B_{12}. Just a few grams can also drastically increase the risk of heart failure. If you experience difficulty in swallowing while taking potassium supplements, consult your physician immediately. If supplements are prescribed, be aware that the absorption of the supplements potassium iodide and potassium chloride is decreased by dairy products, and that both are gastric irritants and should be taken with meals.

Too much salt in your diet can also compromise your body's supply of potassium, as can 1 to 3 ounces per day of licorice candy when made from natural extract. Natural licorice contains glycyrrhizic acid, which causes the retention of sodium and water, counteracting the desired effect of the drug, as well as increasing the excretion of potassium. Only imported licorice usually contains the natural form.

ZINC DEFICIENCY: Another mineral that is excreted at a rapid rate while taking a thiazide diuretic is zinc, and it is conceivable that a deficiency will occur. A shortage of zinc in your system may result in impaired healing of wounds and ulcers, scaly dermatitis of the face and limbs, and anorexia associated with the loss of taste.

Prevention and Treatment: Patients using this drug should be sure to get the Recommended Dietary Allowance of zinc. Animal foods are good sources, with the richest being oysters, herring, milk, and egg yolks. Among plant foods, whole grains are richest in zinc, but it is not as well absorbed from them as from meat. Fiber and phytic acid in the cereal grains hinder its absorption. The recommended intake of 15 mg a day for adults is usually met easily by the diet of the average middle-class person, but deficiencies are more likely if animal protein is underemphasized. As a rule of thumb, two small servings of animal protein a day will provide sufficient zinc.

MAGNESIUM DEFICIENCY: Still another mineral deficiency that could conceivably result from the increased excretion of water is a magnesium deficiency. Magnesium deficiencies are not common because the average American diet contains appreciable amounts of magnesium. However, the high level of magnesium excretion resulting from the use of thiazide makes such a deficiency far more likely.

Clinical signs of magnesium deficiency include muscle weakness, tremors, depression, emotional instability, and irrational behavior.

Prevention and Treatment: A diet containing the four food groups provides the right amount of magnesium. However, if a magnesium depletion is suspected, your diet should feature foods such as nuts (almonds and cashews are highest), meat, fish, milk, whole grains, and fresh greens, since cooking can wash away some magnesium. (See table of Magnesium-Rich Foods, page 300.) Alcohol provokes magnesium excretion, so its intake should be restricted to 2 drinks per day while taking this drug.

IODINE DEFICIENCY: Another problem that could be posed by the thiazide diuretics is hypothyroidism (a sluggish thyroid). It is highly unlikely that this deficiency will occur, but you should be on your guard for such symptoms as a lack of energy, and a tendency to gain weight and retain water, especially in the legs, ankles, and feet. The latter side effect, of course, makes the drug less effective.

An iodine deficiency occurs when the drug creates a critical loss of iodine through excessive excretion. Iodine is essential to normal childhood development and the function of the thyroid gland. If a deficiency of iodine occurs before or shortly after birth, cretinism can occur; so if you are pregnant or nursing, you should be particularly alert to the possibility of this deficiency. Pregnant and lactating women also require greater amounts of iodine than the average person.

Prevention and Treatment: Good sources of iodine such as seafood, fresh fish, and iodized salt should be included in your diet.

Do not, however, eat large amounts of foods that contain goitrogens, such as raw cabbage. Goitrogens are substances that prevent the thyroid's absorption of iodine and thus the manufacture of thyroid hormone. (See table of Goitrogen-Rich Foods, page 298.)

Your iodine needs are small (between 100 and 140 mcg per day is the range of the recommended daily allowances, depending upon age and sex), so it can be reasonably obtained even on a salt-restricted diet. However, if symptoms of hypothyroidism persist, consult your physician.

CALCIUM BALANCE: The thiazide diuretics will cause a calcium depletion due to increased excretion. This may contribute to osteomalacia or osteoporosis. Whenever calcium blood levels are low, the body must liberate the necessary amounts of calcium from the bones, where it is stored, thereby weakening them and making them more susceptible to fractures. This condition, called osteomalacia, is a weakening of the bones as a result of a uniform and steady calcium loss. Prominent symptoms are bone pain in the back, thighs, shoulder region, or ribs; difficulty in walking; and weakness in the muscles of the legs. The condition is reversible once calcium blood levels are raised.

Chronic calcium deficiencies may also lead to osteoporosis, another condition in which the bones are made weak and brittle. However, osteoporosis, the unexplained and rapid loss of calcium from the bones, is irreversible. The first symptoms characteristically are a gradual loss of height, bone pain, and periodontal disease. Fractures often occur in the vertebrae, hip, or wrist.

Prevention and Treatment: Provided that you do not have hypercalcemia, foods rich in calcium (particularly milk, and dairy products such as yogurt and hard cheeses) should be included in the diet. (See table of Calcium-Rich Foods, page 289.) If you have a hypocalcemia condition and find that you must avoid calcium foods because of an intolerance to lactose, the sugar present in dairy products (a problem for an estimated 30 million Americans), a 1,000 mg daily supplement of calcium should be taken. (See Calcium Supplements entry, page 51.) Keep in mind as well that vitamin C assists calcium absorption.

Foods that can decrease the absorption of calcium should be temporarily restricted, such as spinach, cocoa, chocolate, beet greens, tea, and any beverages containing caffeine. A deficiency might arise also if the ratio of phosphorus to calcium in your diet is very high. The ideal ratio is essentially 1 to 1, as in dairy products; when the ratio is 15 or 20 to 1, as in meat, very little calcium is absorbed. Carbonated beverages tend to have a very high phosphorus level and should be avoided. High-fiber foods may contribute to a calcium deficiency, since fiber binds to calcium and passes it out in the stool.

Since there is little calcium in strict vegetarian diets (those that avoid dairy products as well as meat), vegetarians are at greater risk of a deficiency. Those who take magnesium- or aluminum-based antacids are also more prone to calcium deficiencies, because both magnesium and aluminum impair calcium absorption.

It has been observed that oral contraceptives seem to help calcium absorption.

BLOOD GLUCOSE LEVELS: It is conceivable that the thiazide diuretics will reduce your blood glucose levels below normal. This condition is called hypoglycemia. When there is too little blood sugar (that is, if your blood sugar levels drop to below 30 mg/100 ml of blood where a normal level is 100 mg/100 ml), you may become mentally confused due to a lack of glucose reaching the brain. Other early symptoms are headaches, hunger, and an overall sensation that resembles mild drunkeness.

Prevention and Treatment: While taking thiazide diuretics, you should eat five or six small meals a day rather than two or three large ones. Also, you should include plenty of complex carbohydrates, such as starches, vegetables, and cereals, and avoid simple sugars, such as honey and refined sugars. (See table of Simple and Complex Carbohydrates, page 305.)

SODIUM DEPLETION: Thiazide diuretics can lead to an excess excretion of sodium, which may cause the sodium concentration of the blood to drop below normal. Common symptoms caused by this condition are anorexia, nausea, vomiting, and muscle weakness.

Prevention and Treatment: To avoid this, an attempt should be made to avoid excess fluid intake (more than 10 glasses of fluid per day). These symptoms are more common in the elderly, where in very severe cases of sodium deficiency, grand mal seizures and impairment of the senses may be experienced.

OTHER ADVICE: These drugs may upset the gastrointestinal system, so they should be taken with meals or milk to prevent an upset stomach. They are also better absorbed with food.

Alcohol can increase the blood-pressure-lowering effect of this drug and cause abnormally low blood pressures and dizziness when the user stands up.

Thiazides frequently elevate uric acid levels in the blood, which can increase the risk of gout in susceptible people.

These drugs also cause hyperglycemia (abnormally high blood glucose levels) and can aggravate a preexisting diabetic condition.

THIORIDAZINE AND THIORIDAZINE HYDROCHLORIDE

DRUG FAMILY: Anti-psychotic, anti-depressant

BRAND NAME: Mellaril

HOW TO TAKE THIORIDAZINE: As directed by your physician

FOODS TO AVOID: All alcoholic beverages; large amounts of alkaline foods such as milk, buttermilk, cream, almonds, chestnuts, coconuts, all vegetables except corn and lentils, and all fruits except cranberries, prunes, and plums

POSSIBLE SIDE EFFECTS: Constipation, dry mouth, nausea, vomiting, diarrhea, and loss of appetite

ACTION OF THIORIDAZINE: This drug is used in the management of psychotic maladies (including agitation, anxiety, depressed mood, tension, insomnia, and fears in the elderly). It is also used in short-term treatments of moderate to marked depression. In children, its uses are in treating behavioral problems and—in short-term application—hyperactive children.

HIGH-RISK GROUPS: Anyone who takes this drug

NUTRITIONAL INTERACTIONS

ALCOHOL INTERACTION: The effect of thioridazine is likely to be enhanced by alcohol.

Central nervous system depression may be increased, in some cases with severe respiratory failure. Thioridazine can also enhance the effects of alcohol in inhibiting driving skills, with a consequent increase in the chance of motor accidents.

Prevention and Treatment: Alcohol should not be consumed concurrently with this drug.

ALKALINE URINE: Because thioridazine hydrochloride is alkaline, it is excreted at a normal rate only if your urine is acidic. However, if the quantity of alkaline foods in your diet is high, your urine will lose its acidity, and the excretion of this drug will be slowed. A hazardous buildup could conceivably result. The symptoms of such a buildup or overdose are drowsiness, involuntary movements, dryness of the mouth, low blood pressure (especially on standing), and skin rashes.

Prevention and Treatment: Fruits, vegetables, and dairy products tend to be alkaline, and high-protein foods tend to be acidic. Foods causing the production of alkaline urine include milk, buttermilk, cream, almonds, chestnuts, coconuts, all vegetables except corn and lentils, and all fruits except cranberries, prunes, and plums.

Antacids that neutralize the acid in the stomach will also neutralize the acid in the urine, causing it to turn alkaline. Therefore, you should avoid antacids when taking this drug.

GASTROINTESTINAL DISTRESS: This drug is likely to make you constipated and give you a dry mouth. It also causes nausea, vomiting, diarrhea, and change in appetite in some people.

Prevention and Treatment: If constipation is experienced, increase the bulk in your diet by consuming larger servings of foods rich in fiber, such as whole-grain cereal products, breads, and bran. (See table of Dietary Fiber-Rich Foods, page 293.)

If nausea, vomiting, diarrhea, and a change in appetite occur, you should report the symptoms to your doctor immediately. He will adjust the dosage or give you an alternative medication.

THYROID HORMONES

DRUG FAMILY: Hormone

BRAND NAMES: [GENERIC/Brand] THYROID/ Armour; Cytomel; Euthroid; Levothroid; Proloid; S-P-T; Synthroid; Thyroid Strong; Thyrolar; THYROGLOBULIN/Proloid; THYROXINE/Choloxin; Euthroid; Levothroid; Synthroid; Thyrolar; L-Thyroxine; THYROXINE SODIUM/Choloxin; Synthroid; TRIIODOTHYRONINE/Thyrolar; LIOTRIX/Euthroid; Thyrolar; SODIUM LIOTHYRONINE/Thyrolar; SODIUM LEVOTHYROXINE/Synthroid; Levothroid; Thyrolar

HOW TO TAKE THYROID HORMONES: Usually on getting up in the morning, before eating

FOODS TO AVOID: Large amounts of foods containing goitrogens, such as rutabagas, cabbage, spinach, cauliflower, kale, turnips, soybean products, carrots, brussels sprouts, peaches, and beans

POSSIBLE SIDE EFFECTS: None with correct dosage

ACTION OF THYROID HORMONES: These drugs are used in replacement therapy in people with hypothyroidism (underactive thyroid), myxedema (a resulting condition), and simple goiter.

HIGH-RISK GROUPS: Anyone who takes these drugs

NUTRITIONAL INTERACTIONS

GOITROGEN FOODS: Certain foods contain substances called goitrogens, which prevent the thyroid gland from producing thyroid hormones and cause hypothyroidism. In a patient with hypothyroidism, goitrogens will exacerbate the condition and necessitate raising the therapeutic dose of thyroid hormone.

Prevention and Treatment: People taking thyroid medication should limit their intake of foods containing goitrogens, such as rutabagas, cabbage, spinach, cauliflower, kale, turnips, soybean preparations, carrots, brussels sprouts, peaches, and beans.

TOLAZAMIDE

DRUG FAMILY: Anti-diabetic

BRAND NAME: Tolinase

HOW TO TAKE TOLAZAMIDE: With milk or immediately after eating

FOODS TO AVOID: All alcoholic beverages and foods containing alcohol

POSSIBLE SIDE EFFECTS: Hypoglycemia, flatulence, diarrhea, nausea, and indigestion

ACTION OF TOLAZAMIDE: This drug is a member of the sulfonylurea family and is used to reduce blood glucose levels by stimulating the pancreas to produce insulin.

HIGH-RISK GROUPS: The elderly; heavy drinkers

NUTRITIONAL INTERACTION

HYPOGLYCEMIA AND HYPERGLYCEMIA: Too much or too little of tolazamide could conceivably cause hypoglycemia or hyperglycemia, respectively. Hypoglycemia is a condition in which there is too little sugar (glucose) in the blood. If your blood sugar levels drop to below 30 mg/100 ml of blood (a normal level is 100 mg/100 ml of blood), you may become mentally confused due to a lack of glucose reaching the brain. Other early symptoms are headaches, hunger, and a general sensation resembling mild drunkenness. Below 10 mg/100 ml, you could go into a diabetic coma. If the situation is not corrected within a few minutes, permanent brain damage may occur.

If too little tolazamide is taken, you will experience the opposite problem, hyperglycemia, from too much sugar in the blood. This condition is the result of the drug causing the pancreas to release amounts of insulin insufficient to allow the cells in the body to absorb glucose, which starves the cells of the energy they need. In this instance, as well, coma can result.

Alcohol and aspirin enhance the blood-glucose-lowering activity and can also cause the glucose levels to drop so low that the brain is starved of glucose and energy, and you can go into a coma.

Prevention and Treatment: If you are diabetic, you should carefully monitor your food intake to avoid an excess of carbohydrates in the form of simple sugars, such as cookies, candies, sodas, honey, and table sugar. These foods are absorbed very rapidly and will increase your blood sugar to very high levels. If you are diabetic, such high blood sugar levels are dangerous because the limited amount of insulin produced by the pancreas may not be sufficient to bring the levels back into the normal range. A preferred diet is low in fats, but with plenty of complex carbohydrates, such as starches, cereals, and vegetables. (See table of Simple and Complex Carbohydrate Foods, page 305.)

Recent studies have demonstrated that a high-fiber diet may cause a slower and more sustained release of glucose from the gastrointestinal tract into the bloodstream, preventing the wide swings in blood sugar levels. A high-fiber diet also increases the efficiency with which glucose is absorbed by the body. For the diabetic, it is recommended that you remain physically active and exercise daily, because by doing so the cells are made more susceptible to the insulin available. Finally, a change in eating schedule from the standard three meals per day to five or six smaller meals will also help keep blood sugar levels within the normal range.

PARKINSON'S DISEASE: Tolazamide is sometimes prescribed for nondiabetics suffering from Parkinson's disease, a nervous disorder involving a rhythmic tremor, rigidity of muscle action, and slowing of body motion. The elderly seem to be sensitive to this drug, and in some cases have developed hypoglycemia. In very rare instances, they have succumbed to coma.

Prevention and Treatment: If you are an elderly patient on tolazamide, you should carry sugar cubes or candy in the event you experience hypoglycemia.

ALCOHOL INTERACTION: Tolazamide inhibits the breakdown of acetaldehyde, which is produced when alcohol is broken down in the body. This causes a number of unpleasant symptoms. If alcohol is consumed after this drug is taken, severe headaches, flushing, nausea, vomiting, hypertension, weakness, vertigo, blurred vision, and convulsions may occur. The reaction begins within 5 to 10 minutes of one's drinking alcohol and in some people may be caused by a few sips of an alcohol-containing beverage. Even wine-flavored sauces, desserts containing liquor, or wine vinegar may cause the reaction.

Prevention and Treatment: No alcohol should be consumed while taking this drug.

OTHER ADVICE: Tolazamide sometimes irritates the gastrointestinal tract, causing nausea, indigestion, flatulence, and loose stools or diarrhea. It is recommended that it be taken with milk or immediately after eating to minimize gastric irritation.

TOLAZOLINE HYDROCHLORIDE

DRUG FAMILY: Vasodilator

BRAND NAME: Priscoline Hydrochloride

HOW TO TAKE TOLAZOLINE: With meals

FOODS TO AVOID: Large amounts of tyramine- and dopamine-containing foods, such as aged cheese, raisins, avocados, liver, bananas, eggplant, sour cream, alcoholic beverages, salami, meat tenderizers, chocolate, and soy sauce; foods containing alcohol; licorice candy made from natural extract; foods containing monosodium glutamate, and other salty foods such as pickled foods, luncheon meat, snack chips, and processed cheeses

POSSIBLE SIDE EFFECTS: Stomach hyperacidity, nausea, vomiting, and diarrhea

ACTION OF TOLAZOLINE: This drug dilates blood vessels and reduces high blood pressure.

HIGH-RISK GROUPS: Anyone who takes this drug

NUTRITIONAL INTERACTIONS

GASTROINTESTINAL DISTRESS: This drug increases the secretion of acid in the stomach and may lead to nausea, vomiting, and diarrhea.

Prevention and Treatment: Tolazoline should always be taken with meals to prevent an upset stomach.

TYRAMINE-RICH FOODS: Tyramine, a food substance, tends to raise blood pressure and so will reduce the effectiveness of this drug.

Prevention and Treatment: Tyramine-containing foods must be restricted while you are being treated with this drug. Tyramine is common in many foods, but it is found in the greatest amounts in high-protein foods that have undergone some decomposition, such as aged cheese. Tyramine is also found in chicken and beef livers, bananas, eggplant, sour cream, alcoholic beverages, salami, meat tenderizers, chocolate, yeast, and soy sauce. (See table of Tyramine-Rich Foods, page 307.) Raisins and avocados should also be avoided, because

they contain dopamine, which has the same effect as tyramine.

OTHER ADVICE: The drug prevents the complete breakdown of alcohol, leading to a buildup of acetaldehyde (a product arising from the partial breakdown of alcohol) which involves such uncomfortable symptoms as headache, flushing, breathing difficulties, gastrointestinal disturbances, and confusion. Consequently, foods and beverages containing alcohol should not be consumed by people taking tolazoline.

Other food substances that cause hypertension will tend to decrease the activity of the drug. For example, as little as 1 ounce of licorice candy containing natural licorice extract can cause sodium and water retention, and as a result high blood pressure. Hence, licorice should be avoided when you are on this drug. Usually, only imported licorice contains the natural extract. Check the package.

Concentrated sources of dietary sodium should also be eliminated, such as monosodium glutamate and obviously salty foods. Sodium causes water retention in some people, particularly in combination with a low potassium intake. Water retention increases the volume of fluid in the arteries, which is responsible for the elevated blood pressure. To limit the problems of water retention, your diet should contain natural diuretics, foods rich in potassium, such as citrus fruits, bananas, almonds, dates, dairy products, apricots, and bamboo shoots. (See table of Potassium-Rich Foods, page 302.) As many as 15 percent of all Americans have a genetic susceptibility to the effects of excess sodium. We only need about 220 mg of sodium each day, but the average American consumes 6 to 8 grams of salt per day, or 3 to 4 teaspoons.

No salt should be added at the table, but up to 1 teaspoon can be added per day during cooking. Pickled foods, such as sauerkraut, and extremely salty foods, such as luncheon meats, snack chips, and processed cheeses, should be eliminated altogether.

Be alert to the sodium content of food products; read the list of ingredients that appears on the label of all packaged foods. Sodium can be present in a food either as common salt (sodium chloride) or as any other sodium-containing compound, monosodium glutamate being a common one. If sodium appears as one of the first ingredients on the label, the food contains a significant amount of it. If, on the other hand, it appears very near the end of the list (as in bread), then it need not be a concern. Recent evidence points to a protective value for calcium against the harmful effects of sodium, so eat plenty of calcium-containing foods such as dairy products.

You should limit your intake of sodium to 2 to 3 grams per day, watch your weight, and exercise.

TOLBUTAMIDE

DRUG FAMILY: Anti-diabetic

BRAND NAMES: Orinase; SK-Tolbutamide

HOW TO TAKE TOLBUTAMIDE: With milk or immediately after eating

FOODS TO AVOID: All alcoholic beverages and foods containing alcohol

POSSIBLE SIDE EFFECTS: Hypoglycemia, flatulence, nausea, diarrhea, and indigestion

ACTION OF TOLBUTAMIDE: This drug is a member of the sulfonylurea family and is used to reduce blood glucose levels by stimulating the pancreas to produce insulin.

HIGH-RISK GROUPS: The elderly; heavy drinkers

NUTRITIONAL INTERACTION

HYPOGLYCEMIA AND HYPERGLYCEMIA: Too much or too little tolbutamide can cause hypoglycemia or hyperglycemia, respectively. Hypoglycemia is a condition in which there is too little glucose in the blood. If your blood sugar levels drop to below 30 mg/100 ml of blood (a normal level is 100 mg/100 ml of blood), you may become mentally confused due to a lack of glucose reaching the brain. Other early symptoms are headaches, hunger, and a general sensation resembling mild drunkenness. Below 10 mg/100 ml, you could go into a diabetic coma. If the situation is not corrected within a few minutes, permanent brain damage may occur.

If too little tolbutamide is taken, you will experience hyperglycemia, the opposite problem, from too much sugar in the blood. This condition is the result of the drug causing the pancreas to release amounts of insulin insufficient to allow the cells in the body to absorb glucose, which starves the cells of the energy they need. In this instance, as well, coma can result.

Prevention and Treatment: If you are diabetic, you should carefully monitor your food intake to avoid an excess of carbohydrates in the form of simple sugars, such as cookies, candies, sodas, honey, and table sugar. These foods are absorbed very rapidly and will increase your blood sugar to very high levels. If you are diabetic, such high blood sugar levels are dangerous because the limited amount of insulin produced by the pancreas may not be sufficient to bring the levels back into the normal range. A preferred diet is low in fats, but with plenty of complex carbohydrates, such as starches, cereals, and vegetables. (See table of Simple and Complex Carbohydrate Foods, page 305.)

Recent studies have demonstrated that a high-fiber diet may cause a slower and more sustained release of glucose from the gastrointestinal tract into the bloodstream, preventing the wide swings in blood sugar levels. Such a diet also causes the body to absorb glucose more efficiently. For the diabetic, it is recommended that you remain physically active and exercise daily, because in this way the cells are made more susceptible to the insulin available. Finally a change in eating schedule from the standard three meals per day to five or six smaller meals will also help keep blood sugar levels within normal range.

PARKINSON'S DISEASE: Tolbutamide is sometimes prescribed for nondiabetics suffering from Parkinson's disease, a nervous disorder involving a rhythmic tremor, rigidity of muscle action, and slowing of body motion. The elderly seem to be sensitive to this drug, and in some cases have developed hypoglycemia while taking it. In rare instances, some have succumbed to coma.

Prevention and Treatment: If you are an elderly patient on tolbutamide, you should carry sugar cubes or candy in the event you experience hypoglycemia.

OTHER ADVICE: Tolbutamide sometimes irritates the gastrointestinal tract, causing flatulence and loose stools, or diarrhea. It is recommended that it be taken with milk or immediately after eating to minimize gastric irritation.

Alcohol decreases the potency of the drug by accelerating its rate of breakdown in the body. Because of this, tolbutamide is frequently unsuccessful in the treatment of alcoholic diabetics. It is urged that you not drink while taking this drug.

Tolbutamide also prevents the complete breakdown of alcohol, leading to a buildup of acetaldehyde (a product of the partial breakdown of alcohol) which leads to headache, flushing, breathing difficulties, confusion, and gastrointestinal disturbances; this is another good reason not to drink while taking this drug.

TRIAMTERENE

DRUG FAMILY: Diuretics

BRAND NAMES: Dyazide; Dyrenium

HOW TO TAKE TRIAMTERENE: After meals or with milk

FOODS TO AVOID: None. (Note that you should not restrict your intake of sodium unless specifically told to do so by your physician.)

POSSIBLE SIDE EFFECTS: Potassium buildup; calcium and folic acid deficiencies; upset stomach

ACTION OF TRIAMTERENE: This diuretic increases the excretion of water and also of sodium and chloride.

HIGH-RISK GROUPS: The elderly, heavy drinkers, users of oral contraceptives, smokers, vegetarians.

NUTRITIONAL INTERACTIONS

POTASSIUM BUILDUP: Triamterene reduces the body's ability to excrete normal levels of potassium. If people with kidney disease, who have problems in excreting potassium, take triamterene, it could conceivably lead to a buildup of potassium to toxic levels in the body. An irregular heart rate is the primary symptom of this condition. In extreme cases, this condition can lead to muscular weakness and paralysis.

Prevention and Treatment: Potassium supplements should never be taken by people on triamterene. If a toxicity should arise, it needs to be treated by drugs that remove the excess potassium from the body, such as penicillamine. Consult your physician.

CALCIUM DEFICIENCY: Triamterene increases the amount of calcium excreted from the body, which could conceivably lead to a deficiency. Whenever calcium blood levels are low, the body will liberate the necessary amounts of calcium from the bones, where it is stored, thereby weakening them and making them more susceptible to fractures. A condition called osteomalacia can result. This is more likely after middle age, since in older people the body uses dietary calcium less efficiently.

Osteomalacia is a weakening of the bones as a consequence of uniform and steady calcium loss. This disease affects millions of older Americans, but also many younger people. In fact, one out of every four postmenopausal women suffers from this problem. Prominent symptoms are bone pain in the back, thighs, and shoulder region, or ribs; difficulty in walking; and weakness in the muscles of the legs. The condition is reversible once blood calcium levels are raised.

A chronically low intake of calcium may lead to osteoporosis, another condition in which the bones are made weak and brittle. However, osteoporosis, an unexplained and rapid loss of calcium from the bones, is irreversible. Here the first symptoms are backache, a gradual loss of height, and periodontal disease. In cases of osteoporosis, fractures of the vertebrae, hip and wrist occur frequently, sometimes spontaneously.

Approximately 7 percent of women fifty years of age and older have osteoporosis, and certain observers believe that the incidence of this disease is on the rise; between 15 and 20 million Americans are said to have osteoporosis today. In some 30 percent of people over sixty-five, the disease is severe enough to result in fractures. By age eighty, virtually all women experience some degree of osteoporosis; early menopause is a strong predictor of the disease. One out of five cases of the disease is found in men, but generally men get it at a later age and less severely than women.

Prevention and Treatment: The Recommended Dietary Allowance for calcium is 800 mg, and all women should consume at least 1,200 mg of calcium per day. The average intake in the United States, however, is only 450 to 550 mg. For the elderly, and women who have already reached menopause or are about to, this should be increased to 1,500 mg by the consumption of foods rich in calcium, particularly milk, dairy products (including yogurt and hard cheeses), and, to a lesser extent almonds. Three 8-ounce glasses of milk, for example, provide 1,500 mg of calcium. (See table of Calcium-Rich Foods, page 289.)

If calcium foods must be avoided because of an intolerance to lactose, the sugar found in dairy products (a problem for an estimated 30 million Americans), a 1,000 mg daily supplement of calcium should be taken. The best-absorbed supplement is calcium carbonate. (See Calcium Supplements entry, page 51.) If magnesium is included in the supplement, the calcium is slightly better absorbed and any tendency to constipation is reduced. The supplement should be taken in two 500 mg doses, one of which should be consumed before bedtime because most of the calcium loss from your body occurs while you sleep.

Cigarette smoking increases calcium losses from the body, while vitamin C assists calcium absorption. Excessive alcohol consumption also hinders absorption. Foods that can decrease the absorption of calcium should be temporarily restricted, such as kale, rhubarb, spinach, cocoa, chocolate, beet greens, tea, and coffee. A deficiency might also arise if the ratio of phosphorus to calcium in your diet is very high; processed foods, especially carbonated beverages, are particularly high in phosphorus. The ideal ratio is essentially 1 to 1, as in dairy products; when the ratio is 15 or 20 to 1, as in meat, very little calcium is absorbed. High-fiber foods may contribute to a calcium deficiency, since fiber binds to calcium and passes it out in the stool. Excess fat and protein in the diet also hinder absorption.

Since there is little calcium in strict vegetarian diets (those that avoid all dairy products as well as meat) vegetarians are at greater risk of a calcium deficiency. People who take magnesium- or aluminum-based antacids are also more prone to calcium deficiencies, because both magnesium and aluminum in excess impair calcium absorption.

Besides a change in dietary habits and the use of calcium supplements, it is recommended that anyone at risk of this deficiency adopt an exercise regimen that causes the bones to support the weight of the body, to strengthen the bones and to counteract the loss of bone density. A regular walking or jogging program, for example, can help prevent the bone degeneration of the spine, hips, and legs. Note, however, that swimming, though good for the heart as an aerobic exercise, is not especially beneficial for bone buildup.

It has been observed that oral contraceptives help calcium absorption, and that during pregnancy the body absorbs calcium more effectively, making the mother's bones actually stronger, despite the calcium needs of the fetus.

FOLIC ACID DEFICIENCY: Triamterene could conceivably cause you to experience a folic acid deficiency, since it prevents the vitamin from being converted into its active form (tetrahydrofolate).

The first sign of a folic acid or folacin deficiency is likely to be inflamed and bleeding gums. The symptoms that follow are a sore, smooth tongue; diarrhea; forgetfulness; apathy; irritability; anemia; and a reduced resistance to infection. Despite the fact that folacin is found in a variety of foods, folacin deficiency is still the most common vitamin deficiency in the United States.

In adults, deficiencies are limited almost exclusively to the elderly and women, 30 percent of whom have intakes below the recommended daily allowance, and 5 to 7 percent of whom also have severe anemia. There are several factors that account for this bias, but one of the most obvious reasons is that oral contraceptive use decreases the absorption of folic acid. Constant dieting also limits folacin intake, and alcohol interferes with the body's absorption and use of folic acid, as well. Folacin is not stored by the body in any appreciable amounts, so an adequate supply must be consumed on a daily basis.

Folic acid is crucial to the normal metabolism of proteins. In addition, it is essential to the making of new cells. Consequently, a deficiency of this vitamin during pregnancy can lead to birth defects.

Prevention and Treatment: To counteract a deficiency in folic acid, your diet should contain liver, yeast, and leafy vegetables such as spinach, kale, parsley, cauliflower, brussels sprouts, and broccoli. The fruits that are highest in folic acid are oranges and cantaloupes. To a lesser degree, folacin is found in almonds and lima beans, corn, parsnips, green peas, pumpkins, sweet potatoes, bran, peanuts, rye, and whole grain wheat. (See table of Folacin-Rich Foods, page 297.) Approximately one half of the folic acid you consume is absorbed by your body.

Normal cooking temperatures (110 to 120 degrees for 10 minutes) destroy 65 percent of the folacin in your food. Your daily diet, therefore, should include some raw vegetables and fruits. Cooking utensils made out of copper speed up folacin's destruction.

The recommended daily consumption of folacin is 400 mcg. Oral contraceptive users should consume 800 mcg daily.

OTHER ADVICE: It should also be noted that triamterene is frequently prescribed in combination with thiazide diuretics and indomethacin, which deplete the body of potassium and reduce the risk of potassium toxicity. Indomethacin and digitoxin (another drug frequently used in combination with triamterene) also tend to decrease calcium excretion, countering another of the undesirable effects of triamterene.

Triamterene is a gastric irritant, and its use can lead to an upset stomach. It should be taken with meals or milk to reduce the chances of gastrointestinal discomfort.

TRICYCLIC ANTI-DEPRESSANTS

DRUG FAMILY: Anti-depressant

BRAND NAMES: [GENERIC/Brand] AMITRIPTYLINE HYDROCHLORIDE/Elavil; Endep; Etrafon; Limbitrol; Triavil; DESIPRAMINE HYDROCHLORIDE/Norpramin; Pertofrane; DOXEPIN HYDROCHLORIDE/Adapin; Sinequan; IMIPRAMINE HYDROCHLORIDE/Janimine Filmtab; SK-Pramine; Tofranil; NORTRIPTYLINE HYDROCHLORIDE/Aventyl Hydrochloride; Pamelor; PROTRIPTYLINE HYDROCHLORIDE/Vivactil

HOW TO TAKE TRICYCLIC ANTI-DEPRESSANTS: As directed by your physician

FOODS TO AVOID: All alcoholic beverages; large amounts of alkaline foods such as milk, buttermilk, cream, almonds, chestnuts, coconuts, all vegetables except corn and lentils, and all fruits except cranberries, plums, and prunes

POSSIBLE SIDE EFFECTS: Less frequent urination than normal; constipation; dry mouth; sour or metallic taste in the mouth; increased appetite

ACTION OF TRICYCLIC ANTI-DEPRESSANTS: These drugs are taken for the treatment of anxiety or depression.

HIGH-RISK GROUPS: The elderly, heavy drinkers, vegetarians

NUTRITIONAL INTERACTIONS

URINARY PROBLEMS: When taking tricyclic anti-depressants, you tend to urinate less frequently. This does not do physical damage to the body, but it can be distressing, particularly to the elderly, who may be worried by changes in their usual toilet routine.

TOXIC BUILDUP: The effect of these drugs is prolonged by alkaline urine, which slows down the rate at which the drug is excreted from the body. This is unlikely to happen as a result of diet alone, except with chronic, excessive ingestion of foods causing the production of alkaline urine, such as milk, buttermilk, cream, almonds, chestnuts, coconuts, all vegetables except corn and lentils, and all fruits except cranberries, prunes, and plums. In the event that a buildup does occur, however, the potency of these drugs can be doubled, further increasing the risk of adverse side effects. The concurrent consumption of large amounts of antacids can also produce a buildup. Symptoms of such

a hazardous buildup or overdose are dizziness, rapid heart rate, palpitations, blurred vision, weakness, fatigue, muscle tremors, a tendency to become very excited, low blood pressure, and impotence, as well as a worsening of the nutrient interactions listed.

Vegetarians are most at risk and should inform their physicians of their dietary habits.

Antacids that neutralize the acid in the stomach will also neutralize the acid in the urine, making it alkaline. Therefore, avoid antacids while taking tricyclic anti-depressants.

CONSTIPATION: The tricyclic anti-depressants slow down the rate at which the stomach empties its contents into the intestine, which can result in constipation in some patients, especially the elderly.

Prevention and Treatment: Constipation is usually safely remedied by an increase in the bulk in the diet. This means increasing the servings of oatmeal and other whole grain foods (brown rice, whole wheat breads, and cereals). It is not necessary to purchase products that claim "extra fiber" has been added to them. Exercise also will help, for not only does it tune up the muscles in the arms and legs, but it also strengthens the muscles lining the gastrointestinal tract that propel the food through the intestine.

Persistent constipation may also be relieved by doubling the amount of fluid consumed each day. Bran, if used, should be added to the diet gradually, and fluid should be increased by at least ¾ cup per teaspoon of bran. (See table of Dietary Fiber-Rich Food, page 293.)

If your doctor has prescribed acidic compounds, such as sodium warfarin, iron, thyroid preparations, tetracycline, or thiazide diuretics, they should be taken at least 1 hour before tricyclic anti-depressants.

OTHER ADVICE: Since alcohol enhances the effects of the drug, you should not drink while taking it.

Some users of tricyclic anti-depressants experience a dry mouth. Too little saliva is secreted, reducing one's ability to digest carbohydrates (since the saliva contains an enzyme that breaks down starches in the mouth to facilitate their digestion), and making swallowing more difficult (the saliva also lubricates the food for ease of swallowing). Whole grain products rich in fiber should be well represented in the diet since they stimulate salivary flow by mechanical stimulation of the salivary glands.

A shortage of saliva also makes the mouth more susceptible to the growth of bacteria, and that can be responsible for tooth decay and gum disease. You should take special care to brush and floss your teeth often.

You should avoid consuming more than 8 to 10 glasses of fluid per day if you are taking amitriptyline, since it can cause sufficient water retention to dilute blood sodium to abnormally low concentrations. This can lead to loss of appetite, nausea, vomiting, and muscle weakness, especially in the elderly.

Tricyclic anti-depressants can cause a sour or metallic taste in the mouth that detracts from the pleasure of eating. Most people taking these drugs, however, find that this does not effect their food intake, since there is a tendency for the drug to increase the appetite, which leads to weight gain.

TRIFLUOPERAZINE HYDROCHLORIDE

DRUG FAMILY: Anti-psychotic; anti-anxiety

BRAND NAME: Stelazine

HOW TO TAKE TRIFLUOPERAZINE HYDROCHLORIDE: As directed by your physician

FOODS TO AVOID: All alcoholic beverages; large amounts of alkaline foods such as milk, buttermilk, cream, almonds, chestnuts, coconut, all vegetables except corn and lentils, and all fruits except cranberries, prunes, and plums

POSSIBLE SIDE EFFECTS: Nausea, constipation, and a dry mouth

ACTION OF TRIFLUOPERAZINE HYDROCHLORIDE: This drug is used to control psychotic disorders. It is also used to control the excessive anxiety, tension, and agitation of neuroses.

HIGH-RISK GROUPS: Anyone who takes this drug

NUTRITIONAL INTERACTIONS

ALCOHOL INTERACTION: The effect of trifluoperazine hydrochloride is likely to be enhanced by alcohol. Central nervous system depression may be increased, in some cases with severe respiratory failure. Trifluoperazine hydrochloride can also enhance the effects of alcohol in inhibiting driving skills, with a consequent increase in the chances of motor accidents.

Prevention and Treatment: Alcohol should not be consumed concurrently with this drug.

ALKALINE URINE: Because trifluoperazine hydrochloride is alkaline, it is excreted at a normal rate only if your urine is acidic. However, if the quantity of alkaline foods in your diet is high, your urine will lose its acidity, and the excretion of this drug will be slowed. A hazardous buildup could conceivably result. The symptoms of such a buildup or overdose are involuntary movements, dry mouth, nasal congestion, headache, impotence, and distorted vision.

Prevention and Treatment: Fruits, vegetables, and dairy products tend to be alkaline, and high-protein foods tend to be acidic. Foods causing the production of alkaline urine include milk, buttermilk, cream, almonds, chestnuts, coconuts, all vegetables except corn and lentils, and all fruits except cranberries, prunes, and plums.

Antacids that neutralize the acid in the stomach will also neutralize the acid in the urine, causing it to turn alkaline. Therefore, you should avoid antacids while taking this drug.

GASTROINTESTINAL DISTRESS: This drug is likely to cause you to experience nausea, constipation, and a dry mouth.

Prevention and Treatment: If constipation occurs, increase the bulk in the diet by consuming larger servings of foods rich in fiber, like whole-grain cereals, breads, and bran. (See table of Dietary Fiber-Rich Foods, page 293.) Remember that bran will only be beneficial in this respect if you consume ¾ cup of fluid for every teaspoon of bran you eat.

TRIHEXYPHENIDYL AND TRIHEXYPHENIDYL HYDROCHLORIDE

DRUG FAMILY: Anti-Parkinsonism

BRAND NAME: Artane

HOW TO TAKE TRIHEXYPHENIDYL: Preferably before meals, but it should be taken immediately following meals if it tends to cause nausea.

FOODS TO AVOID: None

POSSIBLE SIDE EFFECTS: Drying of the mouth, nausea, vomiting, and constipation

ACTION OF TRIHEXYPHENIDYL: This drug is used in conjunction with levodopa to treat Parkinson's disease. It inhibits the action of the chemical messenger in the brain (the neurotransmitter) that causes the tremor or rigidity.

HIGH-RISK GROUPS: Anyone who takes this drug

NUTRITIONAL INTERACTIONS

GASTROINTESTINAL DISTURBANCES: This drug is likely to make your mouth feel excessively dry. It sometimes causes nausea, vomiting, and constipation.

Prevention and Treatment: Because of the drying of the mouth, trihexyphenidyl should be taken before meals, unless it causes nausea, which would inhibit appetite. Should nausea occur, the drug should be taken after meals, and the thirst can be allayed with water, mints, or chewing gum.

Constipation can be treated by increasing the bulk in the diet by adding more fruit, vegetables, and whole-grain cereal products. (See table of Dietary Fiber-Rich Foods, page 293.) Persistent constipation may also be relieved by doubling the amount of fluid consumed each day. Bran, if used, should be added to the diet gradually, and fluid should be increased by at least ¾ cup per teaspoon of bran.

TRIMETHAPHAN CAMSYLATE

DRUG FAMILY: Vasodilator

BRAND NAME: Arfonad

HOW TO TAKE TRIMETHAPHAN CAMSYLATE: Injection

FOODS TO AVOID: Alcoholic beverages

POSSIBLE SIDE EFFECTS: Constipation

ACTION OF TRIMETHAPHAN CAMSYLATE: This potent dilator of blood vessels is used in the treatment of hypertensive emergencies— that is, when there is a sudden jump in blood pressure.

HIGH-RISK GROUPS: Anyone who consumes alcohol, the elderly

NUTRITIONAL INTERACTIONS

GASTROINTESTINAL DISTRESS: Trimethaphan camsylate reduces the contractions of the intestines, so it is likely to cause constipation.
Prevention and Treatment: If constipation occurs, seek advice from your physician.

OTHER ADVICE: Alcohol enhances its effect by dilating blood vessels and reducing blood pressure. As little as 6 ounces of sherry or 10 ounces of table wine is likely to have a blood-pressure-lowering effect that lasts up to 4 hours. Alcohol should not be consumed for 24 hours after this drug has been taken. If alcohol has already been consumed, this is not the drug of choice.

TRIMETHOPRIM

DRUG FAMILY: Anti-malarial

BRAND NAMES: Bactrim DS; Bactrim I.V.; Bactrim Pediatric; Cotrim; Cotrim D.S.; Proloprim; Septra DS; Septra I.V.; Sulfamethoxazole & Trimethoprim; Sulfamethoxazole w/Trimethoprim (Double Strength); Sulfamethoxazole & Trimethoprim Pediatric; Sulfamethoxazole w/Trimethoprim DS; Sulfamethoxazole w/Trimethoprim SS; Sulfatrim & Sulfatrim D/S; Trimpex

HOW TO TAKE TRIMETHOPRIM: Immediately after meals

FOODS TO AVOID: None

POSSIBLE SIDE EFFECTS: Folic acid deficiency, nausea, vomiting, and diarrhea

ACTION OF TRIMETHOPRIM: This drug is used as an anti-malarial, and as an anti-bacterial agent for certain urinary infections.

HIGH-RISK GROUPS: Users of oral contraceptives, heavy drinkers, children, pregnant women, teenagers, the elderly

NUTRITIONAL INTERACTIONS

FOLIC ACID DEFICIENCY: Trimethoprim is a potent folacin antagonist, since it prevents folacin from being converted to its active form.

If the drug is taken over an extended period or in doses in excess of 25 mg daily, then a deficiency of the vitamin is likely.

Often the first sign of a folic acid or folacin deficiency is inflamed and bleeding gums. The symptoms that follow are a sore, smooth tongue; diarrhea; forgetfulness; apathy; irritability; anemia; and a reduced resistance to infection. Despite the fact that folacin is found in a variety of foods, folacin deficiency is still the most common vitamin deficiency in the United States.

In adults, deficiencies are limited almost exclusively to the elderly and women, 30 percent of whom have intakes below the recommended daily allowance, and 5 to 7 percent of whom also have severe anemia. There are several factors that account for this bias, but one of the most obvious is that oral contraceptive use decreases the absorption of folic acid. Constant dieting also limits folacin intake, and alcohol interferes with the body's use of folic acid, as well. Folacin is not stored by the body in any appreciable amounts, so an adequate supply must be consumed on a daily basis.

Folic acid is essential for the synthesis of new cells, so a folic acid deficiency during pregnancy can lead to birth defects. Pregnant women should always take a folacin supplement with trimethoprim. Folic acid is also crucial to the normal metabolism of proteins.

Prevention and Treatment: To counteract a deficiency in folic acid, your diet should contain liver, yeast, and leafy vegetables such as spinach, kale, parsley, cauliflower, brussels sprouts, and broccoli. The fruits that are highest in folic acid are oranges and cantaloupes. To a lesser degree, folacin is found in almonds and lima beans, corn, parsnips, green peas, pumpkins, sweet potatoes, bran, peanuts, rye, and whole grain wheat. (See table of Folacin-Rich Foods, page 297.) Approximately one half of the folic acid you consume is absorbed by your body.

Normal cooking temperatures (110 to 120 degrees for 10 minutes) destroy up to 65 percent of the folacin in your food. Your daily diet, therefore, should include some raw vegetables and fruits. Cooking utensils made out of copper speed up folacin's destruction.

The recommended daily consumption of folacin is 400 mcg. Pregnant women and oral contraceptive users should consume 800 mcg daily.

If you are taking doses of trimethoprim greater than 25 mg per day, you should also take a supplement of 800 mcg of folic acid per day. This means that an average person needs 1,200 mcg per day, and a pregnant woman requires about 1,600 mcg daily.

GASTROINTESTINAL DISTURBANCES: Trimethoprim sometimes causes nausea, vomiting, and occasionally diarrhea.

Prevention and Treatment: The drug should be taken immediately following meals.

VINCRISTINE SULFATE

DRUG FAMILY: Anti-cancer

BRAND NAME: Oncovin

HOW TO TAKE VINCRISTINE SULFATE: Injection

FOODS TO AVOID: None

POSSIBLE SIDE EFFECTS: Malabsorption of all nutrients, sodium deficiency, constipation

ACTION OF VINCRISTINE SULFATE: This drug acts by preventing cells from multiplying.

HIGH-RISK GROUPS: Anyone who takes this drug

NUTRITIONAL INTERACTIONS

NUTRIENT MALABSORPTION: This drug can lead to atrophy of the lining of the intestines and to general malabsorption, especially of sodium. Sodium deficiency, called hyponatremia (low blood sodium levels), is characterized by a loss of appetite, nausea, vomiting, and muscle weakness. This hyponatremia is made worse by the fact that vincristine sulfate causes water retention, which further reduces the concentration of blood sodium. Your physician will attempt to control this water retention with other medications.

Prevention and Treatment: If you are taking vincristine sulfate, you should not simultaneously be on a low-salt diet. Because of the general malabsorption, you should also take a supplement that contains the recommended daily allowances of vitamins and minerals.

OTHER ADVICE: Most users of this drug also become severely constipated. To minimize this problem, your diet should have a plentiful supply of roughage, including dried or fresh fruit, salad vegetables, radishes, oatmeal, and whole grain foods (brown rice, whole wheat breads, and cereals). Persistent constipation may also be relieved by doubling the amount of fluid consumed each day. Bran, if used, should be added to the diet gradually, and your fluid intake should be increased by at least ¾ cup per teaspoon of bran. (See table of Dietary Fiber-Rich Foods, page 293.)

WARFARIN

DRUG FAMILY: Anti-coagulant

BRAND NAMES: Coumadin; Panwarfin; Warfarin Sodium

HOW TO TAKE WARFARIN: As directed by your physician

FOODS TO AVOID: Large amounts of foods rich in vitamin K, such as kale, spinach, cabbage, cauliflower, other leafy green vegetables, and liver; use alcohol only sparingly

POSSIBLE SIDE EFFECTS: Minor bleeding from such sites as the gums and vagina; bruising

ACTION OF WARFARIN: Commonly referred to as a blood thinner, warfarin decreases the rate at which blood clots. Warfarin is taken by patients who suffer from arteriosclerosis, because their blood tends to clot more readily than normal, which can lead to the blockage of blood vessels. If this happens in the brain or heart, a stroke or heart attack will occur.

HIGH-RISK GROUPS: The elderly; heavy drinkers

NUTRITIONAL INTERACTIONS

VITAMIN K DEFICIENCY: An improper balance of warfarin and vitamin K in the body is likely to cause interrelated problems. These drugs can prevent vitamin K from producing blood-clotting substances in the liver, but a diet that features excess amounts of vitamin K-rich foods can actually reduce the effectiveness of the drug.

People with an abnormally low dietary intake of vitamin K are at risk of hemorrhaging with unusual ease if they use this drug for a long period of time. Bleeding may take place in the gastrointestinal tract (causing black or blood-stained stools), in the urinary tract (causing blood in the urine), and in the uterus (causing blood loss at times other than the normal menstrual periods). Excessive blood loss may result from an injury or surgery. Another sign of deficiency of this vitamin is more frequent and more visible bruising than normal.

Women who have had several pregnancies or whose menstrual periods are heavy are at high risk of a vitamin K deficiency. Many of the elderly should also be careful because they have a problem of poor fat absorption, and vitamin K, a fat-soluble vitamin, must be accompanied by sufficient dietary fat to be properly absorbed.

Prevention and Treatment: You should not consume large amounts of foods rich in vitamin K. In particular, you should avoid eating large quantities of such foods as kale, spinach, cabbage, cauliflower, leafy green vegetables, and liver (especially pork liver) while taking warfarin. However, one should not go to the extreme and risk a hemorrhage by cutting out all such foods. Moderation is the key here.

Vitamin E supplements should not be taken while you are on warfarin, since vitamin E reduces the absorption of vitamin K and may cause bleeding; neither should a user take vitamin K supplements, which counteract the effects of the drug. Do not drink alcohol concurrently with this medication. Alcohol and drugs are broken down in the the liver by the same mechanism; if there is a high level of alcohol present, less of the drug is broken down. Hence, higher levels of this anti-coagulant build up in the body and can be extremely dangerous.

ZINC SULFATE

DRUG FAMILY: Mineral supplement

BRAND NAMES: ACE + Z; Besta; Eldercaps; Eldertonic; Glutofac; Hemocyte Plus; Mediplex; Vicon Forte; Vicon-C; Vicon-Plus; Vio-Bec Forte; Vi-Zac; Zinc-220; Zinckel-220

HOW TO TAKE ZINC SULFATE: With meals

FOODS TO AVOID: Milk or dairy products should not be consumed within 2 hours of consuming zinc sulfate

POSSIBLE SIDE EFFECTS: Copper deficiency, nausea, and diarrhea

ACTION OF ZINC SULFATE: This drug is used to treat people suffering from a zinc deficiency. It is also the drug of choice for treating the rare acrodermatitis enteropathica, a genetic disease that manifests itself after an infant has been weaned from breast milk. A child with this disease develops diarrhea and a severe rash that usually begins around the body's orifices. The child will not thrive, infections will occur, and, if the disease is not treated, the child will eventually die.

HIGH-RISK GROUPS: Children, heart patients, vegetarians

NUTRITIONAL INTERACTIONS

COPPER DEFICIENCY: A copper deficiency could conceivably be precipitated by the use of zinc supplements. The symptoms of this deficiency are anemia, neurological disturbances, abnormalities of connective tissues, and bruising.

Prevention and Treatment: Your mineral status should be monitored carefully while you are taking this drug. If necessary, a copper supplement of 3 mg of elemental copper should be taken at 2 or 3 hours' distance from the administration of the zinc sulfate. However, since excess copper also lowers high-density lipoprotein cholesterol (HDL, the good cholesterol), the copper supplements should also be carefully monitored; a reduction in HDL can increase the risk of heart disease.

OTHER ADVICE: Since absorption of zinc sulphate is reduced by milk or dairy products, it should not be taken with them.

Zinc supplements tend to be gastric irritants, and cause nausea and mild diarrhea in some people. To reduce the risk of these side effects, the supplements should be taken with meals.

Excess zinc tends to raise blood cholesterol levels; thus, people on long-term therapy should be carefully monitored since raised cholesterol levels increase the risk of heart disease.

Appendix I: Food Tables

ACIDIC FOODS

These foods produce acid when broken down in the body; this acid is excreted by the kidneys and contributes to the acidity of the urine. Acidic urine tends to increase the potency of drugs that are naturally acidic and decrease the potency of drugs that are naturally basic (alkaline). Although soft drinks, fruit juices, and wine are acidic foods, in that they contain acid which can irritate the stomach, they do not actually produce acid when broken down in the body and generally do not contribute to the acidity of urine.

Bacon	Fish
Brazil nuts	Lentils
Breads	Macaroni
Cakes	Meat
Cereals	Noodles
Cheese	Peanut Butter
Cookies	Peanuts
Corn	Plums
Crackers	Poultry
Cranberries	Prunes
Eggs	Spaghetti
Filberts	Walnuts

ALKALINE FOODS

These foods produce alkali when broken down in the body; this alkali is excreted by the kidneys and contributes to the alkalinity of the urine. Alkaline urine will tend to increase the potency of drugs that are naturally basic (alkaline) and decrease the potency of drugs that are naturally acidic.

> Almonds
> Buttermilk
> Chestnuts
> Coconuts
> Cream
> Fruits (all except cranberries, prunes, and plums)
> Milk
> Vegetables (all except corn and lentils)

CALCIUM-RICH FOODS

Calcium is needed to build bones and teeth, and to maintain bone strength. Approximately 99 percent of the body's calcium is found in these structures. They also form a reservoir of the mineral to maintain blood calcium at a constant level. The remaining 1 percent of body calcium helps to maintain cell membranes, keep cells in close association with one another, transport substances into and out of cells, and pass messages around the nervous system as well as to and from the muscles. It is also necessary for normal blood clotting and the activation of many enzymes.

Food	Serving	Calcium (mg)
Almonds	1 cup	500
Amaranth	4 ounces	500
Brewer's yeast	14 tablespoons	500
Broccoli	2¼ cups	500
Cheese, cottage	12 ounces	500
Cheese, sandwich	1½ to 2 ounces	500
Collard greens	1 cup	500
Custard	1 cup	500
Dandelion greens	1¼ cups	500
Ice cream	1⅔ cups	500
Kelp	1½ ounces	500

Food	Serving	Calcium (mg)
Mackerel, canned	3½ ounces	500
Milk, whole, low-fat, or buttermilk	8 ounces	500
Mustard greens	1½ cups	500
Oysters	12	500
Salmon, canned	5½ ounces	500
Sardines, canned	3½ ounces	500
Soybean curd	8 ounces	500
Yogurt	¾ cup	500

CHOLESTEROL-RICH FOODS

Blood cholesterol levels are closely related to what you eat. It has been shown that the levels of both cholesterol and fat in your blood can be changed by altering the amount and type of fat in your diet. In general, *saturated fats* (found in butter, lard, dairy products, fatty meats, chicken, coconut, egg yolk, and vegetable shortening) increase the level of cholesterol in your blood. On the other hand, *polyunsaturated fats* (found in liquid vegetable oils like corn, safflower, and soybean oils, along with walnuts, almonds, fish, and margarine) and *monounsaturated fats* to a lesser degree (found in avocados, cashews, olives, and peanuts) decrease cholesterol levels.

Cholesterol moves through the blood attached to specific blood proteins. The two main ones are low-density lipoproteins (LDL) and high-density lipoproteins (HDL); it should be said that LDL is "bad" and HDL is "good." The higher the level of LDL, the greater the risk of arteriosclerosis. HDL, on the other hand, carries cholesterol away from the tissues—including the linings of the arteries—back to the liver, and so it reduces the risk of heart disease.

The ratio of total cholesterol in your body to HDL cholesterol seems to be the best predictor of a future heart attack. This ratio also explains why so many people remain healthy with a total cholesterol level that could cause heart attacks in others. Conversely, your total cholesterol levels might be relatively low but with too great an LDL component, and you would be an excellent candidate for heart disease.

Three quarters of the heart attacks in this country happen among people with cholesterol levels between 150 and 300. Half occur in men with levels below 250. Recent studies indicate that anyone whose ratio of total cholesterol to HDL cholesterol is higher than 4.50 to 1 should be treated to lower that figure. A person with a total cholesterol level of 200 and an HDL level of 35 would have a ratio of 5.7 to 1—the one typically found in Americans who develop heart disease.

MEN AND WOMEN—IS THERE REALLY A DIFFERENCE?

This ratio effect goes a long way toward explaining why men have so many more heart attacks than women. Men and women start out with the same cholesterol levels, but at about puberty boys experience a 20 to 25 percent drop in protective HDL—leaving men with an average HDL level of 45 mg per 100 ml of blood, as opposed to the average 55 mg per 100 ml of blood found in women. This difference is believed to be the reason why there are 60 percent fewer deaths from heart attacks among American women than among American men.

After menopause, however, women lose this advantage. Their HDL levels fall, and their total cholesterol levels go up. You might think, then, that women after menopause are at an even higher risk than men, as their total cholesterol levels are higher—30 percent of women in this country and 25 percent of men have total levels above 240. However, this is *not* the case, because it merely means that there are more older women living than older men—and as we have seen, bad cholesterol levels rise with advancing age. Because a woman's blood cholesterol levels do not go up until after menopause, it takes quite a while before these elevated levels cause enough arteriosclerosis to result in deaths from heart attacks or strokes.

Many people have talked about how estrogen, the female hormone, protects women against heart disease. And although estrogen does seem to keep HDL at high levels in premenopausal women, too much estrogen also appears to be very harmful. Women taking oral contraceptives are actually at a greater risk for suffering from a heart attack than women who are pill-free. This is because oral contraceptives tend to cause clots in the blood vessels, which lead to heart attacks and strokes. (There is also evidence that the risk of clotting increases with the amount of estrogen taken—so it is important to keep the dose of the pill you are using as low as possible; you need just enough to prevent pregnancy and menstrual irregularities.)

Cigarette smoking by users of the pill increases the risk of adverse effects on the heart and blood vessels further. This risk accelerates with age and the amount smoked. Fifteen cigarettes a day or more in women over the age of thirty-five can have lethal effects.

People who are overweight show low levels of HDL. Weight loss increases these levels. So women who are above their ideal weight are not well-protected against cholesterol clogging, even if they do not use the pill and are still premenopausal.

THE BEST WAYS TO LOWER HARMFUL LEVELS

The diet, along with exercise, is the key to lowering harmful LDL levels, sometimes just by raising HDL levels. Several types of fiber appear to lower LDL and raise HDL. Pectin—which forms the pith of oranges and the major portion of the flesh of apples and root vegetables (like turnips)—is one such fiber. One to 2 ounces of pectin a day can lower some people's cholesterol by as much as 10 percent. To get this amount of pectin into your system, you have to eat five good-sized apples a day—it might be easier simply to buy the pure compound in your pharmacy and add it to your desserts.

Eating oatmeal, oat bran, and beans can also significantly reduce harmful levels—by as much as 10 to 20 percent—especially in people with high levels from the start. When you consider that a 1 percent drop in blood cholesterol levels reduces the risk of heart disease by 2 percent, you can see why these fiber-rich diets reduce the overall risk of getting the disease by 20 to 40 percent. And that's significant!

Other ways have been found to lower harmful levels. Japanese fishermen and Eskimos (who eat a lot of fish) rarely die of coronary artery disease. These groups seem to be protected by the high amount of fish oil in their diets—or rather, the eicosa-pentaenoic acid (EPA) it contains. Nobody knows yet why EPA protects the body against heart disease. It appears to reduce the amount of LDL in the blood, while raising HDL levels at the same time. It may also prevent the disk-shaped cells called platelets from sticking to the walls of the blood vessels at the areas of cholesterol deposits, which makes arteriosclerosis worse. (Incidentally, taking 1 aspirin every 2 days will have the same anti-sticking effect.) The moral here is that you should develop a taste for fish—the fattier the better. Mackerel is especially rich in EPA. Shellfish, which was recently thought to be harmful, is no longer carrying around its bad name—it also comes out on top. Original studies showed shellfish to be rich in cholesterol and so off-limits for heart patients. Newer analytical methods have shown that they contain enough of the beneficial EPA to compensate for the cholesterol they contain.

CHOLESTEROL-RICH FOODS

Food	Serving Size	Cholesterol (mg)
Bacon	2 ounces	33
Beef, cooked	4 ounces	94

Food	Serving Size	Cholesterol (mg)
Brie cheese	2 ounces	41
Butter	1 tablespoon	32
Caviar	1 tablespoon	48
Cheddar	2 ounces	40
Chicken, cooked	4 ounces	109
*Cod, cooked	4 ounces	68
*Crab, cooked	4 ounces	114
Heavy cream	1 tablespoon	21
Egg	1 medium	210
*Herring, cooked	4 ounces	111
Lamb, cooked	4 ounces	126
Liver, cooked	4 ounces	377
*Lobster, cooked	4 ounces	171
*Mackerel	4 ounces	90
Milk, whole	1 cup	34
Pork, cooked	4 ounces	126
Processed cheese	2 ounces	50
*Salmon, smoked	4 ounces	80
*Sardines, canned	4 ounces	114
*Shrimp, cooked	4 ounces	229
*Sole, cooked	4 ounces	68
Stilton cheese	2 ounces	69
Sweetbread, cooked	4 ounces	433
*Trout, cooked	4 ounces	91
*Tuna, packed in oil	3 ounces	56
Turkey, cooked	4 ounces	92

*Foods rich in EPA (see above)

DIETARY FIBER-RICH FOODS

Dietary fiber or roughage promotes good digestion and also helps to prevent the onset of many gastrointestinal diseases. Fiber is indigestible and passes through the digestive tract unchanged and so increases the bulk of the stool. This prevents constipation and development of diverticulosis. It also reduces the risk of developing cancer of the large intestine. Fiber derived from cereal is most effective for increasing the bulk of the stool. Thirty to 40 grams of pectin, the fiber found in the pith of oranges, the flesh of apples, and root vegetables (like turnips), reduces blood cholesterol levels by up to 10 percent. A comparable amount of fiber from oatmeal can reduce cholesterol levels by 10 to 20 percent in some people. This is important since a 1 percent drop in cholesterol levels reduces the risk of heart disease by 2 percent.

Food	Serving Size	Fiber (grams)
Apple, with skin	1 medium	2.0
Beans, baked	½ cup	7.3
Bran	½ cup	15.4
Bread, rye	1 slice	.13
Bread, whole wheat	1 slice	.4
Broccoli, cooked	1 cup	4.1
Brussels sprouts, cooked	1 cup	2.9
Cabbage, cooked	¾ cup	2.1
Carrots, cooked	¾ cup	3.7
Cereal, All-Bran	1 cup	19
Cereal, Grape-Nuts	½ cup	4.7
Cereal, Shredded Wheat	1 biscuit	3
Corn, cooked	1 ear	6.6
Corn, canned	½ cup	7.3
Cornflakes	1 cup	2.8
Lettuce, raw	1 cup	.75
Oatmeal	½ cup	8.4
Orange, raw	1 medium	2.6
Peach, with skin	1 medium	1.4
Peanuts, roasted	½ cup	5.8
Pear, with skin	1 medium	2.7
Peas, canned	½ cup	5.3
Pineapple, raw	1 cup	1.9
Plum, with skin	1 medium	1.4
Potatoes, baked	1	3
Raisins	½ ounce	1
Spinach	½ cup	3
Strawberries	1 cup	3.3
Tomatoes, raw	1	1.9
Turnips, boiled	3 ounces	2.2
Walnuts	½ cup	3.1

FAT COMPOSITION OF COMMONLY USED FATS AND OILS

In general, saturated fats increase blood cholesterol levels, while polyunsaturated fats and, to a much lesser extent, monounsaturated fats decrease blood cholesterol levels. The average American diet is high in saturated fats. Therefore, most people should try to include in their daily diets about 2 tablespoons of a vegetable oil with a high polyunsaturated-fat to saturated-fat ratio (see chart) to counteract the effects of their high saturated-fat diet.

	Saturated (grams)	Monounsaturated (grams)	Polyunsaturated (grams)
Butter, 1 tablespoon	9	5	trace
Coconut oil, 1 tablespoon	11	1	trace
Corn oil, 1 tablespoon	2	4	7
Cottonseed oil, 1 tablespoon	4	3	7
Margarine, 1 tablespoon hard (vegetable oils only)	5	7	2
soft (vegetable oils only)	5	6	3
Palm oil, 1 tablespoon	7	6	1
Peanut oil, 1 tablespoon	3	7	4
Olive oil, 1 tablespoon	2	10	2
Rape oil, 1 tablespoon	1	8	5
Safflower oil, 1 tablespoon	2	2	11
Sesame oil, 1 tablespoon	2	5	5
Soybean oil, 1 tablespoon	2	4	8
Sunflower oil, 1 tablespoon	2	5	7

FATTY FOODS

Large quantities of fatty animal foods should be avoided because animal fat tends to raise blood cholesterol levels. However, certain drugs must be dissolved in fat in the gastrointestinal tract if they are to be properly absorbed. Such drugs should be taken with regular milk, which is rich in fat, or some other food with a high fat content. Fat generally delays the emptying of the stomach and consequently slows down the movement of drugs into the small intestine, where the principal absorption occurs. Therefore, it is recommended that when you want a drug to work quickly, it should be taken on an empty stomach.

Food	Serving Size	Fat (grams)
Almonds	1 ounce	15
Avocado	1 (10 ounce)	37
Bacon	2 slices	8
Beef, cooked, lean or fat	3 ounces	16
Beef, ground, cooked	3 ounces	13
Beef, sirloin steak, cooked, lean or fat	3 ounces	27
Buttermilk	1 cup	8
Calves liver, fried	3 ounces	11
Cheese, blue	1 ounce	8
Cheese, cheddar	1 ounce	9
Cheese, cottage, creamed	1 cup	10
lowfat (2 percent)	1 cup	4
Cheese, American	1 ounce	9
Chocolate milk	1 cup	8
Corned beef	3 ounces	10
Egg	1	6
Ice cream, regular	1 cup	14
soft	1 cup	23
Lamb chop	3 ounces	31
Milk, whole	1 cup	8
Peanuts, roasted	1 ounce	14
Pork loin, cooked	3 ounces	28
Sardines	3 ounces	9
Sunflower seeds	1 ounce	14
Tuna, canned in oil, drained	3 ounces	7
Tuna salad	1 cup	22
Veal cutlet, cooked	3 ounces	9

FOLACIN-RICH FOODS

This vitamin is needed for the manufacture of nucleic acids—RNA and DNA, the genetic material found in all cells—as well as for the normal metabolism of certain amino acids (food proteins). In addition, it is necessary for the replacement of worn-out red blood cells, and hence for the prevention of anemia.

Food	Serving Size	Folic acid (mcg)
Apple	1 medium	5–20
Beans, green	1 cup	20–50
Beef, lean	6 ounces	5–20
Bread	1 slice	5–20
Brewer's yeast	1 tablespoon	100–150
Broccoli	2 stalks	100–150
Carrot	1 medium	5–20
Cheese, hard	1 ounce	5–20
Corn	1 medium ear	5–20
Cucumber	1 small	20–50
Egg	1 large	20–50
Grapefruit	½ medium	5–20
Kidney	3 ounces	20–50
Liver	3 ounces	100–150
Milk	8 ounces	5–20
Mushrooms	3 large	5–20
Orange juice	6 ounces	100–150
Pork, lean	6 ounces	5–20
Potato	1 medium	5–20
Sesame seeds	1 tablespoon	5–20
Shellfish	6 ounces	20–50
Spinach	4 ounces	100–150
Squash	⅔ cup	20–50
Strawberries	1 cup	20–50
Veal, lean	6 ounces	5–20
Yogurt	8 ounces	20–50

GOITROGEN-RICH FOODS

Goitrogens are substances that prevent the thyroid gland from producing thyroid hormones, causing goiter (thyroid hormone deficiency) if eaten regularly in large quantities. Although these substances cannot be prevented from acting by iodine, a good supply of dietary iodine (see table of Iodine-Rich Foods) can offer some protection against goitrogen-induced goiter. Cooking goitrogen-rich foods also greatly reduces the likelihood of goiter.

Brussels sprouts
Cabbage
Carrots
Cassava (from which tapioca pudding is made)
Cauliflower
Kale
Kelp, brown and green
Peaches
Pears
Rutabagas
Soybeans
Spinach
Turnips

IODINE-RICH FOODS

The thyroid gland needs iodine to enable it to produce thyroid hormone (thyroxine), which controls the rate at which the cells in the body work, as well as the rate of growth and the development of children.

Food	Serving Size	Iodine (mcg)
Baked goods	3 ounces	9
Cheese	2 ounces	8

Food	Serving Size	Iodine (mcg)
Egg	1 medium	7
Kelp	3 ounces	36
Meat	4 ounces	20
Milk	1 cup	34
Salt, iodized	1 gram	74
Seafood	4 ounces	62
Vegetables	3 ounces	24

IRON-RICH FOODS

This mineral is an integral part of hemoglobin in the blood and myoglobin in the muscles, which carry oxygen to the cells, and is also a part of many enzymes and proteins.

Food	Serving Size	Iron (mg)
Amaranth	3½ ounces	2.0–4
Apricots, dried	6 large halves	1.5–2
Barley	½ cup	1.5–2
Beans, green	1 cup	1.5–2
Beans, cooked	½ cup	2.0–4
Beef, lean	3 ounces	4.0–5
Berries	1 cup	.7–1.4
Bologna	3 to 4 ounces	1.5–2
Bread	1 slice	.3–.7
Brewer's yeast	1 tablespoon	1.5–2
Broccoli	1 cup	.7–1.4
Buckwheat	½ cup	1.5–2
Bulgur wheat, dry	2 tablespoons	.7–1.4
Carrots	1 cup	.7–1.4
Chicken, all cuts	3 to 4 ounces	1.5–2
Collards	1 cup	.7–1.4
Corn grits	1 cup	.3–.7
Cream of Wheat	1 cup	.7–1.4
Eggplant	½ cup	.3–.7

Food	Serving Size	Iron (mg)
Figs, dried	3 medium	2.0–4
Fruits, including apples, bananas, cherries, melons, citrus, pineapple, etc.	1 piece	.3–.7
Ham	2 ounces	1.5–2
Lamb, lean	4 ounces	4.0–5
Liver, calf's	1 ounce	4.0–5
Molasses, blackstrap	1 tablespoon	2.0–4
Mushrooms	⅓ cup	.3–.7
Oatmeal	1 cup	1.5–2
Pasta	½ cup	.3–.7
Peanut butter	2 tablespoons	.3–.7
Peas, cooked	½ cup	2.0–4
Popcorn (popped)	1 cup	.3–.7
Potato	1 medium	.7–1.4
Pumpkin seeds	1 to 2 tablespoons	.7–1.4
Raisins	½ cup	4.0–5
Rice, cooked, white or brown	1 cup	.7–1.4
Tomato	1 small	.3–.7
Soybean curd	4 ounces	2.0–4
Tortilla	6-inch diam.	.7–1.4
Wheatena	⅔ cup	.7–1.4

MAGNESIUM-RICH FOODS

This mineral helps in building bones, in the manufacture of body proteins, in the release of energy from carbohydrates, and in the conduction of nerve impulses to the muscles.

Food	Serving Size	Magnesium (mg)
Almonds	1 ounce	77
Avocado	3 ounces	39
Beet greens, raw	1 cup	154
Bran	1 ounce	140

Food	Serving Size	Magnesium (mg)
Brazil nuts	1 ounce	65
Cashews	1 ounce	76
Cereal, whole grain	1 ounce	38
Cheese	2 ounces	27
Chocolate	2 ounces	167
Hazelnuts	1 ounce	53
Lima beans, cooked	1 cup	91
Peanuts	1 ounce	50
Pecans	1 ounce	41
Pistachios	1 ounce	45
Shrimp, cooked	4 ounces	58
Soybean curd	3 ounces	95
Spinach, cooked	1 cup	113
Walnuts	1 ounce	37
Wheat germ	1 ounce	96

OXALATE-RICH FOODS

This substance, if taken in large enough quantities, can lead to the formation of kidney stones in susceptible people.

Beans, baked	Mustard greens
Beans, green	Okra
Beets	Parsley
Blueberries	Peppers, green
Celery	Raspberries
Chocolate	Soybean curd
Cocoa	Spinach
Collard greens	Squash, summer
Dandelion greens	Strawberries
Eggplant	Tangerines
Grapes	Tea
Kale	Watercress
Lemon peel	Wheat germ

PHOSPHORUS-RICH FOODS

The mineral phosphorus is needed by the body to help keep the acidity of the blood at a normal level, to help build strong bones and teeth, for the release of energy from carbohydrates, proteins, and fats, and for the formation of nucleic acids, cell membranes, and many enzymes.

Food	Serving Size	Phosphorus (mg)
Almonds	1 ounce	126
Apricots, dried	3 ounces	102
Brains, cooked	4 ounces	389
Bran	1 ounce	257
Brazil nuts	1 ounce	169
Cereal, whole grain	1 ounce	97
Cheese	2 ounces	163–432
Chocolate, milk	3 ounces	119–206
Cocoa	1 gram	189
Fish, cooked	4 ounces	143–572
Kidneys, cooked	4 ounces	411
Liver, cooked	4 ounces	212
Milk	1 cup	226
Peanuts	1 ounce	107
Peas, cooked	1 cup	86
Walnuts	1 ounce	146

POTASSIUM-RICH FOODS

This mineral is needed for proper muscle contraction (including the heart muscle), and for the maintenance of the correct fluid balance and correct level of alkali in the body. It also aids in the transmission of nerve impulses, along with the release of energy from carbohydrate and protein.

Food	Serving Size	Potassium (mg)
Apricots, dried	1 cup	1,273
Avocado, Florida	1	1,836
Banana	1 small	440
Beans, lima	1 cup	724
Brussels sprouts, fresh cooked	1 cup	423
Carrots, cooked	1 cup	344
Chicken, broiled	6 ounces	483
Clams, soft	3 ounces	225
Dates, pitted	10	518
Flounder	6 ounces	1,000
Milk, skim	1 cup	406
Orange juice	1 cup	496
Potato, baked	1 medium	782
Prunes, dried and pitted	5 large	298
Spinach, chopped and cooked	1 cup	688
Sweetbreads	3 ounces	433
Tomato, raw	1 medium	300
Tuna, salt-free, canned	1 small container	327
Yogurt, plain	1 container	531

PURINE-RICH FOODS

In susceptible people, consuming large amounts of foods containing purine will increase their chances of contracting gout.

40 to 125 mg per 3 ounces	125 to 700 mg per 3 ounces
Beans, dry	
Fish	Anchovies
Lentils	Brains
Meats	Kidneys
Peas, dry	Liver
Poultry	Meat extracts
Seafood	Sardines
Spinach	Sweetbreads

PROTEIN-RICH FOODS

Foods rich in protein tend to delay the emptying of the stomach and delay the movement of drugs into the small intestine, where the principal absorption occurs. Hence it is often better to take a drug on an empty stomach when you want it to work quickly. Foods rich in protein can produce an acidic urine. An acidic urine decreases the excretion of acidic drugs, permitting them to remain in the blood for longer periods of time and thereby increasing their potency. By contrast, alkaline drugs are excreted more rapidly and, for that reason, become less potent. Sometimes foods rich in protein can complement the action of a drug, as is the case with certain antibiotics given for urinary tract infections, because bacterial growth is impaired in acidic urine.

Food	Serving Size	Protein (grams)
Baked beans	1 ounce	13
Beef, cooked		
lean or fat	3 ounces	23
Beef, ground, cooked	3 ounces	22
Beef, sirloin steak, cooked,		
lean or fat	3 ounces	20
Bluefish, cooked	3 ounces	22
Calves liver, fried	3 ounces	25
Cheese, blue	1 ounce	7
Cheese, cheddar	1 ounce	6
Cheese, cottage, creamed	1 cup	28
lowfat (2 percent)	1 cup	31
Cheese, Swiss	1 ounce	8
Cheese, American	1 ounce	6
Chicken, breast, cooked	3 ounces	28
drumstick, boned, cooked	3 ounces	28
Clams, raw (meat only)	3 ounces	11
Egg	1	6
Lamb chop, cooked	3 ounces	18
Lentils, cooked	1 cup	16
Lima beans, cooked	1 cup	16
Milk, whole	1 cup	8
Milk, lowfat (2 percent)	1 cup	8
Pork, loin, cooked	3 ounces	21
Peanuts, roasted	1 ounce	8

Food	Serving Size	Protein (grams)
Salmon, cooked	3 ounces	17
Shrimp, cooked	3 ounces	21
Sunflower seeds	1 ounce	7
Tuna, canned in oil, drained	3 ounces	24
Veal cutlet, cooked	3 ounces	23
Yogurt, low fat, fruit flavored	8 ounces	10

SIMPLE AND COMPLEX CARBOHYDRATE FOODS

A simple carbohydrate, like the refined sugar in your coffee, has no nutrient value. All it contains is empty calories. But complex carbohydrates are found in foods like potatoes and many other vegetables, and are rich in nutrients and essential to good health.

Simple	Complex
Cakes	Beans
Candies	Breads
Cookies	Carrots
Corn syrup	Cereals
Fruits, dried	Corn
Fruits, fresh	Crackers
Honey	Nuts
Jams	Parsnips
Jellies	Pasta
Molasses	Peas
Soda	Potatoes
Sugar, maple	Sweet potatoes
Sugar, table	Winter squash

SODIUM-RICH FOODS

This mineral is needed for proper muscle contraction, and for the maintenance of the correct fluid balance and correct level of alkali in the body. It also aids in the transmission of nerve impulses. However, excess intake can lead to hypertension, so you should restrict the sodium in your diet to the level your physician recommends.

Food	Serving Size	Sodium (mg)
Bacon, broiled	3 ounces	875
Beans, baked	1 cup	862
Beans, lima	1 cup	192
Beets, canned	1 cup	378
Bread, cracked wheat	1 slice	132
Bread, raisin	1 slice	91
Bread, rye	1 slice	139
Bread, white	1 slice	127
Bread, whole wheat	1 slice	148
Butter, salted	1 ounce	282
Buttermilk	1 cup	319
Cheese, cheddar	2 ounces	400
Cheese, creamed cottage	2 ounces	131
Chicken, cooked	4 ounces	73–98
Clams, cooked	4 ounces	137
Corn, canned	1 cup	496
Corn, sweet	1 cup	25
Cornflakes	1 ounce	287
Crab, cooked	4 ounces	1,140
Egg, cooked	1 medium	61
Fish, cooked	4 ounces	125–202
Ham, cooked	4 ounces	1,063
Liver, cooked	4 ounces	210
Lobster, cooked	4 ounces	239
Margarine, regular	1 ounce	282
Margarine, unsalted	1 ounce	3
Olives, green	4 medium	384
Parmesan	2 ounces	419
Peanut butter	1 ounce	173
Peas, canned	1 cup	401
Pickles, dill	1	857

Food	Serving Size	Sodium (mg)
Pickles, sweet	1	79
Pretzels	1	269
Salad dressing	1 tablespoon	96–335
Sardines, cooked	4 ounces	938
Sausage, cooked	4 ounces	1,095
Scallops, cooked	4 ounces	302
Shrimp, cooked	4 ounces	212
Tomato catsup	1 tablespoon	201
Tomato juice	1 cup	486
Turkey, roast	4 ounces	148
Veal, roast	4 ounces	91

TYRAMINE-RICH FOODS

People suffering from severe depression are sometimes treated with drugs called monoamine-oxidase (MAO) inhibitors, which block the action of the enzyme monoamine-oxidase. Tyramine, a substance found in some foods, normally undergoes conversion in the body to an inactive form through the action of this enzyme. When MAO inhibitors are administered, tyramine remains active and causes the release of the chemical norepinephrine, which leads to constriction of the blood vessels. As a result, the patient can develop severe hypertension and headaches. In extreme cases, the blood pressure can even rise to a fatal level.

> Alcoholic beverages (especially sherry, beer, and
>   such wines as Chianti)
> Bananas
> Bologna
> Broad beans
> Canned Figs
> Cheeses: processed American, Boursault, blue
>   (including Stilton, Roquefort, etc.), Brie,
>   Camembert, cheddar, Gruyère, Mozzarella,
>   Parmesan, and Romano
> Chocolate
> Eggplant

Hot dogs
Liver (chicken and beef)
Meat tenderizers
Pepperoni
Pickled herring
Pineapple
Plums
Salami
Soy sauce
Yeast extracts

VITAMIN A-RICH FOODS

This vitamin is needed for the health of the skin and the epithelial tissues (inner lining of the body). It helps to maintain the structure of cell membranes and is necessary for the healthy functioning of the immune system. Vitamin A is also needed for the maintenance and growth of teeth, hair, eyes, bones, and glands. It occurs in two main forms in nature—as retinol, found only in animal sources, and certain carotenoids, found only in vegetables. Carotenoids are one third as potent as retinol.

Food	Serving Size	Vitamin A (IU)
Apricots, dried	6 halves	2,540
Asparagus	½ cup	605
Beans, green	½ cup	340
Broccoli	½ cup	2,363
Brussels sprouts	½ cup	405
Cantaloupe	½ cup	6,540
Carrots	½ cup	7,610
Corn	1 small ear	310
Egg	1 medium	590
Liver, beef	4 ounces	60,560
Milk, whole	1 cup	350
Orange juice	½ cup	270
Peach	1 medium	1,320
Peas, green	½ cup	430
Potato, sweet	½ cup	8,500

Food	Serving Size	Vitamin A (IU)
Pumpkin	½ cup	8,207
Squash, summer	½ cup	410
Squash, winter	½ cup	4,305
Tomato juice	½ cup	970
Yogurt	½ cup	340

VITAMIN B₁ (THIAMIN)-RICH FOODS

Vitamin B_1 (thiamin) is needed for the metabolism of carbohydrates, for muscle coordination, and for the maintenance of nerve tissue.

Food	Serving Size	Vitamin B₁ (mg)
Asparagus	½ cup	.12
Beans, dried	½ cup	.13
Beef liver	4 ounces	.31
Cereal	½ cup	.10
Collard greens	½ cup	.14
Dandelion greens	½ cup	.12
Ham	4 ounces	.53
Lamb, leg of	4 ounces	.17
Lima beans	½ cup	.16
Macaroni, enriched	½ cup	.10
Milk, 2 percent fat fortified	1 cup	.10
Orange	1 medium	.13
Orange juice	½ cup	.11
Oysters	¾ cup	.25
Pork, lean roast	4 ounces	1.21
Rice, enriched	½ cup	.12
Spaghetti, enriched	½ cup	.10
Veal, roast	4 ounces	.15

VITAMIN B₂ (RIBOFLAVIN)-RICH FOODS

Vitamin B_2 (riboflavin) helps the body convert proteins, fats, and carbohydrates into energy. It is needed for building and maintaining body tissues, and for protecting the body against many skin and eye disorders.

Food	Serving Size	Vitamin B₂ (mg)
Asparagus	½ cup	.13
Beef, lean roast	4 ounces	.25
Broccoli	⅓ cup	.12
Brussels sprouts	½ cup	.11
Cheese, creamed cottage	½ cup	.30
Chicken, skinless	4 ounces	.21
Collard greens	½ cup	.19
Egg	1 medium	.15
Ham	4 ounces	.21
Hamburger	4 ounces	.24
Lamb, leg of	4 ounces	.31
Liver, beef	4 ounces	4.8
Milk, 2 percent fat fortified	1 cup	.52
Milk, skim	1 cup	.44
Milk, whole	1 cup	.41
Salmon, canned	3 ounces	.16
Sardines	4 ounces	.23
Spinach	½ cup	.11
Squash, winter	½ cup	.14
Tuna, canned	3 ounces	.11
Veal, roast	4 ounces	.35
Yogurt	½ cup	.19

VITAMIN B₃ (NIACIN)-RICH FOODS

This vitamin is found in all cells of the body and is essential for many metabolic processes, such as the conversion of food into energy, the manufacture of fat, protein metabolism, and the use of oxygen by the tissues. The term "niacin" really refers to two compounds, nicotinic acid and nicotinamide (also called niacinamide). Consuming large amounts of nicotinic acid, but not nicotinamide, can produce dilation of the blood vessels or a "flushing" effect.

Food	Serving Size	Niacin (mg)
Asparagus, cooked	1 cup	1.9
Banana	1 small	.7
Beef	4 ounces	5.7
Bread, enriched	1 slice	.5
Bread, whole wheat	1 slice	.8
Chicken	4 ounces	8
Corn muffin	1	1.3
Corn, sweet	1 cup	2.4
Lamb	4 ounces	5.7
Liver, cooked	4 ounces	18.2
Peaches, fresh	1 medium	1
Peanut butter	1 tablespoon	2.5
Peas, fresh or frozen, cooked	1 cup	3.2
Pork	4 ounces	5.7
Potato, boiled	1 medium	1.6
Rice, long-grain, cooked	1 cup	2.1
Swordfish, cooked	4 ounces	11.4
Tuna, canned	3 ounces	12.7
Turkey	4 ounces	8
Veal	4 ounces	8

VITAMIN B$_6$ (PYRIDOXINE)-RICH FOODS

Vitamin B$_6$ (pyridoxine) is needed for amino acid metabolism, the formation of certain proteins, and the proper functioning of the nervous system.

Food	Serving Size	Vitamin B$_6$ (mg)
Bananas	1 medium	.61
Beef, cooked	4 ounces	.30
Bran flakes	1 cup	.29
Cabbage, cooked	1 cup	.10
Carrots, cooked	1 cup	.10
Fish, cooked	4 ounces	.23 –.95

Food	Serving Size	Vitamin B$_6$ (mg)
Grape-Nuts cereal	3 ounces	2.41
Lamb cutlets, cooked with bone	4 ounces	.14
Liver, cooked	4 ounces	.83
Milk	1 cup	.10
Oatmeal	1 cup	.29
Peanuts	1 cup	.58
Pork, cooked	4 ounces	.47
Potato, baked	1 medium	.28
Veal, cooked	4 ounces	.36

VITAMIN B$_{12}$-RICH FOODS

Vitamin B$_{12}$ is needed for the normal development of red blood cells and for the healthy functioning of all cells, particularly those in the bone marrow, nervous system, and intestines.

Food	Serving Size	Vitamin B$_{12}$ (mcg)
Beef, cooked	4 ounces	1–2
Cheese	2 ounces	.8
Chicken, cooked	4 ounces	1
Egg, cooked	1 medium	.8
Fish, fatty, cooked	4 ounces	5–28
Lamb, cooked	4 ounces	1–2
Liver, cooked	4 ounces	28–121
Milk	1 cup	.7
Pork, cooked	4 ounces	1–3
Veal, cooked	4 ounces	1.1
Whitefish, cooked	4 ounces	1–5

VITAMIN C-RICH FOODS

Vitamin C (ascorbic acid) is needed for the production of collagen, the intercellular cement that gives structure to the muscles, blood vessels, bones, and cartilage. It also contributes to the health of teeth and gums, and aids in the body's absorption of iron.

Food	Serving Size	Vitamin C (mg)
Broccoli, cooked	1 cup	140
Brussels sprouts, cooked	1 cup	135
Cantaloupe	half, 5-inch diameter	63
Cauliflower, cooked	1 cup	66
Collard greens, cooked	1 cup	87
Cranberry juice	1 cup	81
Grapefruit juice	1 cup	102
Kale, cooked	1 cup	68
Lemon juice	1 cup	112
Mustard greens	1 cup	68
Orange	1 medium	66
Orange juice	1 cup	102
Parsley, raw, chopped	1 cup	68
Papaya	1 cup, cubed	102
Pepper, raw, green	1	94
Pineapple juice	1 cup	80
Spinach, cooked	1 cup	50
Strawberries	1 cup	88
Turnip greens, cooked	1 cup	68

VITAMIN D-RICH FOODS

The major function of this vitamin is to regulate calcium and phosphate metabolism, which is necessary for the development of healthy, strong teeth and bones.

Food	Serving Size	Vitamin D (IU)
Cheese	2 ounces	.5–7.0
Egg, cooked	1 medium	28–36
Herring, broiled	4 ounces	1,003
Liver, calf's, cooked	4 ounces	11.4
Milk	1 quart	400
Salmon, canned	3 ounces	428.6
Sardines, canned in oil	3 ounces	257.1
Tuna, canned in oil	3 ounces	198.9

VITAMIN E-RICH FOODS

Although the role of vitamin E in our bodies is ill defined, everybody agrees it has an important role in protecting our cell membranes from wear and tear. Some evidence indicates that the vitamin can facilitate the healing of burns and wounds when topically applied. Anybody taking drugs that cause mal-absorption of fat should be sure to include in his diet some foods rich in vitamin E, since these drugs will impair the absorption of E.

Food	Serving Size	Vitamin E (mgs)*
Almonds, raw	1 ounce	7
Coconut	1 ounce	1
Cod liver oil	1 tablespoon	3
Corn oil	1 tablespoon	12
Cottonseed oil	1 tablespoon	9
Olive oil	1 tablespoon	2
Palm oil	1 tablespoon	5
Peanuts, raw	1 ounce	5
Pecans, raw	1 ounce	6
Rape oil	1 tablespoon	6
Safflower oil	1 tablespoon	5
Sesame oil	1 tablespoon	4
Soybean oil	1 tablespoon	13
Soybeans, dry	3 ounces	17

Food	Serving Size	Vitamin E (mgs)*
Sunflower oil	1 tablespoon	9
Walnuts, raw	1 ounce	6
Wheat germ oil	1 tablespoon	36

*Expressed as alpha tocopherol. 1 mg of alpha tocopherol is equivalent to 1 IU of vitamin E. The other tocopherols are less potent.

VITAMIN K-RICH FOODS

Vitamin K is needed for the manufacture of certain substances in the liver responsible for blood clotting.

Food	Serving Size	Vitamin K (mcg)
Asparagus, cooked	1 cup	82.7
Bacon, cooked	2 ounces	26.3
Bread, whole wheat	1 slice	4.8
Broccoli, cooked	1 cup	310
Cabbage, cooked	1 cup	87.5
Cheese	2 ounces	20
Lettuce	1 outer, 2 inner, 3 heart leaves	29.4
Liver, beef, cooked	4 ounces	104.9
Oats, rolled	1 cup	48
Spinach, cooked	1 cup	160.2
Turnip greens, cooked	1 cup	942.5
Watercress	1 ounce	16.3

ZINC-RICH FOODS

The mineral zinc is involved in the manufacture of DNA and body protein. It also aids in the proper action of insulin, helps the body's use of vitamin A, and is essential for the normal functioning of the immune system.

Food	Serving Size	Zinc (mg)
Applesauce	1 cup	.2–.5
Beef, lean	3½ ounces	4.0–5.0
Bran	¾ cup	1.0–1.5
Bread, white	2 slices	.5–1
Bread, whole wheat	2 slices	1.0–1.5
Cheddar cheese	1 ounce	.5–1
Chicken breast	3 ounces	.5–1
Clams	3 ounces	1.0–1.5
Cranberry-apple drink	8 ounces	.5–1
Egg	1 medium	.2–.5
Gefilte fish	3½ ounces	.2–.5
Lamb	3½ ounces	4.0–5.0
Liver	3 ounces	4.0–5.0
Mango	½ medium	.2–.5
Milk, whole or skim	8 ounces	.5–1
Oysters, Atlantic	3½ ounces	74.7
Oysters, Pacific	3½ ounces	9.4
Pineapple juice	8 ounces	.2–.5
Popcorn	2 cups	1.0–1.5
Pork, lean	3½ ounces	4.0–5.0
Potato, cooked	1 medium	.2–.5
Puffed wheat	1 ounce	.5–1
Rice, brown	1 cup	1.0–1.5
Rice, white	1 cup	.5–1
Tomato	1 medium	.2–.5
Tuna	3 ounces	.5–1
Wheat germ	1 tablespoon	1.0–1.5

Appendix II: Supplement Tables

RECOMMENDED DIETARY ALLOWANCES (RDA)

The Recommended Dietary Allowance (RDA) values are established by the Food and Nutrition Board of the National Research Council. The RDA are the quantities of each nutrient that should be included in the diet each day.

RDA levels are not minimums. They are designed with a safety margin planned to provide for the needs of various stresses and to make possible other potential improvements in body growth and function. The U.S. RDA, often listed on food labels, takes the highest RDA (whether it is found in the male, female, or child values) and recommends that value to all people.

Age (years)	Weight (kg)	Weight (lbs)	Height (cm)	Height (in)	Protein (g)	(RE)[2] Vitamin A	(mcg)[3] Vitamin D	(mg) Vitamin E	(mg) Vitamin C	(mg) Thiamin	(mg) Riboflavin	(mg equiv.) Niacin[4]	(mg) Vitamin B$_6$	(mcg) Folacin	(mcg) Vitamin B$_{12}$	(mg) Calcium	(mg) Phosphorus	(mg) Magnesium	(mg) Iron	(mg) Zinc	(mcg) Iodine
Infants																					
0.0-0.5	6	13	60	24	kg × 2.2	420	10	3	35	0.3	0.4	6	0.3	30	0.5	360	240	50	10	3	40
0.5-1.0	9	20	71	28	kg × 2.0	400	10	4	35	0.5	0.6	8	0.6	45	1.5	540	360	70	15	5	50
Children																					
1-3	13	29	90	35	23	400	10	5	45	0.7	0.8	9	0.9	100	2.0	800	800	150	15	10	70
4-6	20	44	112	44	30	500	10	6	45	0.9	1.0	11	1.3	200	2.5	800	800	200	10	10	90
7-10	28	62	132	52	34	700	10	7	45	1.2	1.4	16	1.6	300	3.0	800	800	250	10	10	120
Males																					
11-14	45	99	157	62	45	1,000	10	8	50	1.4	1.6	18	1.8	400	3.0	1,200	1,200	350	18	15	150
15-18	66	145	176	69	56	1,000	10	10	60	1.4	1.7	18	2.0	400	3.0	1,200	1,200	400	18	15	150
19-22	70	154	177	70	56	1,000	7.5	10	60	1.5	1.7	19	2.2	400	3.0	800	800	350	10	15	150
23-50	70	154	178	70	56	1,000	5	10	60	1.4	1.6	18	2.2	400	3.0	800	800	350	10	15	150
51 +	70	154	178	70	56	1,000	5	10	60	1.2	1.4	16	2.2	400	3.0	800	800	350	10	15	150

Age (years)	Weight (kg)	(lbs)	Height (cm)	(in)	Protein (g)	(RE)[2] Vitamin A	(mcg)[3] Vitamin D	(mg) Vitamin E	(mg) Vitamin C	(mg) Thiamin	(mg) Riboflavin	(mg equiv.) Niacin[4]	(mg) Vitamin B_6	(mcg) Folacin	(mcg) Vitamin B_{12}	(mg) Calcium	(mg) Phosphorus	(mg) Magnesium	(mg) Iron	(mg) Zinc	(mcg) Iodine
Females																					
11-14	46	101	157	62	46	800	10	8	50	1.1	1.3	15	1.8	400	3.0	1,200	1,200	300	18	15	150
15-18	55	120	163	64	46	800	10	8	60	1.1	1.3	14	2.0	400	3.0	1,200	1,200	300	18	15	150
19-22	55	120	163	64	44	800	7.5	8	60	1.1	1.3	14	2.0	400	3.0	800	800	300	18	15	150
23-50	55	120	163	64	44	800	5	8	60	1.0	1.2	13	2.0	400	3.0	800	800	300	18	15	150
51+	55	120	163	64	44	800	5	8	60	1.0	1.2	13	2.0	400	3.0	800	800	300	10	15	150
Pregnant[1]					+30	+200	+5	+2	+20	+0.4	+0.3	+2	+0.6	+400	+1.0	+400	+400	+150		+5	+25
Lactating[2]					+20	+400	+5	+3	+40	+0.5	+0.5	+5	+0.5	+100	+1.0	+400	+400	+150		+10	+50

[1]Pregnant and lactating women are well advised to take iron supplements as recommended by their physician.
[2]1 RE, = 5 IU
[3]1 mcg = 40 IU
[4]One mg equivalent is equal to 1 mg of niacin or 60 mg of tryptophan.

Reproduced from Recommended Dietary Allowances, 9th ed. (1980), National Academy of Sciences, Washington, D.C.

VITAMIN AND MINERAL SUPPLEMENTS FOR CHILDREN

These are a sampling of popular vitamin and mineral supplements, showing the amounts of essential nutrients they contain.

Only the nutrients discussed in the interactions have been included. The other ingredients have been omitted.

Brand Name:	Bugs Bunny Plus Iron (Miles Labs)	Centrum Junior (Lederle)	Chewable for children (Radiance)
VITAMINS:			
A (IU)	2,500	5,000	4,000
D (IU)	400	400	400

Brand Name:	Bugs Bunny Plus Iron (Miles Lab)	Centrum Junior (Lederle)	Chewable for Children (Radiance)
E (IU)	15	15	3.4
C (mg)	60	60	60
B$_1$ (mg)	1.05	1.5	2
B$_2$ (mg)	1.2	1.7	2.4
B$_6$ (mg)	1.05	2	2
B$_{12}$ (mcg)	4.5	6	10
Niacin (mg)	13.5	20	10
Folacin (mg)	.3	.4	-
MINERALS			
Calcium (mg)	-	-	19
Phosphorus (mg)	-	-	-
Iron (mg)	15	18	12
Potassium (mg)	-	-	4
Magnesium (mg)	-	25	22
Zinc (mg)	-	10	-
Copper (mg)	-	2	.2
Iodine (mcg)	-	50	-

Brand Name	Flintstones Plus Iron (Miles Labs.)	Poly-Vi-Sol w/Iron and Zinc Chewable (Mead Johnson)	Poly-Vi-Sol w/Iron Drops (Mead Johnson)
VITAMINS			
A (IU)	2,500	2,500	1,500
D (IU)	400	400	400
E (IU)	15	15	5
C (mg)	60	60	35
B$_1$ (mg)	1.05	1.05	.5
B$_2$ (mg)	1.2	1.2	.6
B$_6$ (mg)	1.05	1.05	.4
B$_{12}$ (mcg)	4.5	4.5	-
Niacin (mg)	13.5	13.5	8
Folacin (mg)	.3	.3	-

Brand Name:	Flintstones Plus Iron (Miles Labs.)	Poly-Vi-Sol w/Iron and Zinc Chewable (Mead Johnson)	Poly-Vi-Sol w/Iron Drops (Mead Johnson)
MINERALS			
Calcium (mg)	-	-	-
Phosphorus (mg)	-	-	-
Iron (mg)	15	12	10
Potassium (mg)	-	-	-
Magnesium (mg)	-	-	-
Zinc (mg)	-	8	-
Copper (mg)	-	-	-
Iodine (mcg)	-	-	-

Brand Name:	Unicap Chewable (Upjohn)	Vita-Lea Chewables (Shaklee)
VITAMINS		
A (IU)	5,000	2,000
D (IU)	400	400
E (IU)	15	10
C (mg)	60	60
B_1 (mg)	1.5	1.1
B_2 (mg)	1.7	1.2
B_6 (mg)	2	1.5
B_{12} (mcg)	6	3
Niacin (mg)	20	14
Folacin (mg)	.4	.3
MINERALS		
Calcium (mg)	-	130
Phosphorus (mg)	-	100
Iron (mg)	-	10
Potassium (mg)	-	-
Magnesium (mg)	-	60
Zinc (mg)	-	1.5
Copper (mg)	-	0.2
Iodine (mcg)	-	15

VITAMIN AND MINERAL SUPPLEMENTS FOR ADULTS

These are a sampling of popular vitamin and mineral supplements, showing the amounts of essential nutrients they contain.

Only the nutrients discussed in the interactions have been included. The other ingredients have been omitted.

Brand Name:	Centrum A to Zinc (Lederle)
VITAMINS	
A (IU)	5,000
D (IU)	400
E (IU)	30
C (mg)	90
B$_1$ (mg)	2.25
B$_2$ (mg)	2.6
B$_6$ (mg)	3.0
B$_{12}$ (mcg)	9
Niacin (mg)	20
Folacin (mg)	.4
MINERALS	
Calcium (mg)	162
Phosphorus (mg)	125
Iron (mg)	27
Potassium (mg)	7.7
Magnesium (mg)	100
Zinc (mg)	22.5
Copper (mg)	3
Iodine (mcg)	150

Brand Name:	Myadec (Parke-Davis)
VITAMINS	
A (IU)	10,000
D (IU)	400
E (IU)	30

Brand Name:	Myadec (Parke-Davis)
C (mg)	250
B_1 (mg)	10
B_2 (mg)	10
B_6 (mg)	5
B_{12} (mcg)	6
Niacin (mg)	100
Folacin (mg)	.4
MINERALS	
Calcium (mg)	-
Phosphorus (mg)	-
Iron (mg)	20
Potassium (mg)	-
Magnesium (mg)	100
Zinc (mg)	20
Copper (mg)	2
Iodine (mcg)	150

Brand Name:	One-A-Day Plus Iron (Miles Labs.)	One-A-Day Plus Minerals (Miles Labs.)	Poly-Vi-Sol w/Iron Chewable (Mead Johnson)
VITAMINS			
A (IU)	5,000	5,000	2,500
D (IU)	400	400	400
E (IU)	30	30	15
C (mg)	60	60	60
B_1 (mg)	1.5	1.5	1.05
B_2 (mg)	1.7	1.7	1.2
B_6 (mg)	2	2	1.05
B_{12} (mcg)	6	6	4.5
Niacin (mg)	20	20	13.5
Folacin (mg)	.4	.4	.3
K (mcg)	50	50	-

Brand Name:	One-A-Day Plus Iron (Miles Labs.)	One-A-Day Plus Minerals (Miles Labs.)	Poly-Vi-Sol w/Iron Chewable (Mead Johnson)
MINERALS			
Calcium (mg)	-	130	-
Phosphorus (mg)	-	100	-
Iron (mg)	18	18	12
Potassium (mg)	-	37.5	-
Magnesium (mg)	-	100	-
Zinc (mg)	-	15	8
Copper (mg)	-	2	-
Iodine (mcg)	-	150	-

Brand Name:	Stresstabs 600 (Lederle)	Theragran-M (Squibb)
VITAMINS		
A (IU)	-	10,000
D (IU)	-	400
E (IU)	30	15
C (mg)	600	200
B_1 (mg)	15	10
B_2 (mg)	15	10
B_6 (mg)	5	5
B_{12} (mcg)	12	5
Niacin (mg)	100	100
Folacin (mg)	-	-
MINERALS		
Calcium (mg)	-	-
Phosphorus (mg)	-	-
Iron (mg)	-	12
Potassium (mg)	-	-
Magnesium (mg)	-	65
Zinc (mg)	-	1.5
Copper (mg)	-	2
Iodine (mcg)	-	150

Bibliography

Anderson, L., M. S. Dibbie, P. R. Turkki, H. S. Mitchell, and H. J. Rynbergen. *Nutrition in Health and Disease*. Philadelphia: J. B. Lippincott Company, 1982.

Basu, T. K. *Clinical Implications of Drug Use*, Vols. I and II. Boca Raton, Fla.: CRC Press, 1980.

Goodhart, R. S., and M. E. Shils. *Modern Nutrition in Health and Disease*, 6th ed. Philadelphia: Lea and Febiger, 1980.

Goodman, A., L. S. Gilman, and A. Gilman. *The Pharmacological Basis of Therapeutics*, 6th ed. New York: The Macmillan Co., Inc., 1980.

Hathcock, J. N., and J. Coon. *Nutrition and Drug Interactions*. New York: Academic Press, 1978.

Modell, W. *Drugs of Choice, 1984–1985*. St. Louis: C. V. Mosby Co., 1984.

Morgan, B. L. G. *The Lifelong Nutrition Guide*. Englewood Cliffs, N.J.: Prentice-Hall, Inc., 1983.

Nutrition Reviews. Present Knowledge in Nutrition, 5th ed. Washington, D.C.: The Nutrition Foundation, Inc., 1984.

Paul, A. A., and D. A. T. Southgate. *McCance and Widdowson's The Composition of Foods*, 4th ed. London: Her Majesty's Stationery Office, 1978.

Physician's Desk Reference, 38th ed. Oradell, N.J.: Medical Economics Co., Inc., 1984.

Physicians' Desk Reference for Nonprescription Drugs, 5th ed. Oradell, N.J.: Medical Economics Co., Inc., 1984.

Roe, D. A. *Drug-Induced Nutritional Deficiencies*. Westport, Conn.: The AVI Publishing Co., Inc., 1978.

Roe, D. A. *Drugs and Nutrition in the Geriatric Patient*. New York: Churchill Livingstone, 1984.

Tallarida, R. J. *The Top 200 1984: The Most Widely Prescribed Drugs in America*. Philadelphia: W. B. Saunders Co., 1984.

Whitney, E. N., and C. B. Cataldo. *Understanding Normal and Clinical Nutrition*. New York: West Publishing Co., 1983.

Winick, M. *Nutrition and Drugs*. New York: John Wiley and Sons, 1983.

Index of Drugs

GENERIC DRUGS AND DRUG CATEGORIES
APPEAR IN SMALL CAPITAL LETTERS

About the Author

Brian L.G. Morgan was born in England and educated at Queen Elizabeth College, London University, where he obtained his Ph.D. in nutrition. He came to America in 1975 to take a fellowship at the Institute of Human Nutrition, Columbia University, College of Physicians and Surgeons, where he has remained ever since. At present Dr. Morgan holds a joint appointment at the Institute and the Columbia School of Dental and Oral Surgery, and is actively involved in nutrition research and teaching health professionals. He lives in Manhattan with his wife, author Roberta Morgan.

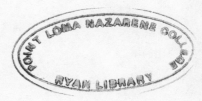